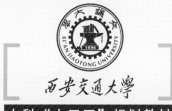

西安交通大学
本科"十三五"规划教材

人体解剖学 图谱
Atlas of Human Anatomy

（第2版）
（Second Edition）

主编 Chief Editors
钱亦华 Qian Yihua
林　奇 Lin Qi

U0303750

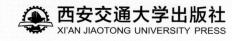

西安交通大学出版社
XI'AN JIAOTONG UNIVERSITY PRESS

图书在版编目（CIP）数据

人体解剖学图谱 = Atlas of Human Anatomy：英文 / 钱亦华，林奇主编. —2版
. — 西安：西安交通大学出版社，2022.9
ISBN 978-7-5693-1854-8

Ⅰ. ①人… Ⅱ. ①钱… ②林… Ⅲ. ①人体解剖学-
图谱 Ⅳ. ①R322-64

中国版本图书馆CIP数据核字（2020）第230504号

书　　名	人体解剖学图谱（第2版）
主　　编	钱亦华　林　奇
责任编辑	赵丹青
责任校对	秦金霞

出版发行	西安交通大学出版社
	（西安市兴庆南路1号　邮政编码　710048）
网　　址	http://www.xjtupress.com
电　　话	（029）82668357　82667874（市场营销中心）
	（029）82668315（总编办）
传　　真	（029）82668280
印　　刷	西安五星印刷有限公司

开　　本	889 mm×1194 mm　1/16	印 张	25.75	字 数	695千字
版次印次	2022年9月第2版　2022年9月第1次印刷
书　　号	ISBN 978-7-5693-1854-8
定　　价	158.00元

如发现印装质量问题，请与本社市场营销中心联系调换。
订购热线：（029）82665248　82667874
投稿热线：（029）82668803
读者信箱：med_xjup@163.com

版权所有　侵权必究

主编简介

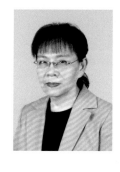

钱亦华，医学博士，三级教授，博士生导师。就职于西安交通大学基础医学院解剖学与组织胚胎学系，从事人体解剖学教学工作37年，主要研究领域为阿尔茨海默病的发病机制与防治。任中国解剖学会理事、中国神经科学学会神经退行性疾病分会委员、陕西省解剖学会副理事长等。曾赴美国、日本、澳大利亚留学和访学。于2013荣获"王宽诚育才奖"；2018年成为首批西安交通大学医学部教学名师。以第一完成人获省科技进步二等奖1项，获省级教学成果特等奖1项（2020-6）。发表教学与科研论文130余篇，SCI收录43篇。编写教材、专著35部，其中主编5部，副主编4部。

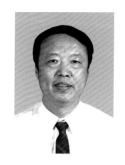

林奇，教授，硕士研究生导师。毕业于原西安医科大学医疗系，曾在基层从事临床医疗工作，1978年调回母校，长期从事人体解剖学教学及科研工作。曾赴美国新墨西哥州大学医学院进修学习。曾任西安交通大学医学三系副主任，社区医学院副院长、院长等。在科研上主要致力于心血管应用解剖学方面的研究。曾获省部级科技进步二等奖、三等奖。发表学术论文13篇，主编教材、专著10余部。

编写人员名单

主编 Chief Editors　　　　　钱亦华 Qian Yihua　　　林　奇 Lin Qi

副主编 Vice Chief Editors　　张玉秋 Zhang Yuqiu　　冯改丰 Feng Gaifeng

　　　　　　　　　　　　　　　陈新林 Chen Xinlin　　凌树才 Ling Shucai

编者 Editorial Staffs　　　　（按姓氏笔画排序）

马延兵 Ma Yanbing	西安交通大学 Xi'an Jiaotong University
王跃秀 Wang Yuexiu	首都医科大学 Capital Medical University
计胜峰 Ji Shengfeng	西安交通大学 Xi'an Jiaotong University
冯改丰 Feng Gaifeng	西安交通大学 Xi'an Jiaotong University
许杰华 Xu Jiehua	西安交通大学 Xi'an Jiaotong University
孙小勇 Sun Xiaoyong	西安培华学院医学院 Medical School of Xi'an Peihua University
李月英 Li Yueying	西安交通大学 Xi'an Jiaotong University
杨　杰 Yang Jie	西安交通大学 Xi'an Jiaotong University
杨维娜 Yang Weina	西安交通大学 Xi'an Jiaotong University
杨蓬勃 Yang Pengbo	西安交通大学 Xi'an Jiaotong University
肖新莉 Xiao Xinli	西安交通大学 Xi'an Jiaotong University
张玉秋 Zhang Yuqiu	复旦大学 Fudan University
张建水 Zhang Jianshui	西安交通大学 Xi'an Jiaotong University
张峰昌 Zhang Fengchang	西安交通大学 Xi'an Jiaotong University
陈新林 Chen Xinlin	西安交通大学 Xi'an Jiaotong University
林　奇 Lin Qi	西安交通大学 Xi'an Jiaotong University
胡　明 Hu Ming	西安交通大学 Xi'an Jiaotong University
贺桂琼 He Guiqiong	重庆医科大学 Chongqing Medical University
贾　宁 Jia Ning	西安交通大学 Xi'an Jiaotong University
钱亦华 Qian Yihua	西安交通大学 Xi'an Jiaotong University
凌树才 Ling Shucai	浙江大学 Zhejiang University
乾永强 Qian Yongqiang	西安交通大学 Xi'an Jiaotong University
韩　华 Han Hua	西安交通大学 Xi'an Jiaotong University
曾俊杰 Zeng Junjie	西安培华学院医学院 Medical School of Xi'an Peihua University
靳　辉 Jin Hui	西安交通大学 Xi'an Jiaotong University

英文校对 English Proofreading

John Bosco Ruganzu　　Mohammad Yasir Rizvi

绘图 Draftsman

林　奇 Lin Qi

摄像 Camera Crew

计胜峰 Ji Shengfeng　　　　段保国 Duan Baoguo　　　　刘国强 Liu Guoqiang

标本制作 Preparing Specimens　（按姓氏笔画排序）

马建国 Ma Jianguo　　　马延兵 Ma Yanbing　　　计胜峰 Ji Shengfeng　　　刘编生 Liu Biansheng

张峰昌 Zhang Fengchang　段保国 Duan Baoguo　　赵顺西 Zhao Shunxi　　　韩　华 Han Hua

序 FOREWORD

人体解剖学是研究正常人体形态结构的学科，它属于自然科学中的形态学范畴，其自身特点决定了通过图片和精练的文字获得所需知识是学习和掌握这门学科的必由之路。尽管人体解剖学属于古老的学科，但从事该学科教学和研究的同仁们并没有放弃对人类自身奥秘的探索，尤其是近年来介入和微创等治疗措施的临床应用、影像学检查设备的更新和数字化技术的引入，使这个所谓的"夕阳学科"又焕发出了青春的光彩，取得了进一步的发展。伴随着这些发展和进步，图片在展示、学习和研究正常人体形态结构方面发挥了越来越重要的作用。

时间过得真快，转眼之间钱亦华教授和林奇教授主编的《人体解剖学图谱》已经出版9年多了！令人感动的是，钱亦华教授和林奇教授及其他编者在该图谱出版之后的这段时间里没有满足，更没有止步，他们不断改进方法，极力追求图片的准确、系统和精美，已经完成了《人体解剖学图谱》（第2版）的编写工作。我有幸提前拜读了该图谱的书稿，深受感染和启发。

为了克服解剖学内容的文字叙述晦涩、抽象、难记等缺陷，图谱能使相关的学习内容变得更为直观、更易理解、更能记牢。即将出版的第2版图谱在保持图谱以往所具备的特点的基础上，着重在以下4个方面进行了改进：①更新并增加了一些标本图，其中包括一些典型的影像图和彩绘图；②文字部分除了修订了临床要点之外，还在部分临床要点中融入了临床典型病例，为帮助学生解决基础学习与临床应用的对接问题提供了便利；③图谱中的标注采用了中英文双语形式，充分体现了现代教育要走向国际化、与国际接轨的趋势；④版面采用大16开，文字直接标在图上。

本书的作者常年工作在人体解剖学教学和科研的第一线，具有丰富的经验。他们根据学习和临床工作需要编写本图谱，将为人体解剖学的学习和教学做出重要贡献。

中国解剖学会　　　　　　　　　理　事　长
《神经解剖学杂志》　　　　　　主　　编
空军军医大学人体解剖与组织胚胎学教研室　教　　授

2021年8月于西安

前 言 PREFACE

人体解剖学是研究正常人体各部分形态结构、位置毗邻及生长发育规律与功能关系的学科，是所有医学生的必修课程，它不仅是基础医学中的支柱学科之一，更是基础医学与临床医学之间的重要桥梁课程。由于人体正常器官形态结构复杂，涉及名词繁多、难学、难记且直观性强，因此解剖学教学必须利用形态结构图来学习。基于此，我们在 2013 年编写出版了第 1 版《人体解剖学图谱》。

在医学教育改革不断深化的驱动下，为加强基础医学与临床医学教育教学贯通融合、医学教育国际化深入发展，以及践行国家"一带一路"战略思想，我们有必要编写第 2 版《人体解剖学图谱》。

《人体解剖学图谱》已使用了 9 年，受到了广大读者的喜爱，同时我们也收到了同行专家、读者、学生的宝贵意见。第 2 版《人体解剖学图谱》将按照继承发展的编写原则，遵循最新版教学大纲的要求，贯彻全国医学教育改革最新理念和精髓，体现医学教育国际化的思想。本书图片主要以真实标本图为主、彩绘图为辅，但个别章节由于内容的特点所限，如脊髓、神经系统传导通路等，使用了比较多的彩绘图。本书共有 550 余幅图，其中，标本照片为 350 余幅，彩绘图为 200 余幅。标本照片经过了必要的软件处理，使其色彩更加真实，结构更加清晰。彩绘图多数是根据真实标本创新绘制的，能与标本图相互取长补短，甚至能示意出标本照片难以表达的结构，在增加了形态结构的表现力的同时，还增添了视觉效果。本次再版在第 1 版的基础上新增了 30 余幅图，使全书内容更加丰富、全面和系统。其中，还精选了部分具有代表性的标本切面解剖图、标本铸型图以及磁共振成像图（MRI），使学生能将完整的实物结构与平面结构、铸型结构以及临床影像结合起来进行学习，以便达到活学活用的目的。本书文字部分穿插在图中，以中英文双语对照的形式展现，并完善了解剖学纲要，丰富充实了临床要点。这主要表现为将重要解剖形态结构纲要性总结，以表格、关系树状图等形式展现，使其具有言简意赅、易读易记的特点，便于学生理解记忆，以及更好地学习、掌握教材中的基本知识点；同时，增设与解剖知识密切相关的临床要点并融入了临床典型病例，以提高学生学习兴趣，做到理论联系实际，贯彻落实"早临床、多临床、反复临床"的医学教育改革理念。

本书仍按系统解剖学的框架编排，内容分为运动系统、内脏学、脉管系统、感觉器、神经与内分泌系统共 5 篇，篇下还列有章和节，方便阅读时查找。本书做到了四个结合，即标本照片与彩绘图结合、图与文字结合、基础与临床结合、中文与英文结合，使书的内容丰富、适用范围扩大。本书不仅可以作为本科生、专科生人体解剖学的教学用书，还可以作为七年制、八年制人体解剖学双语教学及留学生的辅导教材。

本次再版图书的编写得到了复旦大学、浙江大学、首都医科大学、重庆医科大学的教授们的倾心相助，在此表示衷心的感谢！

本书的编写和出版得到西安交通大学出版社及西安交通大学医学部基础医学院人体解剖与组织胚胎学系的支持和帮助。本书获得了 2018 年西安交通大学本科"十三五"规划教材、校级重点教改项目（1810Z）、校教师教学发展中心基础课程质量建设重点教改项目（1902Z-29）及医学部教改项目（2018）支持，在此一并表示衷心感谢！由于作者水平所限，书中难免存在遗漏之处，恳请读者批评和指正，以便再版时修正。

钱亦华，林奇

2022.3.18

目 录 *CONTENTS*

第一篇 运动系统
Part 1 Locomotor System

第一章 骨学
Chapter 1 Osteology

第一节 躯干骨

Section 1 The bones of trunk

第二节　颅骨
Section 2 Skull

第三节　四肢骨

Section 3 Limb bones

第二章　关节学

Chapter 2　Arthrology

第一节　中轴骨的连结

Section 1 Joints of axial skeleton

第二节 四肢骨的连结

Section 2 Joints of limbs

第三章　肌学

Chapter 3　Myology

第一节　肌学总论

Section 1 Introduction of myology

第二节　头肌与颈肌

Section 2 Muscles of head and neck

第三节　躯干肌

Section 3 Muscles of trunk

第四节　上肢肌

Section 4　Muscles of upper limb

第五节　下肢肌

Section 5　Muscles of lower limb

第二篇　内脏学
Part 2 Splanchnology

第四章　消化系统
Chapter 4 Alimentary system

第五章　呼吸系统
Chapter 5 Respiratory system

第六章　泌尿系统
Chapter 6 Urinary system

第七章 生殖系统
Chapter 7 Reproductive system

第八章 腹膜
Chapter 8 Peritoneum

第三篇　脉管系统
Part 3　Angiology System

第九章　心血管系统
Chapter 9　Cardiovascular system

第一节　心
Section 1　Heart

第二节　动脉
Section 2　Artery

第三节 静脉

Section 3 Vein

第四篇 感觉器
Part 4 Sensory Organs

第十一章 视器
Chapter 11 Visual organ

第十二章 前庭蜗器
Chapter 12 Vestibulocochlear organ

第五篇　神经与内分泌系统
Part 5 Nervous and Endocrine System

第十三章　中枢神经系统
Chapter 13 Central nervous system

第一节　脊髓
Section 1 Spinal cord

第二节　脑干
Section 2 Brain stem

第三节　小脑

Section 3　Cerebellum

第四节　间脑

Section 4　Diencephalon

第五节 端脑

Section 5 Telencephalon

第六节　脑和脊髓的被膜、血管及脑脊液循环

Section 6　Meninges, blood vessels, and cerebrospinal fluid circulation of brain and spinal cord

第十四章　周围神经系统

Chapter 14　Peripheral nervous system

第一节　脊神经

Section 1　Spinal nerve

第二节 脑神经

Section 2 Cranial nerve

第三节 内脏神经系统

Section 3 Visceral nervous system

第十五章 神经系统的传导通路
Chapter 15 Conductive pathways of nervous system

第十六章 内分泌系统
Chapter 16 Endocrine system

附录

典型磁共振成像图（MRI）

弥散张量成像（DTI）白质纤维束图

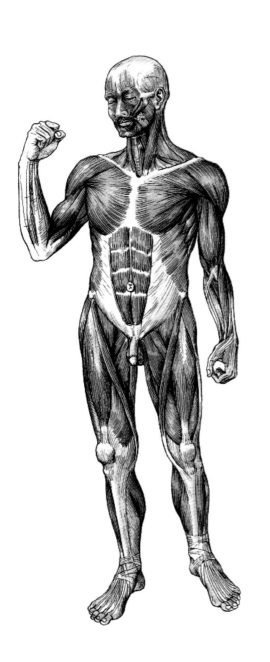

第一篇
运动系统
Part 1 Locomotor System

第一章　骨学
Chapter 1　Osteology

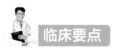

临床要点

骨构造的临床意义

通常5岁以后,长骨骨干内的红骨髓逐渐变为黄骨髓,但在慢性失血过多或重度贫血时,黄骨髓可转化为红骨髓,恢复造血功能。在椎骨、长骨两端的骺及扁骨内终生存在红骨髓。颅骨中扁骨的密质骨分别形成其内、外板,内板薄而松脆,故颅骨骨折多见于内板。外板和内板之间的骨松质,称板障。

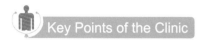

Key Points of the Clinic

Clinical significance of bone structure

Normally, after five years old, the red bone marrow in the long bone diaphysis gradually becomes yellow bone marrow, but in chronic haemorrhage or severe anemia, yellow bone marrow could be transformed into red bone marrow to restore hematopoietic function. However, red bone marrow exists in the vertebrae, the epiphysis at both ends of the long bone and the flattened bone is red bone marrow for life time. The inner and outer plates of the cranium are formed by the dense bone in the flat bone. The inner plate is thin and brittle. Therefore, the fracture of skull is more common in the inner plate. The spongy bone between the two plates, called the diploe.

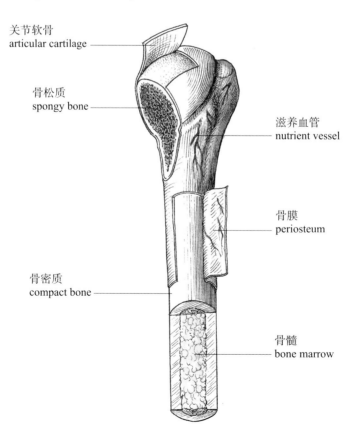

关节软骨
articular cartilage

骨松质
spongy bone

滋养血管
nutrient vessel

骨膜
periosteum

骨密质
compact bone

骨髓
bone marrow

图 1-1　骨的构造
Structure of bone

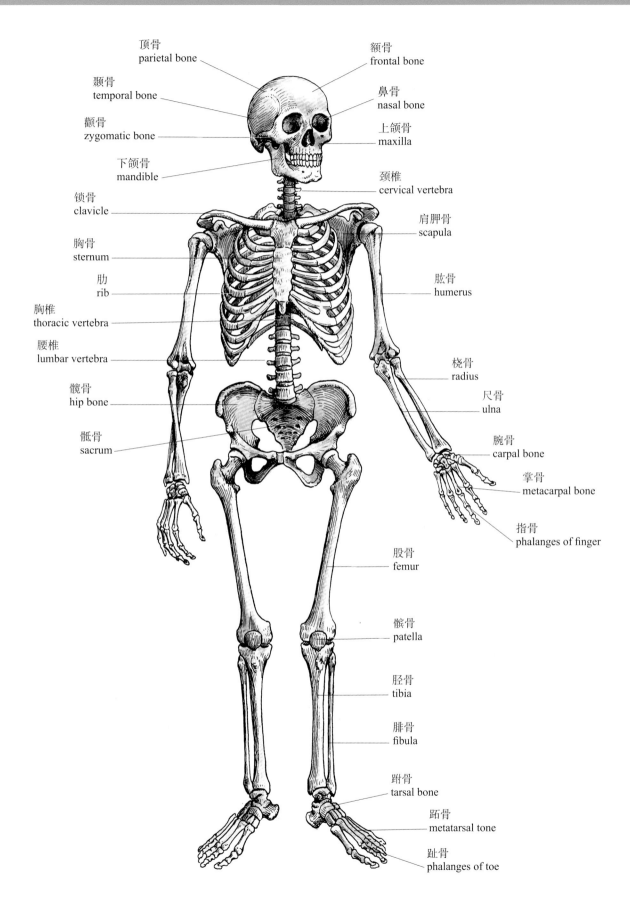

顶骨
parietal bone

额骨
frontal bone

颞骨
temporal bone

鼻骨
nasal bone

颧骨
zygomatic bone

上颌骨
maxilla

下颌骨
mandible

颈椎
cervical vertebra

锁骨
clavicle

肩胛骨
scapula

胸骨
sternum

肋
rib

肱骨
humerus

胸椎
thoracic vertebra

腰椎
lumbar vertebra

桡骨
radius

髋骨
hip bone

尺骨
ulna

骶骨
sacrum

腕骨
carpal bone

掌骨
metacarpal bone

指骨
phalanges of finger

股骨
femur

髌骨
patella

胫骨
tibia

腓骨
fibula

跗骨
tarsal bone

跖骨
metatarsal tone

趾骨
phalanges of toe

图 1-2 全身骨骼
Skeleton

第一节　躯干骨　Section 1　The bones of trunk

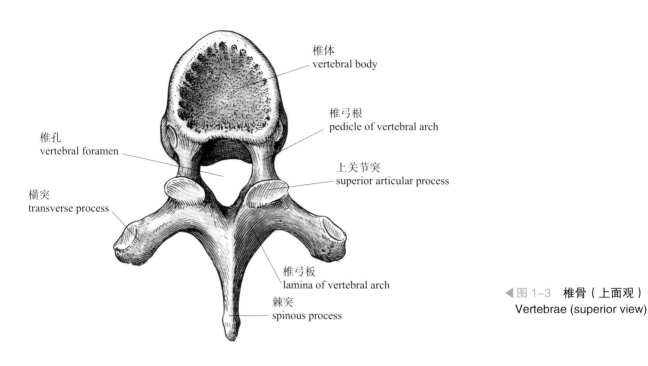

椎体
vertebral body

椎弓根
pedicle of vertebral arch

上关节突
superior articular process

椎孔
vertebral foramen

横突
transverse process

椎弓板
lamina of vertebral arch

棘突
spinous process

◀图 1-3　椎骨（上面观）
Vertebrae (superior view)

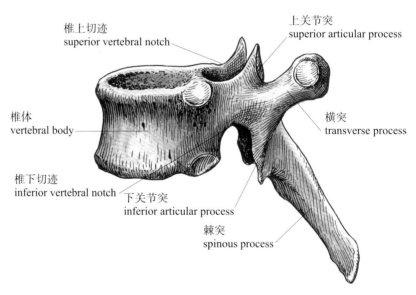

椎上切迹
superior vertebral notch

上关节突
superior articular process

椎体
vertebral body

横突
transverse process

椎下切迹
inferior vertebral notch

下关节突
inferior articular process

棘突
spinous process

▶图 1-4　椎骨（侧面观）
Vertebrae (lateral view)

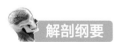 解剖纲要

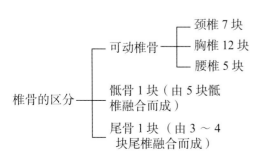

椎骨的区分 ── 可动椎骨 ── 颈椎 7 块
胸椎 12 块
腰椎 5 块

骶骨 1 块（由 5 块骶椎融合而成）

尾骨 1 块（由 3～4 块尾椎融合而成）

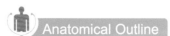 Anatomical Outline

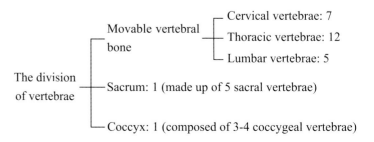

The division of vertebrae ── Movable vertebral bone ── Cervical vertebrae: 7
Thoracic vertebrae: 12
Lumbar vertebrae: 5

Sacrum: 1 (made up of 5 sacral vertebrae)

Coccyx: 1 (composed of 3-4 coccygeal vertebrae)

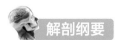 解剖纲要　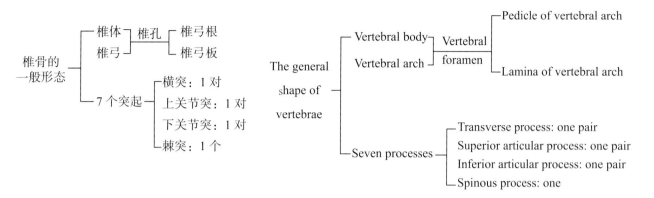 Anatomical Outline

椎骨的一般形态
- 椎体
- 椎弓 — 椎孔 — 椎弓根 / 椎弓板
- 7个突起
  - 横突：1 对
  - 上关节突：1 对
  - 下关节突：1 对
  - 棘突：1 个

The general shape of vertebrae
- Vertebral body
- Vertebral arch — Vertebral foramen — Pedicle of vertebral arch / Lamina of vertebral arch
- Seven processes
  - Transverse process: one pair
  - Superior articular process: one pair
  - Inferior articular process: one pair
  - Spinous process: one

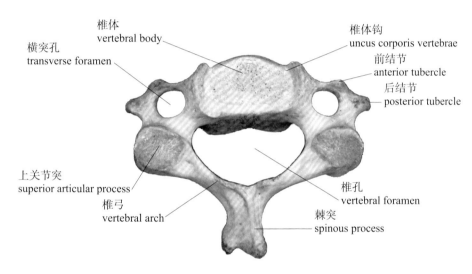

图 1-5　颈椎（上面观）
Cervical vertebra (superior view)

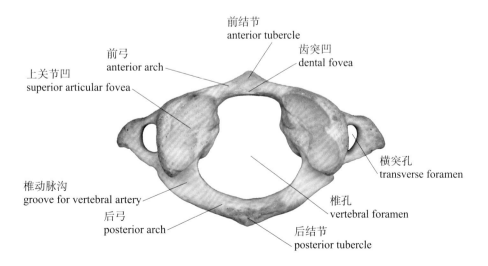

图 1-6　寰椎（上面观）
Atlas (superior view)

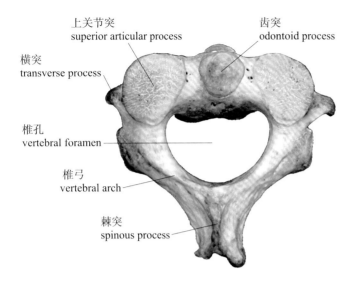

上关节突
superior articular process

齿突
odontoid process

横突
transverse process

椎孔
vertebral foramen

椎弓
vertebral arch

棘突
spinous process

◀ 图 1-7 枢椎（上面观）
Axis (superior view)

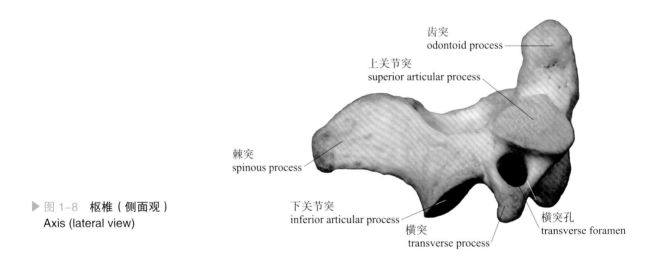

齿突
odontoid process

上关节突
superior articular process

棘突
spinous process

下关节突
inferior articular process

横突
transverse process

横突孔
transverse foramen

▶ 图 1-8 枢椎（侧面观）
Axis (lateral view)

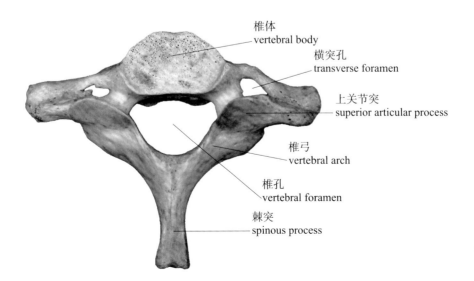

椎体
vertebral body

横突孔
transverse foramen

上关节突
superior articular process

椎弓
vertebral arch

椎孔
vertebral foramen

棘突
spinous process

◀ 图 1-9 隆椎
Prominent vertebra

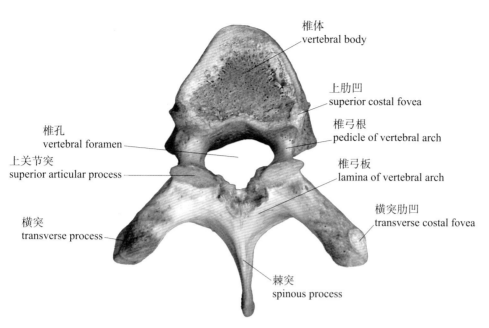

图 1-10 胸椎（上面观）
Thoracic vertebra (superior view)

椎体
vertebral body

上肋凹
superior costal fovea

椎弓根
pedicle of vertebral arch

椎弓板
lamina of vertebral arch

横突肋凹
transverse costal fovea

棘突
spinous process

横突
transverse process

上关节突
superior articular process

椎孔
vertebral foramen

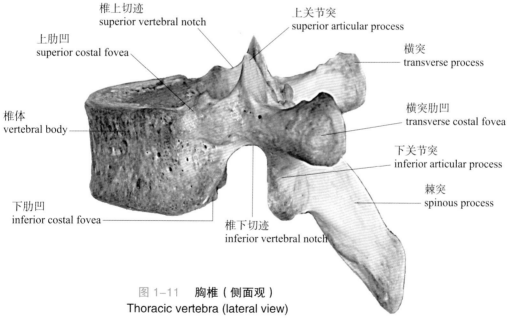

图 1-11 胸椎（侧面观）
Thoracic vertebra (lateral view)

椎上切迹
superior vertebral notch

上关节突
superior articular process

上肋凹
superior costal fovea

横突
transverse process

横突肋凹
transverse costal fovea

下关节突
inferior articular process

棘突
spinous process

椎体
vertebral body

下肋凹
inferior costal fovea

椎下切迹
inferior vertebral notch

解剖纲要

各部椎骨的主要形态特征

结构	颈椎	胸椎	腰椎
椎体	椭圆形、小、有椎体钩	心形、大，侧面有肋凹	肾形、粗大
椎孔	三角形、较大	圆形、较小	卵圆形或三角形、大
横突	有横突孔和前、后结节	伸向后外、有横突肋凹	薄而长、伸向两侧
关节突关节面	近似水平位	近似冠状位	近似矢状位
棘突	短、末端分叉	长、伸向后下，叠瓦状排列	宽板状、水平向后伸

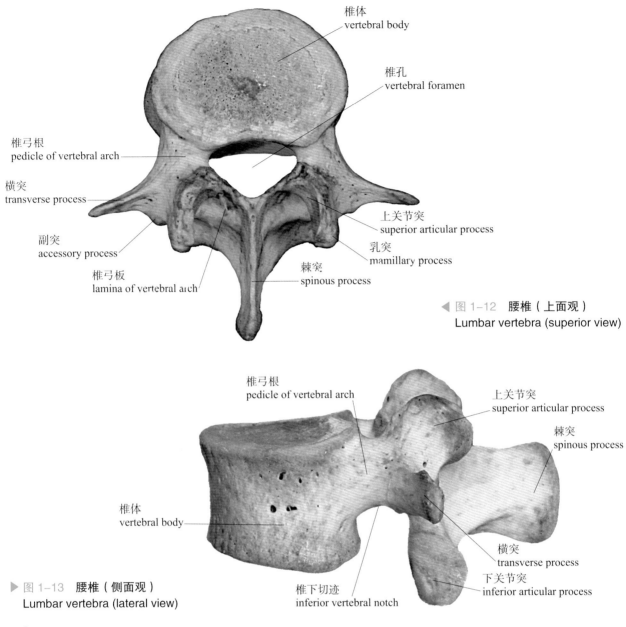

椎体
vertebral body

椎孔
vertebral foramen

椎弓根
pedicle of vertebral arch

横突
transverse process

副突
accessory process

椎弓板
lamina of vertebral arch

棘突
spinous process

上关节突
superior articular process

乳突
mamillary process

◀ 图 1-12　腰椎（上面观）
Lumbar vertebra (superior view)

椎弓根
pedicle of vertebral arch

上关节突
superior articular process

棘突
spinous process

椎体
vertebral body

横突
transverse process

下关节突
inferior articular process

椎下切迹
inferior vertebral notch

▶ 图 1-13　腰椎（侧面观）
Lumbar vertebra (lateral view)

Anatomical Outline

Main morphological characteristics of vertebrae in all parts

Structure	Cervical vertebrae	Thoracic vertebrae	Lumbar vertebrae
Body	Ellipse, small, with vertebral uncus	Heart-shaped, larger, costal fovea on the lateral surface	Kidney- shaped, massive
Vertebral foramen	Triangle, larger	Roundness, smaller	Ovoid or triangle, large
Transverse process	There are transverse foramen and anterior and posterior nodules	Extending backward and lateral, with transverse costal fovea	Thin and long, extending to both sides
Facet of articular process	Approximate horizontal position	Approximate coronal position	Approximate sagittal position
Spinal process	Short, end bifurcation	Long, extended backward and inferior, imbricate arrangement	Wide plate, horizontal backward

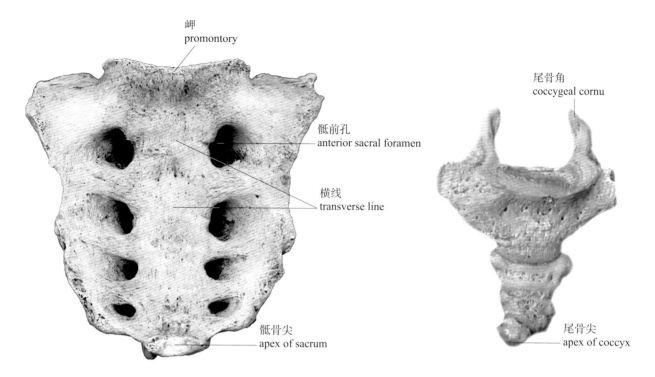

图 1-14 骶骨（前面观）
Sacrum (anterior view)

图 1-16 尾骨（前面观）
Coccyx (anterior view)

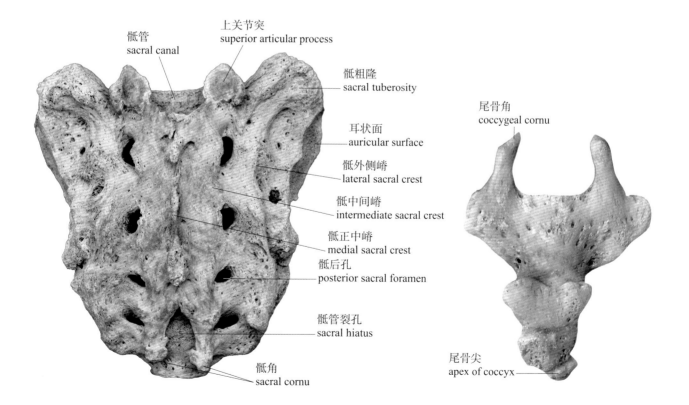

图 1-15 骶骨（后面观）
Sacrum (posterior view)

图 1-17 尾骨（后面观）
Coccyx (posterior view)

锁骨下动脉沟
sulcus for subclavian artery

前斜角肌结节
tubercle for scalenus anterior

锁骨下静脉沟
sulcus for subclavian vein

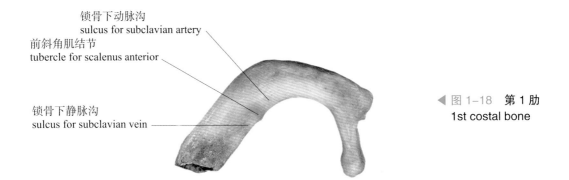

◄ 图 1–18　第 1 肋
1st costal bone

前锯肌粗隆
serratus anterior tuberosity

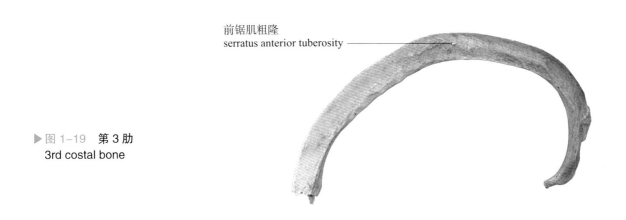

► 图 1–19　第 3 肋
3rd costal bone

肋体
shaft of rib

肋沟
costal groove

肋角
costal angle

肋结节
costal tubercle

肋颈
costal neck

肋头关节面
articular surface of costal head

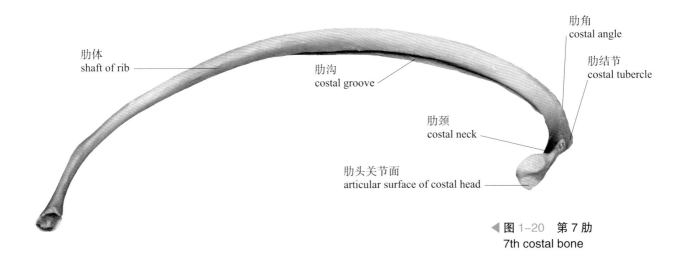

◄ 图 1–20　第 7 肋
7th costal bone

► 图 1–21　第 12 肋
12th costal bone

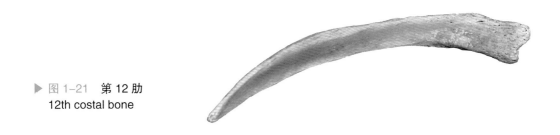

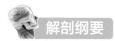 解剖纲要

肋的组成

肋由肋骨和肋软骨组成，共 12 对，可分为 3 类。

1. 真肋：1 ～ 7 肋，直接与胸骨相连。

2. 假肋：8 ～ 10 肋，肋前端借肋软骨与上位肋相连，形成肋弓。

3. 浮肋：11 肋、12 肋，前端游离于腹壁肌肉中。

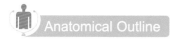 Anatomical Outline

Composition of ribs

The ribs which are composed of costal bone and costal cartilage, are 12 pairs in all and which can be divided into three kinds.

1. True ribs: 1-7 ribs, directly connected to the sternum.

2. False ribs: 8-10 ribs, the front end of rib is connected to the upper rib via the costal cartilage to form the costal arch.

3.Floating ribs: 11 and 12 ribs, the front ends are attached to the abdominal wall muscle.

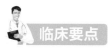 临床要点

胸骨角的标志意义

1. 平对第 4 胸椎体下缘，是上、下纵隔的分界平面。

2. 奇静脉弓位于此平面内，并向前汇入上腔静脉。

3. 为气管分杈平面。

4. 平对主动脉弓的起、止端。

5. 左主支气管在此平面与食管交叉。

6. 胸导管在此平面由右向左行。

7. 平对第 2 肋，为计数肋的标志。

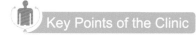 Key Points of the Clinic

The symbolic significance of the sternal angle

1. Sternal angle directly face the lower border of the 4th thoracic vertebra and is the boundary plane of the upper and lower mediastinum.

2. The azygos vein arch is located in this plane and drainage into the superior vena cava anteriorly.

3. It is the plane of trachea bifurcation.

4. Sternal angle directly face the beginning and end of the aortic arch.

5. The left main bronchus intersects with the esophagus at this level.

6. The thoracic duct moves from right to left on this plane.

7. The plane passes through the second sternocostal joint and is a sign of counting ribs.

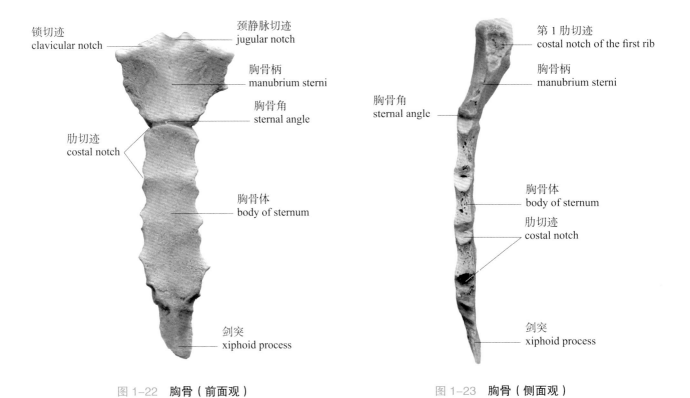

锁切迹
clavicular notch

颈静脉切迹
jugular notch

胸骨柄
manubrium sterni

胸骨角
sternal angle

肋切迹
costal notch

胸骨体
body of sternum

剑突
xiphoid process

图 1-22　胸骨（前面观）
Sternum (anterior view)

第 1 肋切迹
costal notch of the first rib

胸骨柄
manubrium sterni

胸骨角
sternal angle

胸骨体
body of sternum

肋切迹
costal notch

剑突
xiphoid process

图 1-23　胸骨（侧面观）
Sternum (lateral view)

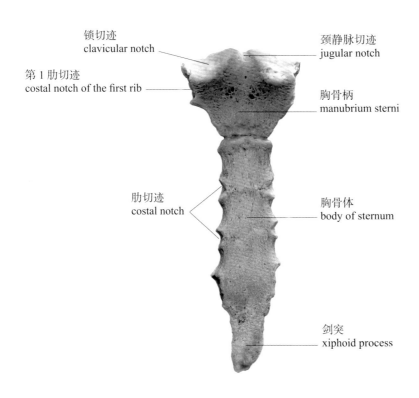

锁切迹
clavicular notch

颈静脉切迹
jugular notch

第 1 肋切迹
costal notch of the first rib

胸骨柄
manubrium sterni

肋切迹
costal notch

胸骨体
body of sternum

剑突
xiphoid process

图 1-24　胸骨（后面观）
Sternum (posterior view)

第二节 颅骨 Section 2 Skull

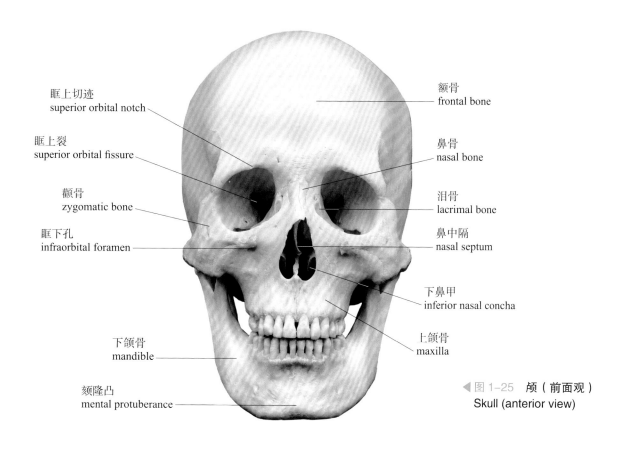

眶上切迹
superior orbital notch

眶上裂
superior orbital fissure

颧骨
zygomatic bone

眶下孔
infraorbital foramen

下颌骨
mandible

颏隆凸
mental protuberance

额骨
frontal bone

鼻骨
nasal bone

泪骨
lacrimal bone

鼻中隔
nasal septum

下鼻甲
inferior nasal concha

上颌骨
maxilla

◀ 图 1-25 颅（前面观）
Skull (anterior view)

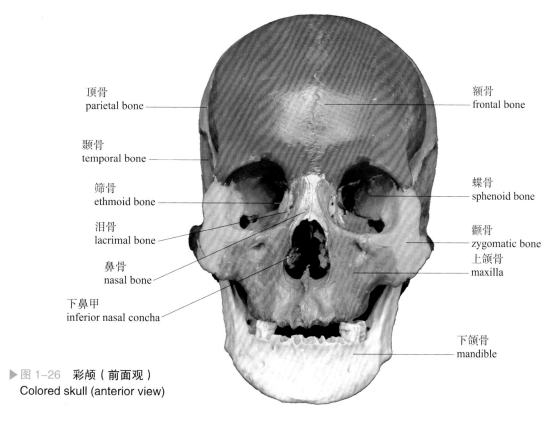

顶骨
parietal bone

颞骨
temporal bone

筛骨
ethmoid bone

泪骨
lacrimal bone

鼻骨
nasal bone

下鼻甲
inferior nasal concha

额骨
frontal bone

蝶骨
sphenoid bone

颧骨
zygomatic bone

上颌骨
maxilla

下颌骨
mandible

▶ 图 1-26 彩颅（前面观）
Colored skull (anterior view)

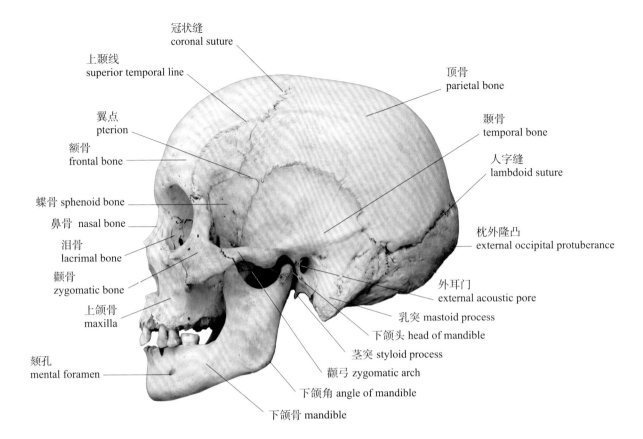

冠状缝
coronal suture

上颞线
superior temporal line

顶骨
parietal bone

翼点
pterion

颞骨
temporal bone

额骨
frontal bone

人字缝
lambdoid suture

蝶骨 sphenoid bone

鼻骨 nasal bone

泪骨
lacrimal bone

枕外隆凸
external occipital protuberance

颧骨
zygomatic bone

外耳门
external acoustic pore

上颌骨
maxilla

乳突 mastoid process

下颌头 head of mandible

颏孔
mental foramen

茎突 styloid process

颧弓 zygomatic arch

下颌角 angle of mandible

下颌骨 mandible

图 1-27 颅（侧面观）
Skull (lateral view)

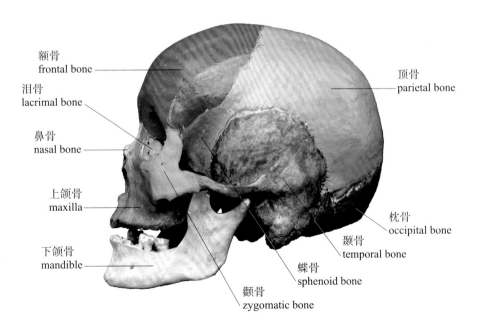

额骨
frontal bone

顶骨
parietal bone

泪骨
lacrimal bone

鼻骨
nasal bone

上颌骨
maxilla

枕骨
occipital bone

颞骨
temporal bone

下颌骨
mandible

蝶骨
sphenoid bone

颧骨
zygomatic bone

图 1-28 彩颅（侧面观）
Colored skull (lateral view)

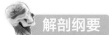 解剖纲要

脑颅
- 单一：额骨、枕骨、蝶骨、筛骨
- 成对：颞骨、顶骨

颅骨的组成
面颅
- 成对：上颌骨、腭骨、颧骨、鼻骨、泪骨、下鼻甲
- 单一：犁骨、下颌骨、舌骨

Anatomical Outline

The composition of the skull

Cerebral cranium
- Unpaired bones: frontal bone, occipital bone, sphenoid bone, ethmoid bone
- Paired bones: temporal bone, parietal bone

Facial cranium
- Paired bones: maxillae, palatine bone, zygomatic bone, nasal bone, lacrimal bone, inferior nasal conchae
- Unpaired bones: vomer, mandible, hyoid bone

解剖纲要

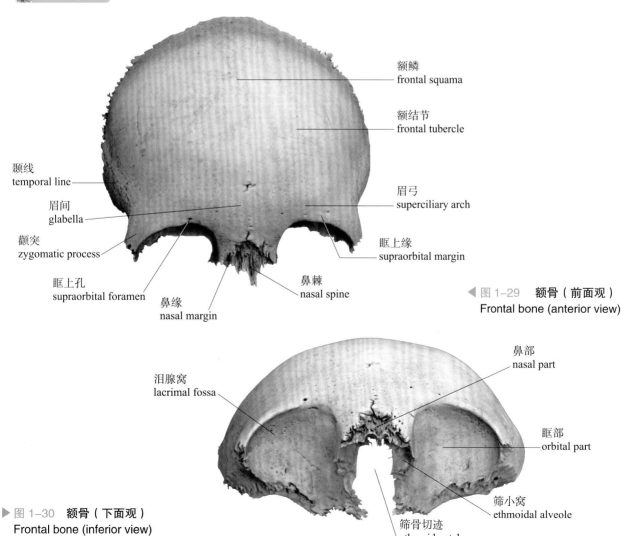

额鳞
frontal squama

额结节
frontal tubercle

颞线
temporal line

眉间
glabella

颧突
zygomatic process

眶上孔
supraorbital foramen

鼻缘
nasal margin

眉弓
superciliary arch

眶上缘
supraorbital margin

鼻棘
nasal spine

◀ 图 1-29　额骨（前面观）
Frontal bone (anterior view)

泪腺窝
lacrimal fossa

鼻部
nasal part

眶部
orbital part

筛小窝
ethmoidal alveole

▶ 图 1-30　额骨（下面观）
Frontal bone (inferior view)

筛骨切迹
ethmoid notch

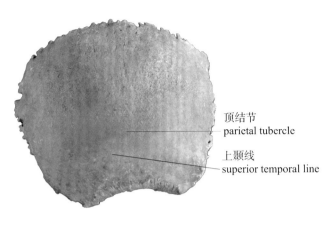

顶结节
parietal tubercle

上颞线
superior temporal line

图 1-31　顶骨（外面观）
Parietal bone (external view)

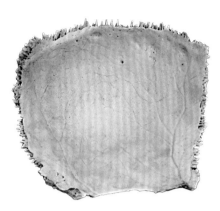

图 1-32　顶骨（内面观）
Parietal bone (internal view)

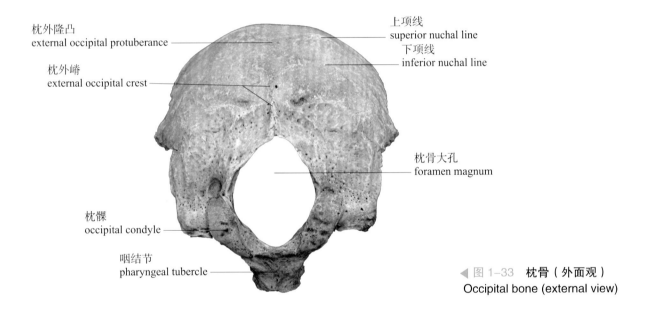

枕外隆凸
external occipital protuberance

枕外嵴
external occipital crest

枕髁
occipital condyle

咽结节
pharyngeal tubercle

上项线
superior nuchal line

下项线
inferior nuchal line

枕骨大孔
foramen magnum

◀ 图 1-33　枕骨（外面观）
Occipital bone (external view)

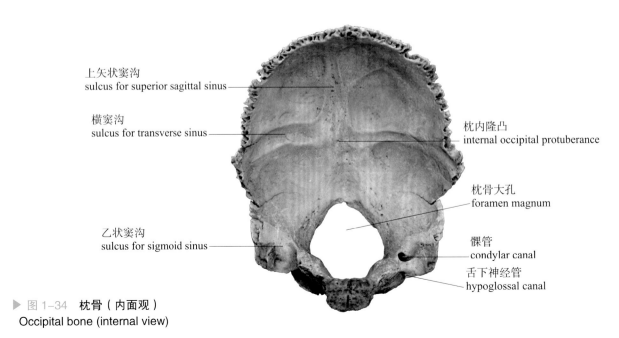

上矢状窦沟
sulcus for superior sagittal sinus

横窦沟
sulcus for transverse sinus

乙状窦沟
sulcus for sigmoid sinus

枕内隆凸
internal occipital protuberance

枕骨大孔
foramen magnum

髁管
condylar canal

舌下神经管
hypoglossal canal

▶ 图 1-34　枕骨（内面观）
Occipital bone (internal view)

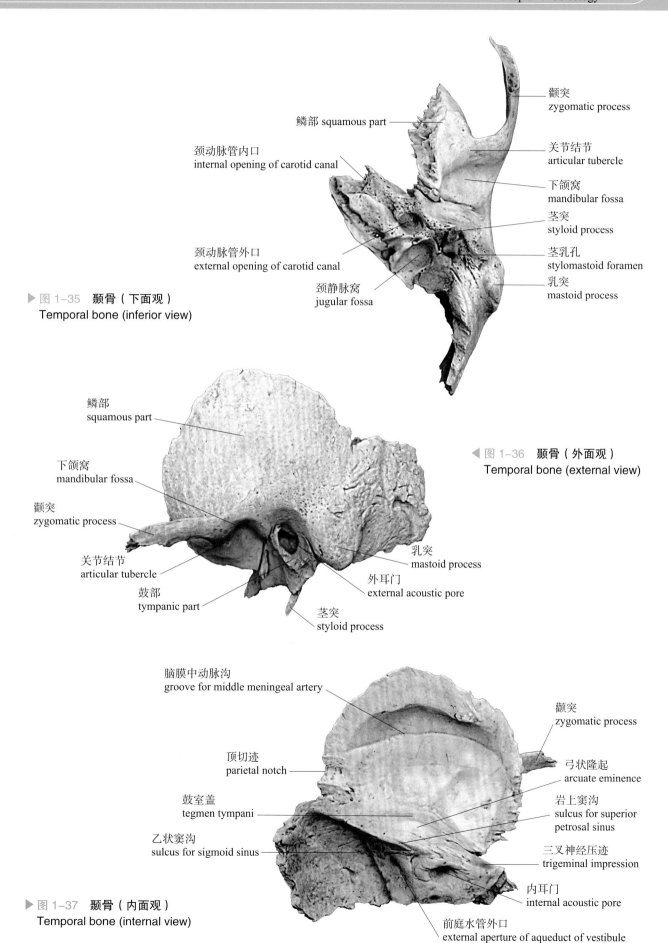

颧突
zygomatic process

鳞部 squamous part

关节结节
articular tubercle

颈动脉管内口
internal opening of carotid canal

下颌窝
mandibular fossa

茎突
styloid process

颈动脉管外口
external opening of carotid canal

茎乳孔
stylomastoid foramen

乳突
mastoid process

颈静脉窝
jugular fossa

▶ 图 1-35 颞骨（下面观）
Temporal bone (inferior view)

鳞部
squamous part

下颌窝
mandibular fossa

颧突
zygomatic process

关节结节
articular tubercle

鼓部
tympanic part

茎突
styloid process

乳突
mastoid process

外耳门
external acoustic pore

◀ 图 1-36 颞骨（外面观）
Temporal bone (external view)

脑膜中动脉沟
groove for middle meningeal artery

颧突
zygomatic process

顶切迹
parietal notch

弓状隆起
arcuate eminence

鼓室盖
tegmen tympani

岩上窦沟
sulcus for superior
petrosal sinus

乙状窦沟
sulcus for sigmoid sinus

三叉神经压迹
trigeminal impression

内耳门
internal acoustic pore

▶ 图 1-37 颞骨（内面观）
Temporal bone (internal view)

前庭水管外口
external aperture of aqueduct of vestibule

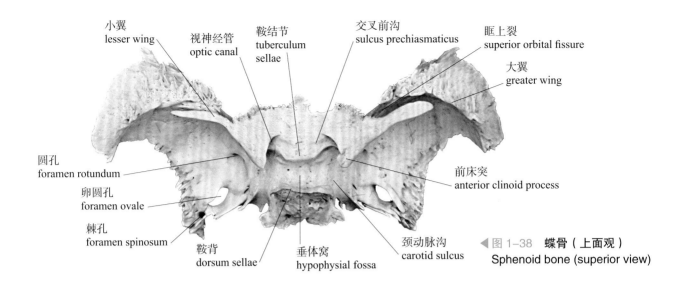

小翼 lesser wing
视神经管 optic canal
鞍结节 tuberculum sellae
交叉前沟 sulcus prechiasmaticus
眶上裂 superior orbital fissure
大翼 greater wing
圆孔 foramen rotundum
卵圆孔 foramen ovale
棘孔 foramen spinosum
鞍背 dorsum sellae
垂体窝 hypophysial fossa
颈动脉沟 carotid sulcus
前床突 anterior clinoid process

◀ 图 1-38　**蝶骨（上面观）**
Sphenoid bone (superior view)

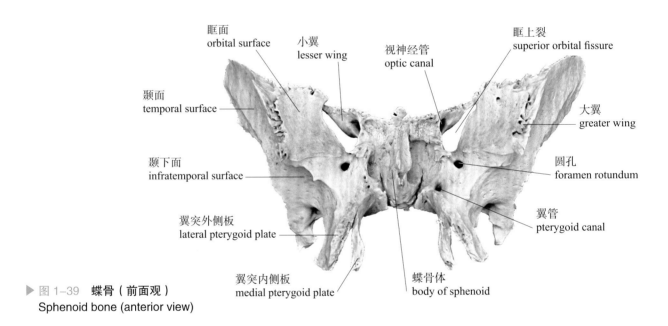

眶面 orbital surface
小翼 lesser wing
视神经管 optic canal
眶上裂 superior orbital fissure
颞面 temporal surface
大翼 greater wing
颞下面 infratemporal surface
圆孔 foramen rotundum
翼突外侧板 lateral pterygoid plate
翼管 pterygoid canal
翼突内侧板 medial pterygoid plate
蝶骨体 body of sphenoid

▶ 图 1-39　**蝶骨（前面观）**
Sphenoid bone (anterior view)

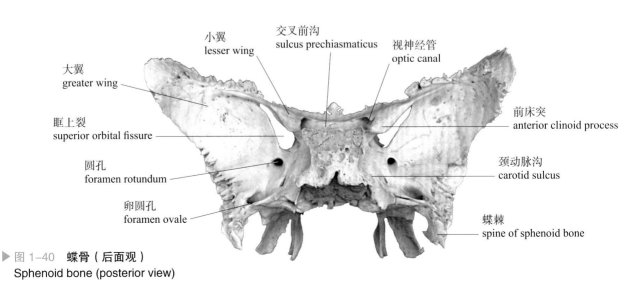

小翼 lesser wing
交叉前沟 sulcus prechiasmaticus
视神经管 optic canal
大翼 greater wing
前床突 anterior clinoid process
眶上裂 superior orbital fissure
圆孔 foramen rotundum
颈动脉沟 carotid sulcus
卵圆孔 foramen ovale
蝶棘 spine of sphenoid bone

▶ 图 1-40　**蝶骨（后面观）**
Sphenoid bone (posterior view)

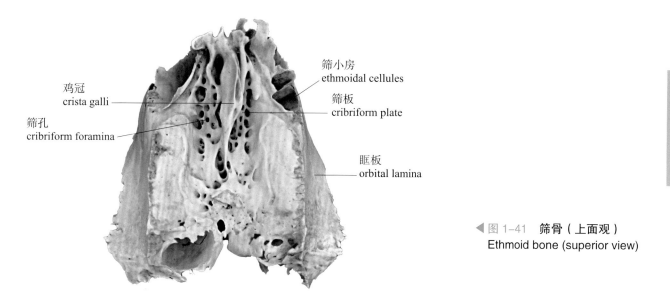

鸡冠
crista galli

筛孔
cribriform foramina

筛小房
ethmoidal cellules

筛板
cribriform plate

眶板
orbital lamina

◀ 图 1-41 筛骨（上面观）
Ethmoid bone (superior view)

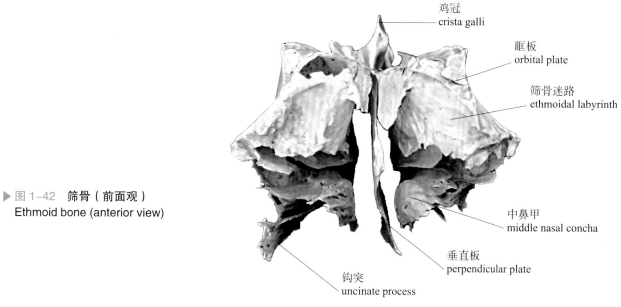

▶ 图 1-42 筛骨（前面观）
Ethmoid bone (anterior view)

鸡冠
crista galli

眶板
orbital plate

筛骨迷路
ethmoidal labyrinth

中鼻甲
middle nasal concha

垂直板
perpendicular plate

钩突
uncinate process

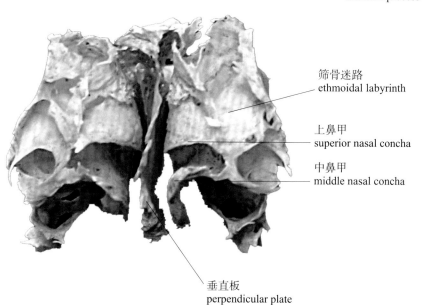

筛骨迷路
ethmoidal labyrinth

上鼻甲
superior nasal concha

中鼻甲
middle nasal concha

◀ 图 1-43 筛骨（后面观）
Ethmoid bone (posterior view)

垂直板
perpendicular plate

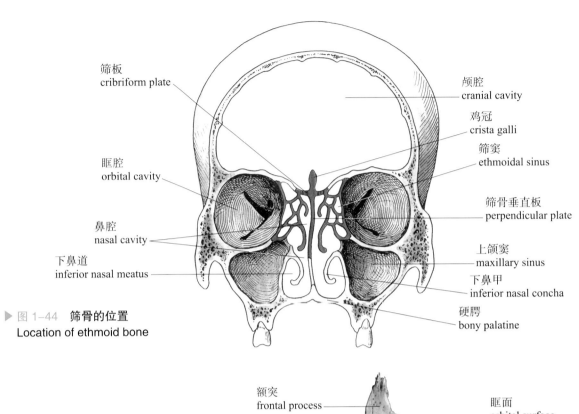

筛板
cribriform plate

颅腔
cranial cavity

鸡冠
crista galli

筛窦
ethmoidal sinus

眶腔
orbital cavity

筛骨垂直板
perpendicular plate

鼻腔
nasal cavity

上颌窦
maxillary sinus

下鼻道
inferior nasal meatus

下鼻甲
inferior nasal concha

硬腭
bony palatine

▶ 图 1-44　筛骨的位置
Location of ethmoid bone

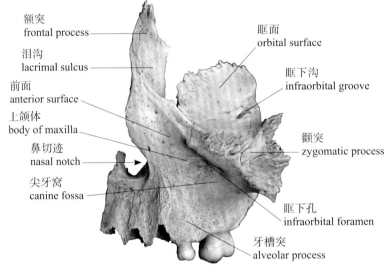

额突
frontal process

眶面
orbital surface

泪沟
lacrimal sulcus

眶下沟
infraorbital groove

前面
anterior surface

上颌体
body of maxilla

颧突
zygomatic process

鼻切迹
nasal notch

尖牙窝
canine fossa

眶下孔
infraorbital foramen

牙槽突
alveolar process

▶ 图 1-45　上颌骨（外侧面）
Maxilla (lateral view)

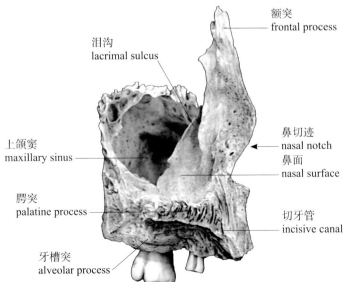

额突
frontal process

泪沟
lacrimal sulcus

上颌窦
maxillary sinus

鼻切迹
nasal notch

鼻面
nasal surface

腭突
palatine process

切牙管
incisive canal

牙槽突
alveolar process

◀ 图 1-46　上颌骨（内侧面）
Maxilla (medial view)

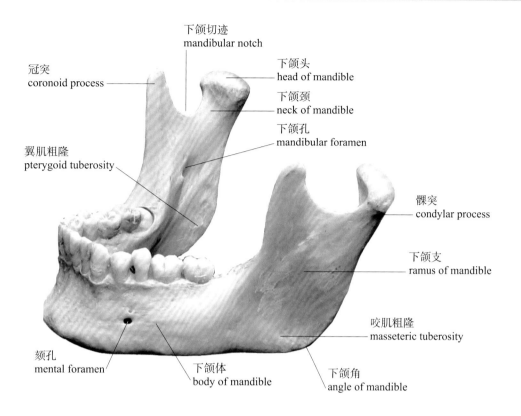

下颌切迹
mandibular notch

下颌头
head of mandible

下颌颈
neck of mandible

下颌孔
mandibular foramen

冠突
coronoid process

翼肌粗隆
pterygoid tuberosity

髁突
condylar process

下颌支
ramus of mandible

咬肌粗隆
masseteric tuberosity

颏孔
mental foramen

下颌体
body of mandible

下颌角
angle of mandible

图 1–47　下颌骨（侧面观）
Mandible (lateral view)

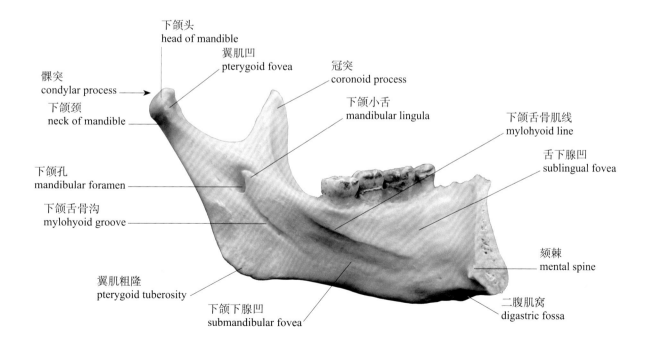

下颌头
head of mandible

翼肌凹
pterygoid fovea

冠突
coronoid process

下颌小舌
mandibular lingula

下颌舌骨肌线
mylohyoid line

髁突
condylar process

下颌颈
neck of mandible

下颌孔
mandibular foramen

舌下腺凹
sublingual fovea

下颌舌骨沟
mylohyoid groove

翼肌粗隆
pterygoid tuberosity

下颌下腺凹
submandibular fovea

颏棘
mental spine

二腹肌窝
digastric fossa

图 1–48　下颌骨（内面观）
Mandible (medial view)

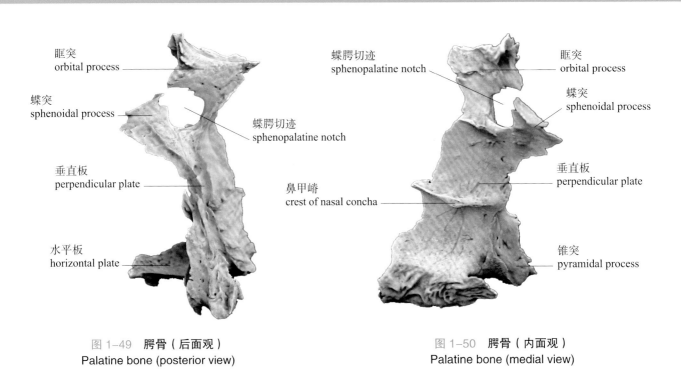

图 1-49　腭骨（后面观）
Palatine bone (posterior view)

图 1-50　腭骨（内面观）
Palatine bone (medial view)

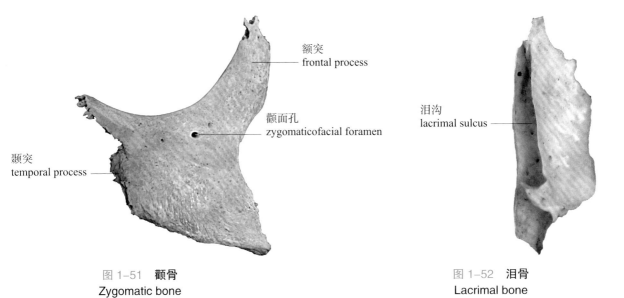

图 1-51　颧骨
Zygomatic bone

图 1-52　泪骨
Lacrimal bone

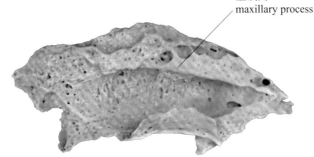

图 1-53　下鼻甲
Inferior nasal conchae

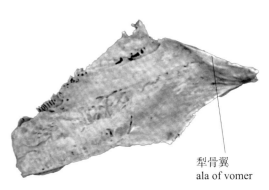

图 1-54　犁骨
Vomer

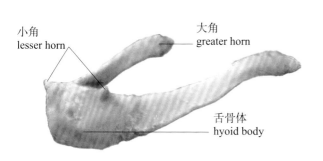

图 1-55 舌骨（侧面观）
Hyoid bone (lateral view)

小角 lesser horn
大角 greater horn
舌骨体 hyoid body

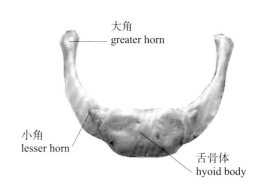

图 1-56 舌骨（上面观）
Hyoid bone (superior view)

大角 greater horn
小角 lesser horn
舌骨体 hyoid body

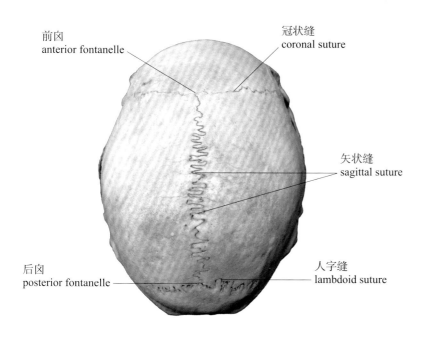

前囟 anterior fontanelle
冠状缝 coronal suture
矢状缝 sagittal suture
后囟 posterior fontanelle
人字缝 lambdoid suture

◀ 图 1-57 颅顶（外面观）
Calvaria (external view)

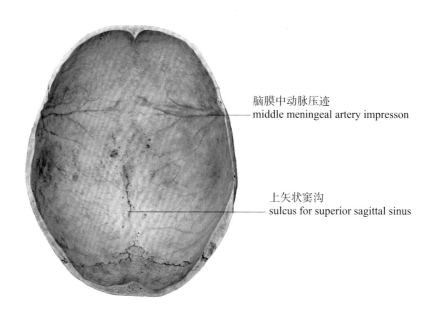

脑膜中动脉压迹 middle meningeal artery impresson
上矢状窦沟 sulcus for superior sagittal sinus

▶ 图 1-58 颅顶（内面观）
Calvaria (internal view)

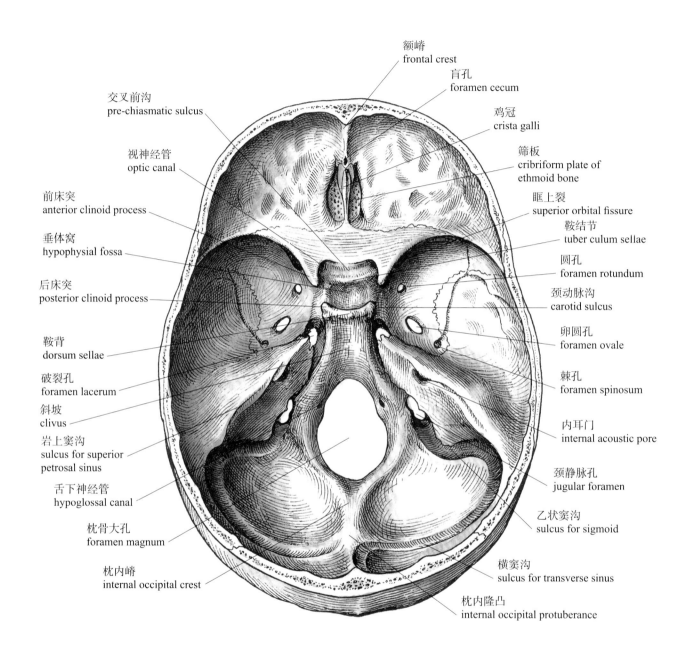

额嵴
frontal crest

盲孔
foramen cecum

鸡冠
crista galli

筛板
cribriform plate of
ethmoid bone

眶上裂
superior orbital fissure

鞍结节
tuber culum sellae

圆孔
foramen rotundum

颈动脉沟
carotid sulcus

卵圆孔
foramen ovale

棘孔
foramen spinosum

内耳门
internal acoustic pore

颈静脉孔
jugular foramen

乙状窦沟
sulcus for sigmoid

横窦沟
sulcus for transverse sinus

枕内隆凸
internal occipital protuberance

交叉前沟
pre-chiasmatic sulcus

视神经管
optic canal

前床突
anterior clinoid process

垂体窝
hypophysial fossa

后床突
posterior clinoid process

鞍背
dorsum sellae

破裂孔
foramen lacerum

斜坡
clivus

岩上窦沟
sulcus for superior
petrosal sinus

舌下神经管
hypoglossal canal

枕骨大孔
foramen magnum

枕内嵴
internal occipital crest

图 1-59　颅底（内面观，模式图）
The base of skull (internal view, diagram)

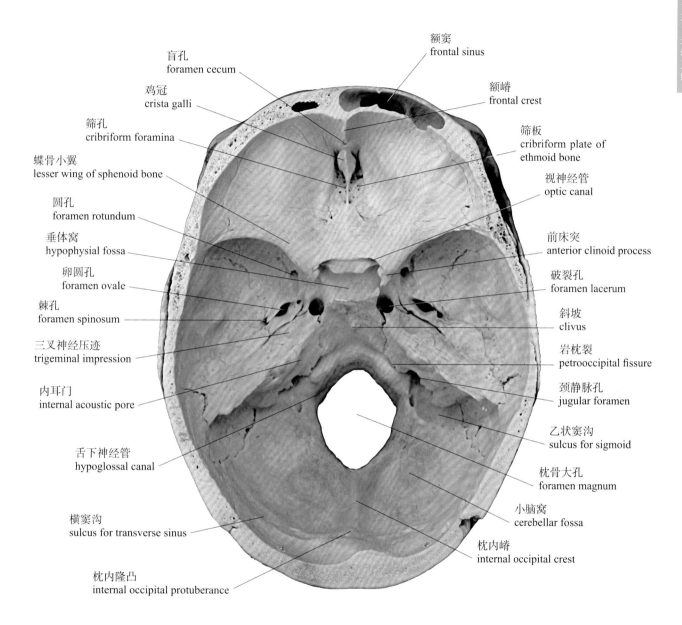

盲孔
foramen cecum

鸡冠
crista galli

筛孔
cribriform foramina

蝶骨小翼
lesser wing of sphenoid bone

圆孔
foramen rotundum

垂体窝
hypophysial fossa

卵圆孔
foramen ovale

棘孔
foramen spinosum

三叉神经压迹
trigeminal impression

内耳门
internal acoustic pore

舌下神经管
hypoglossal canal

横窦沟
sulcus for transverse sinus

枕内隆凸
internal occipital protuberance

额窦
frontal sinus

额嵴
frontal crest

筛板
cribriform plate of
ethmoid bone

视神经管
optic canal

前床突
anterior clinoid process

破裂孔
foramen lacerum

斜坡
clivus

岩枕裂
petrooccipital fissure

颈静脉孔
jugular foramen

乙状窦沟
sulcus for sigmoid

枕骨大孔
foramen magnum

小脑窝
cerebellar fossa

枕内嵴
internal occipital crest

图 1-60 颅底（内面观）
The base of skull (internal view)

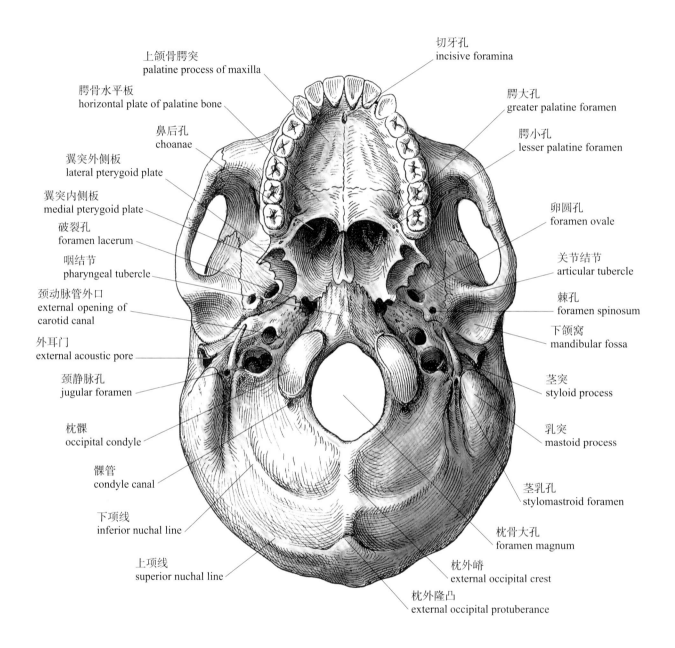

上颌骨腭突
palatine process of maxilla

腭骨水平板
horizontal plate of palatine bone

鼻后孔
choanae

翼突外侧板
lateral pterygoid plate

翼突内侧板
medial pterygoid plate

破裂孔
foramen lacerum

咽结节
pharyngeal tubercle

颈动脉管外口
external opening of
carotid canal

外耳门
external acoustic pore

颈静脉孔
jugular foramen

枕髁
occipital condyle

髁管
condyle canal

下项线
inferior nuchal line

上项线
superior nuchal line

切牙孔
incisive foramina

腭大孔
greater palatine foramen

腭小孔
lesser palatine foramen

卵圆孔
foramen ovale

关节结节
articular tubercle

棘孔
foramen spinosum

下颌窝
mandibular fossa

茎突
styloid process

乳突
mastoid process

茎乳孔
stylomastroid foramen

枕骨大孔
foramen magnum

枕外嵴
external occipital crest

枕外隆凸
external occipital protuberance

图 1-61　颅底（外面观，模式图）
The base of skull (external view, diagram)

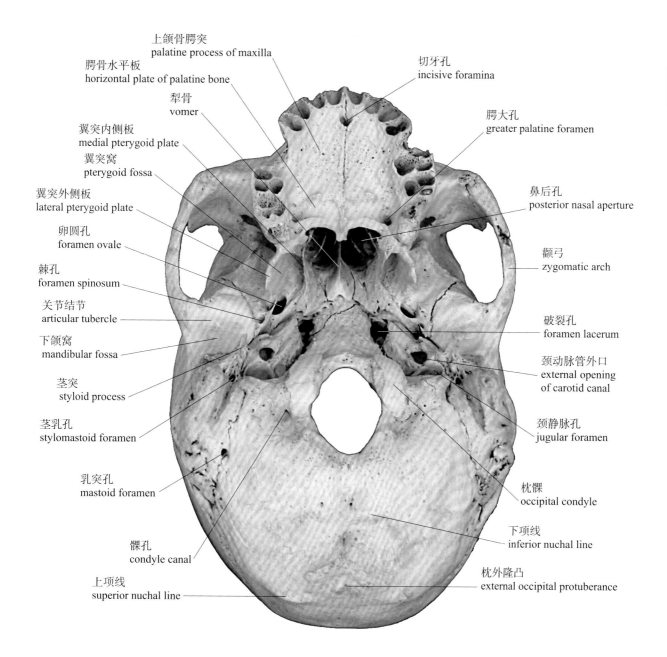

图 1-62 颅底（外面观）
The base of skull (external view)

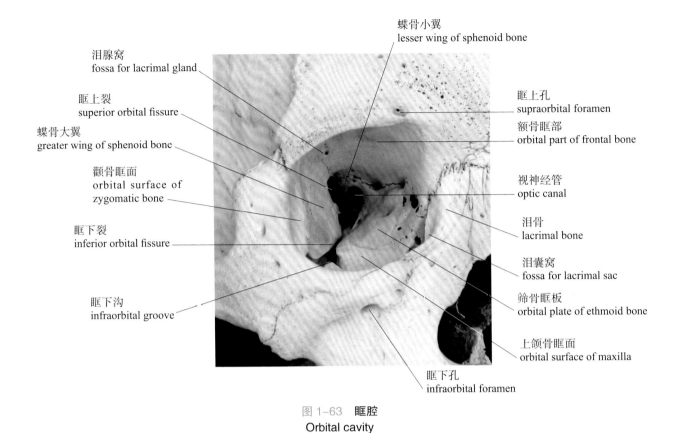

泪腺窝
fossa for lacrimal gland

眶上裂
superior orbital fissure

蝶骨大翼
greater wing of sphenoid bone

颧骨眶面
orbital surface of
zygomatic bone

眶下裂
inferior orbital fissure

眶下沟
infraorbital groove

蝶骨小翼
lesser wing of sphenoid bone

眶上孔
supraorbital foramen

额骨眶部
orbital part of frontal bone

视神经管
optic canal

泪骨
lacrimal bone

泪囊窝
fossa for lacrimal sac

筛骨眶板
orbital plate of ethmoid bone

上颌骨眶面
orbital surface of maxilla

眶下孔
infraorbital foramen

图 1-63 眶腔
Orbital cavity

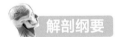 解剖纲要

眶腔的通连

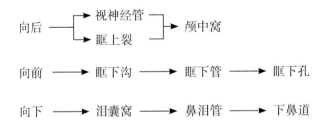

向后 ┬→ 视神经管 ┐
     └→ 眶上裂 ┘ → 颅中窝

向前 → 眶下沟 → 眶下管 → 眶下孔

向下 → 泪囊窝 → 鼻泪管 → 下鼻道

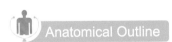 Anatomical Outline

The communication of the orbital cavity

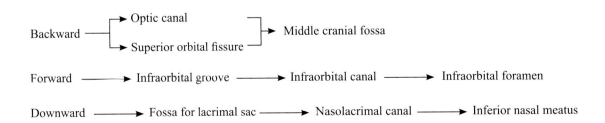

Backward ┬→ Optic canal ┐
         └→ Superior orbital fissure ┘ → Middle cranial fossa

Forward → Infraorbital groove → Infraorbital canal → Infraorbital foramen

Downward → Fossa for lacrimal sac → Nasolacrimal canal → Inferior nasal meatus

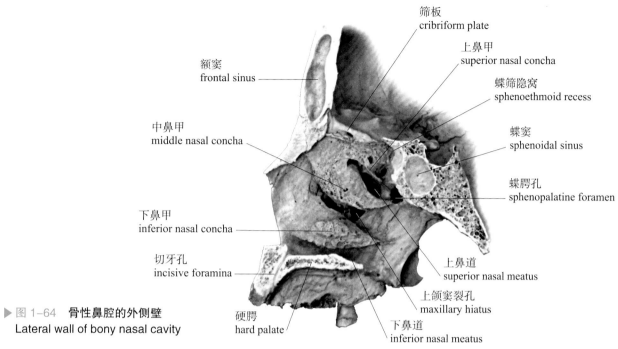

筛板
cribriform plate

额窦
frontal sinus

上鼻甲
superior nasal concha

蝶筛隐窝
sphenoethmoid recess

中鼻甲
middle nasal concha

蝶窦
sphenoidal sinus

蝶腭孔
sphenopalatine foramen

下鼻甲
inferior nasal concha

切牙孔
incisive foramina

上鼻道
superior nasal meatus

上颌窦裂孔
maxillary hiatus

硬腭
hard palate

下鼻道
inferior nasal meatus

▶ 图 1-64　**骨性鼻腔的外侧壁**
Lateral wall of bony nasal cavity

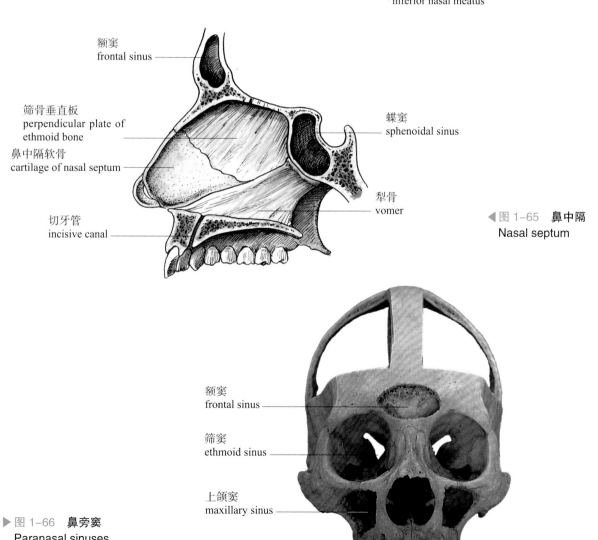

额窦
frontal sinus

筛骨垂直板
perpendicular plate of
ethmoid bone

鼻中隔软骨
cartilage of nasal septum

蝶窦
sphenoidal sinus

犁骨
vomer

切牙管
incisive canal

◀ 图 1-65　**鼻中隔**
Nasal septum

额窦
frontal sinus

筛窦
ethmoid sinus

上颌窦
maxillary sinus

▶ 图 1-66　**鼻旁窦**
Paranasal sinuses

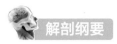 解剖纲要

鼻旁窦的位置、开口部位及临床要点

名称	位置	开口部位	临床意义
额窦	眉弓与眉间深面	中鼻道	鼻旁窦具有丰富的血管，可协助调节吸入空气的温度和湿度；其次对发音起共鸣作用。此部位出现炎症可产生脓鼻涕并影响发音
筛窦	筛骨迷路	前、中群开口于中鼻道，后群开口于上鼻道	
蝶窦	蝶骨体	蝶筛隐窝	
上颌窦	上颌骨体	中鼻道	

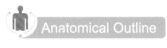 Anatomical Outline

The position, location and clinical significance of paranasal sinus

Name	Position	Opening	Clinical significance
Frontal sinus	Lies deep to superciliary arch and glabella	Middle nasal meatus	The paranasal sinuses are rich in blood vessels and help to regulate the temperature and humidity of the inhaled air. They also resonate with the pronunciation. The inflammation of paranasal sinuses can produce a strong runny nose and affect pronunciation
Ethmoidal sinus	Ethmoidal labyrinth	Anterior and middle groups open to the middle nasal meatus, posterior group open to the superior nasal meatus	
Sphenoid sinus	The body of the sphenoid bone	Sphenoethmoidal recess	
Maxillary sinus	The body of the maxillary	Middle nasal meatus	

第三节　四肢骨　Section 3　Limb bones

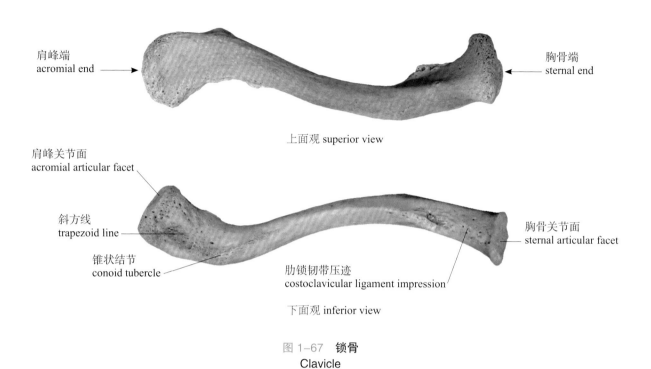

肩峰端
acromial end

胸骨端
sternal end

上面观 superior view

肩峰关节面
acromial articular facet

斜方线
trapezoid line

锥状结节
conoid tubercle

肋锁韧带压迹
costoclavicular ligament impression

胸骨关节面
sternal articular facet

下面观 inferior view

图 1-67　锁骨
Clavicle

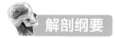 解剖纲要

上肢骨的构成 ┬ 肢带骨：肩胛骨、锁骨
　　　　　　 └ 自由肢骨 ┬ 臂骨：肱骨
　　　　　　　　　　　　 ├ 前臂骨：尺骨、桡骨
　　　　　　　　　　　　 └ 手骨：腕骨（8）、掌骨（5）、指骨（14）

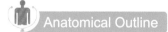 Anatomical Outline

The composition of upper limb bone ┬ Shoulder girdle: scapula, clavicle
　　　　　　　　　　　　　　　　　 └ Bones of free upper limb ┬ Bones of arm: humerus
　　　　　　　　　　　　　　　　　　　　　　　　　　　　　　 ├ Bones of forearm: ulna, radius
　　　　　　　　　　　　　　　　　　　　　　　　　　　　　　 └ Bones of hand: carpal bone (8), metacarpal bones(5), phalanges(14)

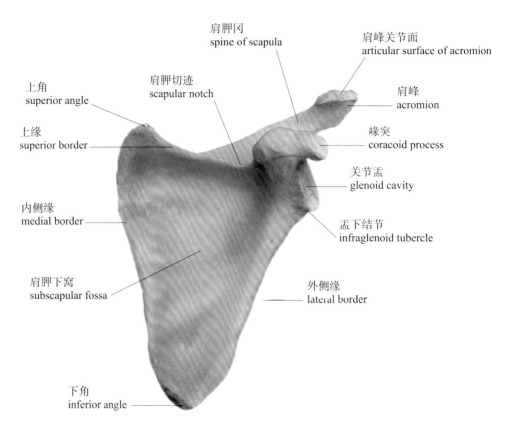

肩胛冈
spine of scapula

肩峰关节面
articular surface of acromion

上角
superior angle

肩胛切迹
scapular notch

肩峰
acromion

上缘
superior border

喙突
coracoid process

关节盂
glenoid cavity

内侧缘
medial border

盂下结节
infraglenoid tubercle

肩胛下窝
subscapular fossa

外侧缘
lateral border

下角
inferior angle

图 1-68　肩胛骨（前面观）
Scapula (anterior view)

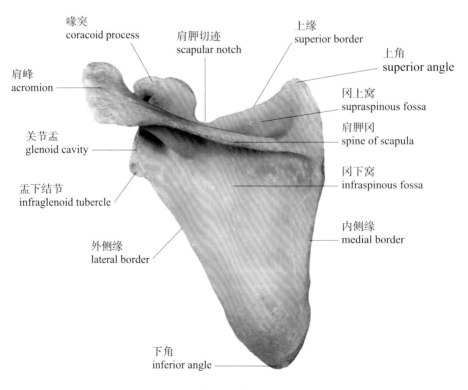

喙突
coracoid process

肩胛切迹
scapular notch

上缘
superior border

上角
superior angle

肩峰
acromion

冈上窝
supraspinous fossa

肩胛冈
spine of scapula

关节盂
glenoid cavity

冈下窝
infraspinous fossa

盂下结节
infraglenoid tubercle

内侧缘
medial border

外侧缘
lateral border

下角
inferior angle

图 1-69　肩胛骨（后面观）
Scapula (posterior view)

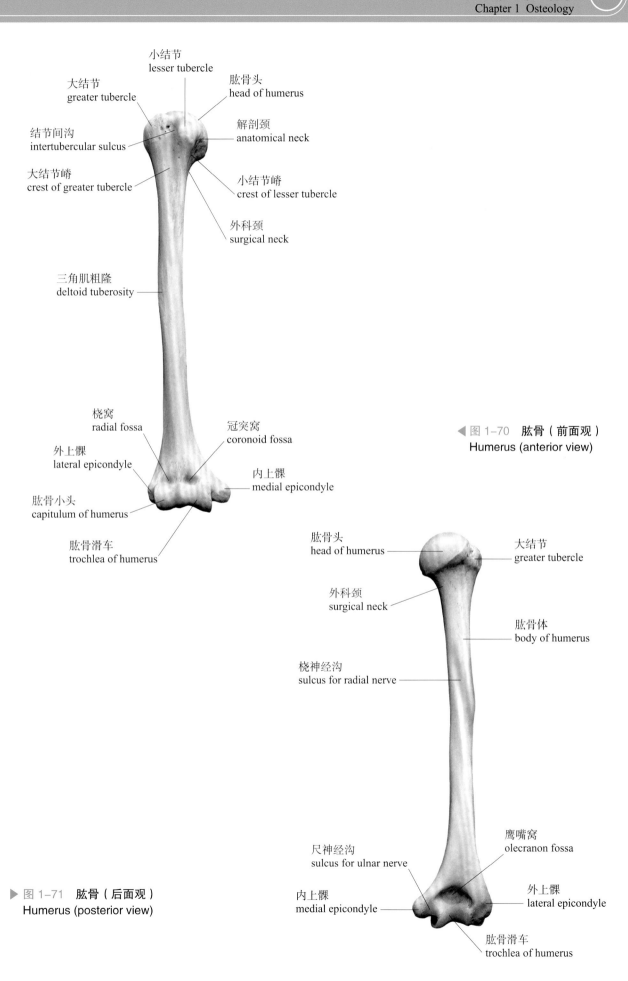

小结节
lesser tubercle

大结节
greater tubercle

肱骨头
head of humerus

结节间沟
intertubercular sulcus

解剖颈
anatomical neck

大结节嵴
crest of greater tubercle

小结节嵴
crest of lesser tubercle

外科颈
surgical neck

三角肌粗隆
deltoid tuberosity

桡窝
radial fossa

冠突窝
coronoid fossa

外上髁
lateral epicondyle

内上髁
medial epicondyle

肱骨小头
capitulum of humerus

肱骨滑车
trochlea of humerus

▶ 图 1-70　肱骨（前面观）
Humerus (anterior view)

肱骨头
head of humerus

大结节
greater tubercle

外科颈
surgical neck

肱骨体
body of humerus

桡神经沟
sulcus for radial nerve

鹰嘴窝
olecranon fossa

尺神经沟
sulcus for ulnar nerve

外上髁
lateral epicondyle

内上髁
medial epicondyle

肱骨滑车
trochlea of humerus

▶ 图 1-71　肱骨（后面观）
Humerus (posterior view)

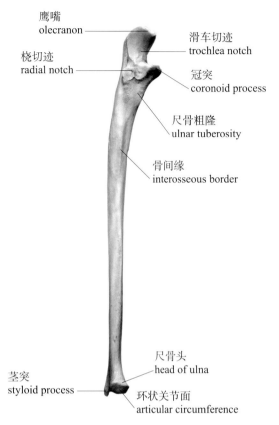

鹰嘴 olecranon

桡切迹 radial notch

滑车切迹 trochlea notch

冠突 coronoid process

尺骨粗隆 ulnar tuberosity

骨间缘 interosseous border

尺骨头 head of ulna

茎突 styloid process

环状关节面 articular circumference

图 1-72　尺骨（前外侧面观）
Ulna (anterolateral view)

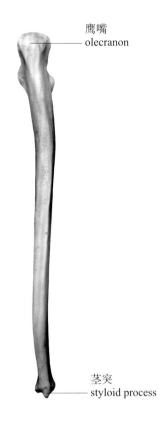

鹰嘴 olecranon

茎突 styloid process

图 1-73　尺骨（后面观）
Ulna (posterior view)

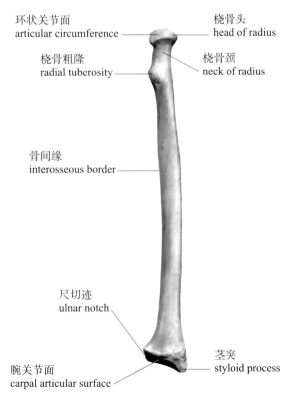

环状关节面 articular circumference

桡骨头 head of radius

桡骨粗隆 radial tuberosity

桡骨颈 neck of radius

骨间缘 interosseous border

尺切迹 ulnar notch

茎突 styloid process

腕关节面 carpal articular surface

图 1-74　桡骨（前面观）
Radius (anterior view)

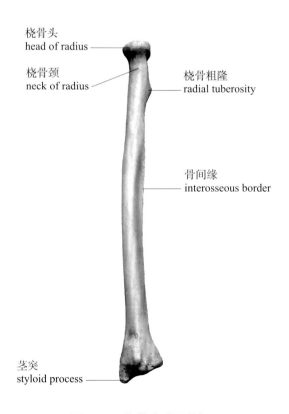

桡骨头 head of radius

桡骨颈 neck of radius

桡骨粗隆 radial tuberosity

骨间缘 interosseous border

茎突 styloid process

图 1-75　桡骨（后面观）
Radius (posterior view)

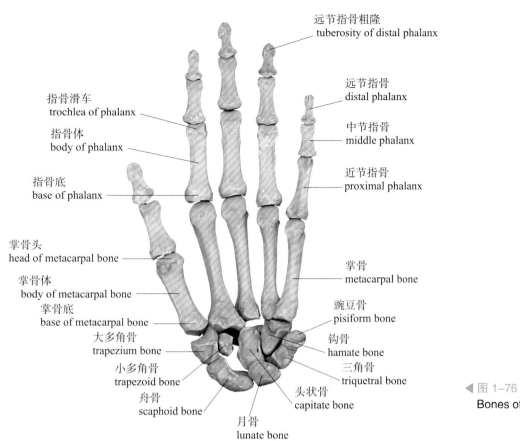

远节指骨粗隆
tuberosity of distal phalanx

远节指骨
distal phalanx

中节指骨
middle phalanx

近节指骨
proximal phalanx

指骨滑车
trochlea of phalanx

指骨体
body of phalanx

指骨底
base of phalanx

掌骨头
head of metacarpal bone

掌骨体
body of metacarpal bone

掌骨底
base of metacarpal bone

大多角骨
trapezium bone

小多角骨
trapezoid bone

舟骨
scaphoid bone

月骨
lunate bone

掌骨
metacarpal bone

豌豆骨
pisiform bone

钩骨
hamate bone

三角骨
triquetral bone

头状骨
capitate bone

◀ 图 1-76 手骨（前面观）
Bones of hand (anterior view)

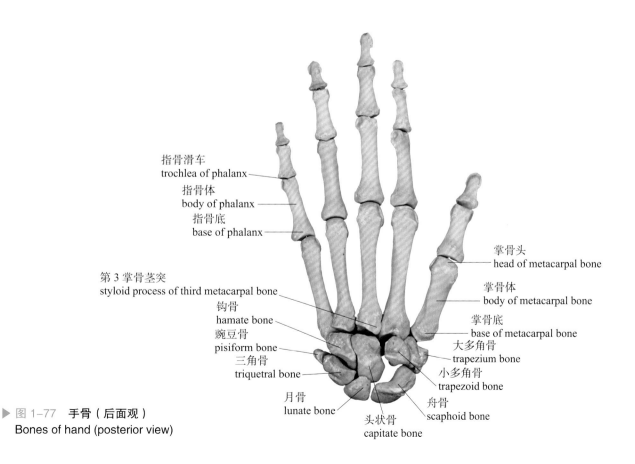

指骨滑车
trochlea of phalanx

指骨体
body of phalanx

指骨底
base of phalanx

第 3 掌骨茎突
styloid process of third metacarpal bone

钩骨
hamate bone

豌豆骨
pisiform bone

三角骨
triquetral bone

月骨
lunate bone

头状骨
capitate bone

掌骨头
head of metacarpal bone

掌骨体
body of metacarpal bone

掌骨底
base of metacarpal bone

大多角骨
trapezium bone

小多角骨
trapezoid bone

舟骨
scaphoid bone

▶ 图 1-77 手骨（后面观）
Bones of hand (posterior view)

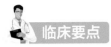

临床要点

上肢骨的临床要点

1. 锁骨由于位置表浅，易发生骨折，一般多见于骨体的内、中 1/3 交界处。

2. 肱骨上端骨折易发生在外科颈处；肱骨中段骨折易伤及桡神经及其伴行血管；肱骨下端骨折易发生在内、外上髁的连线处，临床称为肱骨髁上骨折。

3. 桡骨下端由于突然变宽、骨质较松，成为力学上的弱点，当跌倒手掌触地时较易骨折，临床称为前臂远端骨折或 Colle's 骨折。

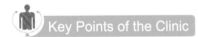

Key Points of the Clinic

Clinical main points of upper limb bone

1. Because of the superficial position of the clavicle, it is easy to be fractured, which is usually found at junction of medial and middle 1/3 of the shaft of clavicle.

2. The fracture of the upper end of humerus is easy to occur in the surgical neck; The fracture occurring in the middle portion of humerus is likely to damage the radial nerve and its accompanying blood vessels; The fracture of the lower end of humerus is easy to occur at the imaginary line between the medial and lateral epicondyles. It is called supracondylar fracture of humerus in clinic.

3. The lower end of radius becomes a dynamical weakness because of its sudden broadening and loosening bone. It is easier to fracture when falling into the palm and touching the ground. It is called distal forearm fracture or Colle's fracture in the clinic.

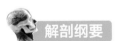

解剖纲要

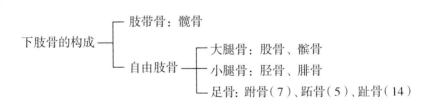

下肢骨的构成 ┬ 肢带骨：髋骨
　　　　　　 └ 自由肢骨 ┬ 大腿骨：股骨、髌骨
　　　　　　　　　　　　 ├ 小腿骨：胫骨、腓骨
　　　　　　　　　　　　 └ 足骨：跗骨（7）、跖骨（5）、趾骨（14）

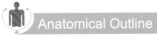

Anatomical Outline

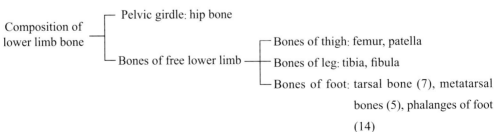

Composition of lower limb bone ┬ Pelvic girdle: hip bone
　　　　　　　　　　　　　　　 └ Bones of free lower limb ┬ Bones of thigh: femur, patella
　　　　　　　　　　　　　　　　　　　　　　　　　　　 ├ Bones of leg: tibia, fibula
　　　　　　　　　　　　　　　　　　　　　　　　　　　 └ Bones of foot: tarsal bone (7), metatarsal bones (5), phalanges of foot (14)

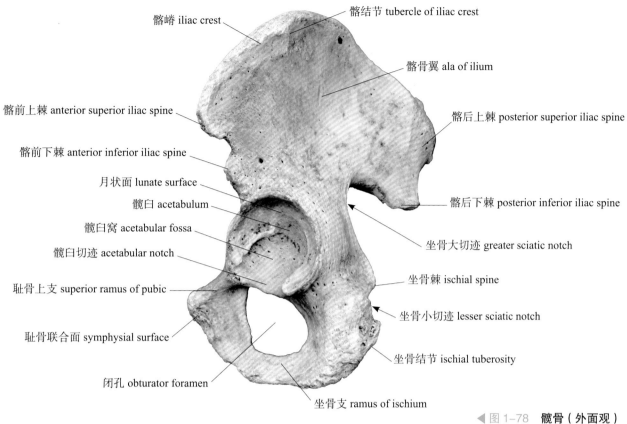

髂嵴 iliac crest

髂结节 tubercle of iliac crest

髂骨翼 ala of ilium

髂前上棘 anterior superior iliac spine

髂后上棘 posterior superior iliac spine

髂前下棘 anterior inferior iliac spine

月状面 lunate surface

髋臼 acetabulum

髂后下棘 posterior inferior iliac spine

髋臼窝 acetabular fossa

坐骨大切迹 greater sciatic notch

髋臼切迹 acetabular notch

耻骨上支 superior ramus of pubic

坐骨棘 ischial spine

坐骨小切迹 lesser sciatic notch

耻骨联合面 symphysial surface

坐骨结节 ischial tuberosity

闭孔 obturator foramen

坐骨支 ramus of ischium

◀ 图 1-78　髋骨（外面观）
Hip bone (external view)

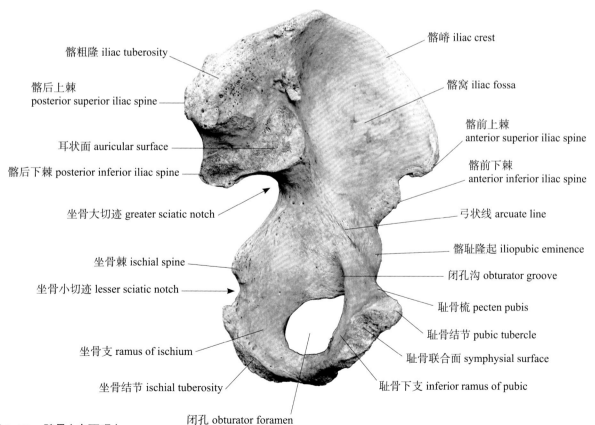

髂粗隆 iliac tuberosity

髂嵴 iliac crest

髂后上棘
posterior superior iliac spine

髂窝 iliac fossa

耳状面 auricular surface

髂前上棘
anterior superior iliac spine

髂后下棘 posterior inferior iliac spine

髂前下棘
anterior inferior iliac spine

坐骨大切迹 greater sciatic notch

弓状线 arcuate line

髂耻隆起 iliopubic eminence

坐骨棘 ischial spine

闭孔沟 obturator groove

坐骨小切迹 lesser sciatic notch

耻骨梳 pecten pubis

耻骨结节 pubic tubercle

坐骨支 ramus of ischium

耻骨联合面 symphysial surface

坐骨结节 ischial tuberosity

耻骨下支 inferior ramus of pubic

闭孔 obturator foramen

▶ 图 1-79　髋骨（内面观）
Hip bone (internal view)

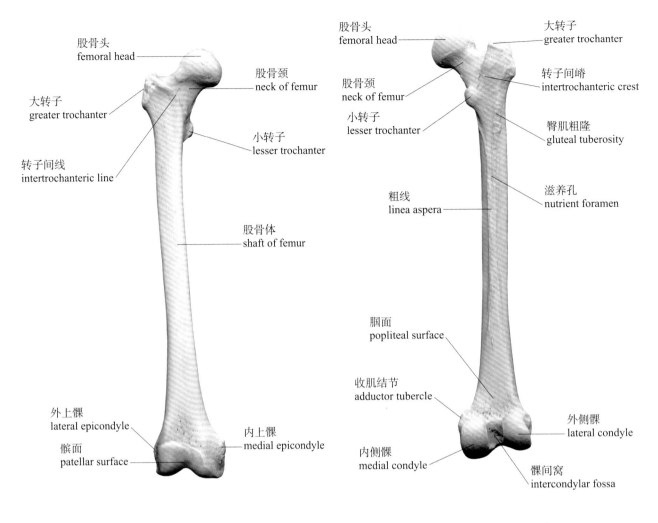

股骨头 femoral head
股骨颈 neck of femur
大转子 greater trochanter
小转子 lesser trochanter
转子间线 intertrochanteric line
股骨体 shaft of femur
外上髁 lateral epicondyle
髌面 patellar surface
内上髁 medial epicondyle

图 1-80 股骨（前面观）
Femur (anterior view)

股骨头 femoral head
大转子 greater trochanter
股骨颈 neck of femur
转子间嵴 intertrochanteric crest
小转子 lesser trochanter
臀肌粗隆 gluteal tuberosity
粗线 linea aspera
滋养孔 nutrient foramen
腘面 popliteal surface
收肌结节 adductor tubercle
外侧髁 lateral condyle
内侧髁 medial condyle
髁间窝 intercondylar fossa

图 1-81 股骨（后面观）
Femur (posterior view)

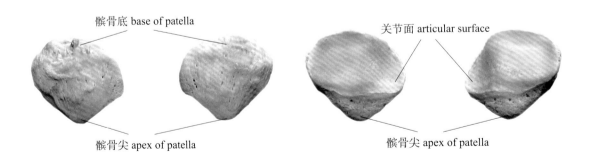

髌骨底 base of patella
髌骨尖 apex of patella

图 1-82 髌骨（前面观）
Patella (anterior view)

关节面 articular surface
髌骨尖 apex of patella

图 1-83 髌骨（后面观）
Patella (posterior view)

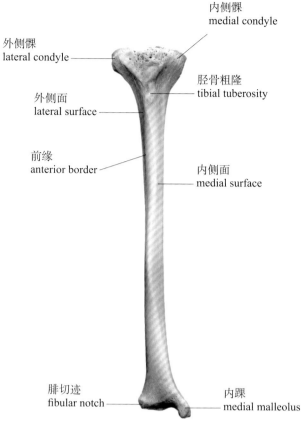

外侧髁
lateral condyle

内侧髁
medial condyle

外侧面
lateral surface

胫骨粗隆
tibial tuberosity

前缘
anterior border

内侧面
medial surface

腓切迹
fibular notch

内踝
medial malleolus

图 1-84 胫骨（前面观）
Tibia (anterior view)

髁间隆起
intercondylar eminence

内侧髁
medial condyle

外侧髁
lateral condyle

比目鱼肌线
soleal line

腓关节面
fibular articular facet

内踝
medial malleolus

腓切迹
fibular notch

图 1-85 胫骨（后面观）
Tibia (posterior view)

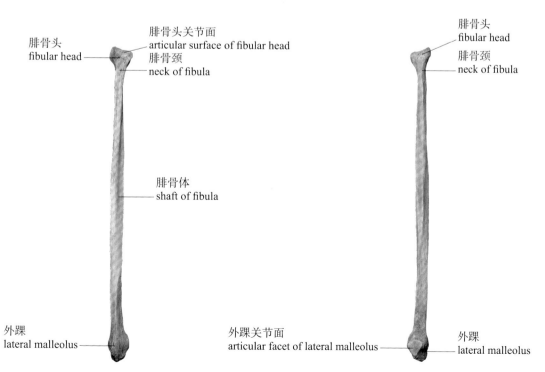

腓骨头
fibular head

腓骨头关节面
articular surface of fibular head

腓骨颈
neck of fibula

腓骨体
shaft of fibula

外踝
lateral malleolus

图 1-86 腓骨（前面观）
Fibula (anterior view)

腓骨头
fibular head

腓骨颈
neck of fibula

外踝关节面
articular facet of lateral malleolus

外踝
lateral malleolus

图 1-87 腓骨（后面观）
Fibula (posterior view)

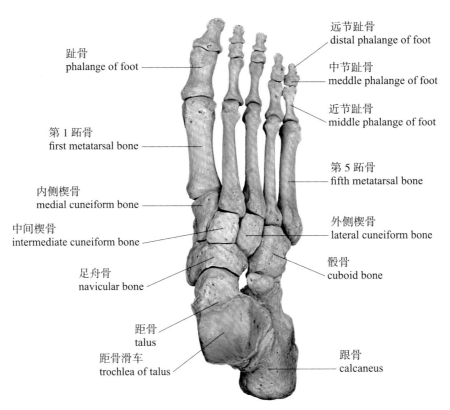

趾骨
phalange of foot

远节趾骨
distal phalange of foot

中节趾骨
meddle phalange of foot

近节趾骨
middle phalange of foot

第 1 跖骨
first metatarsal bone

第 5 跖骨
fifth metatarsal bone

内侧楔骨
medial cuneiform bone

外侧楔骨
lateral cuneiform bone

中间楔骨
intermediate cuneiform bone

骰骨
cuboid bone

足舟骨
navicular bone

距骨
talus

跟骨
calcaneus

距骨滑车
trochlea of talus

图 1-88 足骨（上面观）
Bones of foot (superior view)

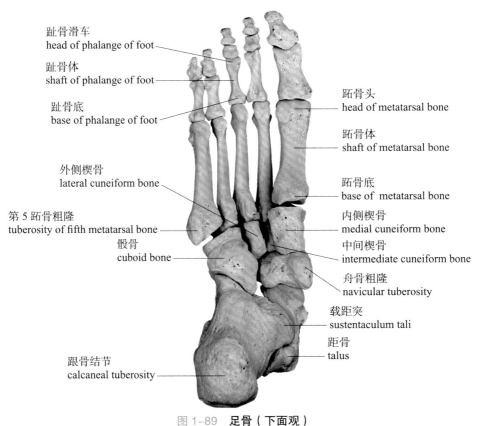

趾骨滑车
head of phalange of foot

趾骨体
shaft of phalange of foot

跖骨头
head of metatarsal bone

趾骨底
base of phalange of foot

跖骨体
shaft of metatarsal bone

外侧楔骨
lateral cuneiform bone

跖骨底
base of metatarsal bone

第 5 跖骨粗隆
tuberosity of fifth metatarsal bone

内侧楔骨
medial cuneiform bone

骰骨
cuboid bone

中间楔骨
intermediate cuneiform bone

舟骨粗隆
navicular tuberosity

载距突
sustentaculum tali

距骨
talus

跟骨结节
calcaneal tuberosity

图 1-89 足骨（下面观）
Bones of foot (inferior view)

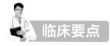 临床要点

下肢骨的临床要点

1. 股骨颈骨折常见于老年人，因老年人骨质疏松，受外力创伤易引起骨折。

2. 髌骨位置表浅，可因外力直接打击而发生粉碎性骨折，也可因间接暴力致横行骨折。

3. 胫骨的横切面呈三角形，下 1/3 呈四边形，故在中 1/3 与下 1/3 交界处，骨的形态转变，易发生骨折。

4. 踝关节背屈时，距骨与踝部密切接触、无活动余地，但在跖屈时，距骨可向两侧轻微活动，所以踝关节往往在跖屈位容易扭伤。

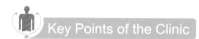 Key Points of the Clinic

Clinicale main points of lower limb bone

1. Femoral neck fractures are common in the elderly, mainly due to osteoporosis in the elderly, which can cause fractures with minor violence.

2. The position of the patella is superficial, which can be caused by comminuted fracture or transverse fracture induced by indirect violence.

3. The transverse section of the tibia is triangular, and the lower 1/3 is quadrilateral, so at the junction of middle and lower 1/3, the bone morphology changes and is prone to fracture.

4. During ankle dorsiflexion, the talus contacts with the ankle closely, and there is no space for movement, but in metatarsal flexion, the talus can move slightly to both sides, so the ankle is often sprained in metatarsal flexion.

第二章　关节学
Chapter 2　Arthrology

第一节　中轴骨的连结　Section 1　Joints of axial skeleton

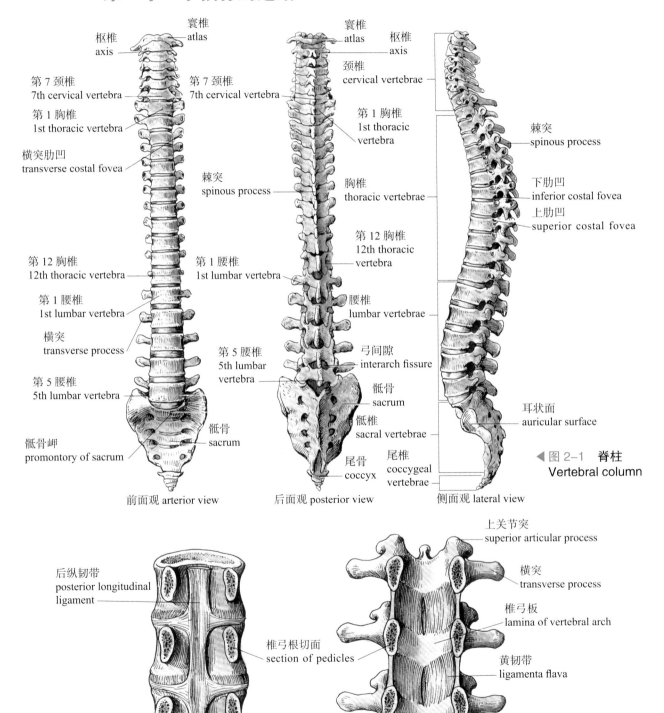

枢椎 axis
寰椎 atlas
第 7 颈椎 7th cervical vertebra
第 1 胸椎 1st thoracic vertebra
横突肋凹 transverse costal fovea
第 12 胸椎 12th thoracic vertebra
第 1 腰椎 1st lumbar vertebra
横突 transverse process
第 5 腰椎 5th lumbar vertebra
骶骨岬 promontory of sacrum

前面观 anterior view

寰椎 atlas
枢椎 axis
第 7 颈椎 7th cervical vertebra
棘突 spinous process
第 1 腰椎 1st lumbar vertebra
第 5 腰椎 5th lumbar vertebra
骶骨 sacrum
尾骨 coccyx

后面观 posterior view

枢椎 axis
颈椎 cervical vertebrae
第 1 胸椎 1st thoracic vertebra
胸椎 thoracic vertebrae
第 12 胸椎 12th thoracic vertebra
腰椎 lumbar vertebrae
弓间隙 interarch fissure
骶骨 sacrum
骶椎 sacral vertebrae
尾椎 coccygeal vertebrae

棘突 spinous process
下肋凹 inferior costal fovea
上肋凹 superior costal fovea
耳状面 auricular surface

侧面观 lateral view

◀ 图 2-1　脊柱
Vertebral column

后纵韧带 posterior longitudinal ligament
椎弓根切面 section of pedicles

后纵韧带 posterior longitudinal ligament

上关节突 superior articular process
横突 transverse process
椎弓板 lamina of vertebral arch
黄韧带 ligamenta flava
下关节突 inferior articular process

黄韧带 ligamenta flara

图 2-2　椎骨的连结（冠状切面，模式图）
Joints of vertebrae (coronal section, diagram)

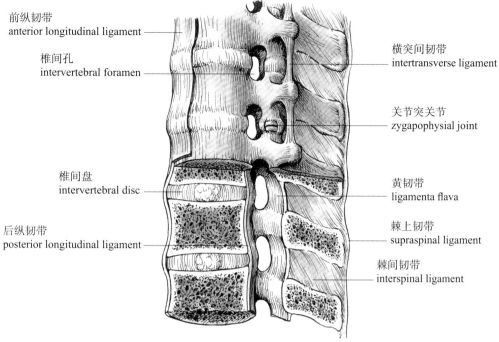

前纵韧带
anterior longitudinal ligament

椎间孔
intervertebral foramen

椎间盘
intervertebral disc

后纵韧带
posterior longitudinal ligament

横突间韧带
intertransverse ligament

关节突关节
zygapophysial joint

黄韧带
ligamenta flava

棘上韧带
supraspinal ligament

棘间韧带
interspinal ligament

图 2-3　椎骨的连结（矢状切面，模式图）
Joints of vertebrae (sagittal section, diagram)

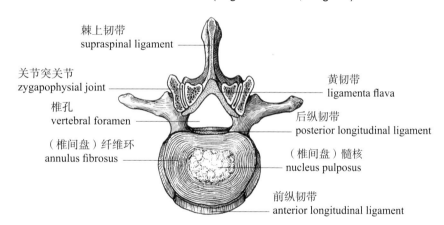

棘上韧带
supraspinal ligament

关节突关节
zygapophysial joint

椎孔
vertebral foramen

（椎间盘）纤维环
annulus fibrosus

黄韧带
ligamenta flava

后纵韧带
posterior longitudinal ligament

（椎间盘）髓核
nucleus pulposus

前纵韧带
anterior longitudinal ligament

图 2-4　椎骨的连结（水平切面，模式图）
Joints of vertebrae (horizontal section, diagram)

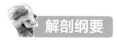 解剖纲要

椎骨连结

　　椎骨之间的连结方式有软骨连结、韧带连结和关节连结，所有椎骨借其连结装置相连，形成脊柱。椎骨的连结包括椎体间连结和椎弓间连结。椎体间连结有椎间盘、前纵韧带和后纵韧带，椎弓间连结包括黄韧带、横突间韧带、棘间韧带、棘上韧带和关节突关节。

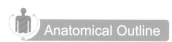 Anatomical Outline

The joints of vertebrae

　　The articulations between the vertebrae include the cartilages, ligaments and joints. All the vertebrae together with their articulations form the vertebral column. The articulations of the vertebrae exist between vertebral bodies and between vertebral arches. The articulations between vertebral bodies include intervertebral discs, anterior and posterior longitudinal ligaments, while the articulations between vertebral arches include the flava ligaments, intertransverse ligaments, interspinal ligaments, supraspinal ligaments and zygapophyseal joints.

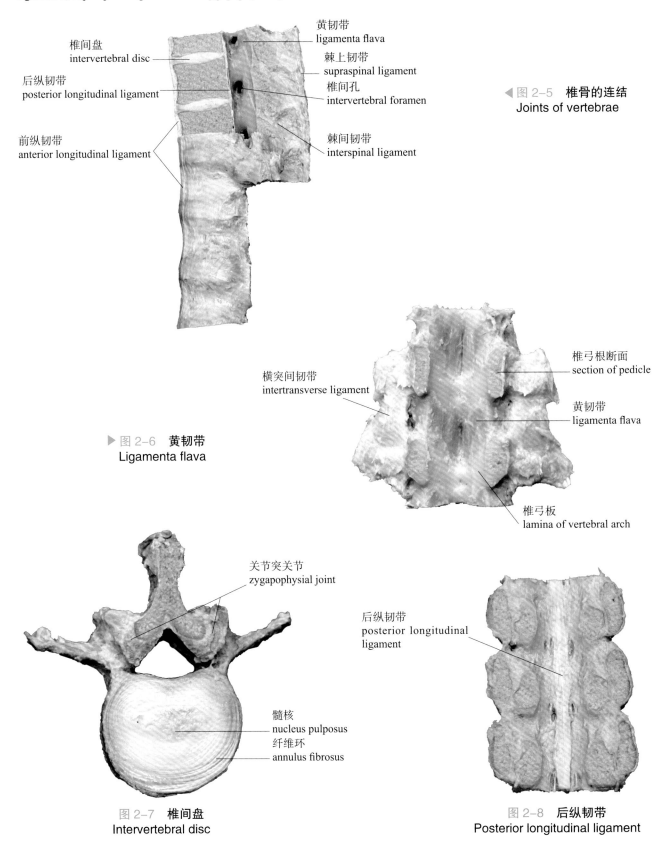

椎间盘
intervertebral disc

后纵韧带
posterior longitudinal ligament

前纵韧带
anterior longitudinal ligament

黄韧带
ligamenta flava

棘上韧带
supraspinal ligament

椎间孔
intervertebral foramen

棘间韧带
interspinal ligament

◀ 图 2-5　椎骨的连结
Joints of vertebrae

横突间韧带
intertransverse ligament

椎弓根断面
section of pedicle

黄韧带
ligamenta flava

椎弓板
lamina of vertebral arch

▶ 图 2-6　黄韧带
Ligamenta flava

关节突关节
zygapophysial joint

髓核
nucleus pulposus
纤维环
annulus fibrosus

后纵韧带
posterior longitudinal
ligament

图 2-7　椎间盘
Intervertebral disc

图 2-8　后纵韧带
Posterior longitudinal ligament

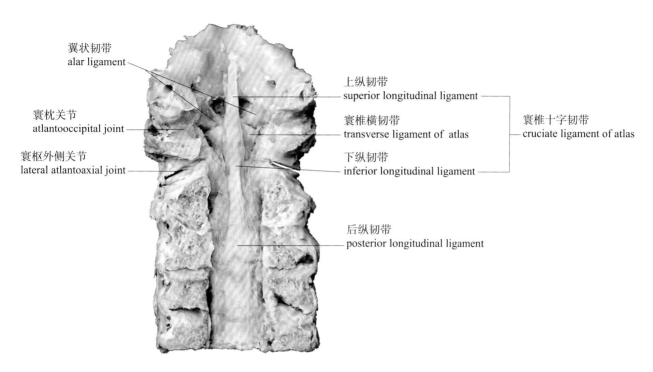

翼状韧带
alar ligament

寰枕关节
atlantooccipital joint

寰枢外侧关节
lateral atlantoaxial joint

上纵韧带
superior longitudinal ligament

寰椎横韧带
transverse ligament of atlas

下纵韧带
inferior longitudinal ligament

寰椎十字韧带
cruciate ligament of atlas

后纵韧带
posterior longitudinal ligament

图 2-9　寰枕关节与寰枢关节（后面观）
Atlantooccipital and atlantoaxial joints (posterior view)

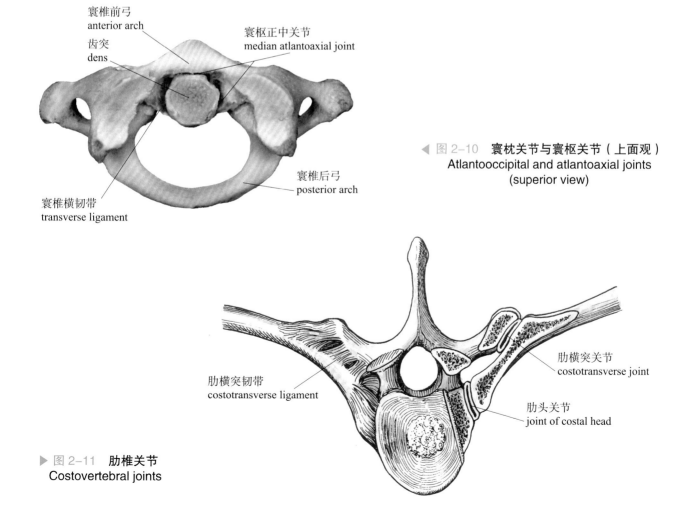

寰椎前弓
anterior arch

齿突
dens

寰枢正中关节
median atlantoaxial joint

寰椎横韧带
transverse ligament

寰椎后弓
posterior arch

◀ 图 2-10　寰枕关节与寰枢关节（上面观）
Atlantooccipital and atlantoaxial joints
(superior view)

肋横突韧带
costotransverse ligament

肋横突关节
costotransverse joint

肋头关节
joint of costal head

▶ 图 2-11　肋椎关节
Costovertebral joints

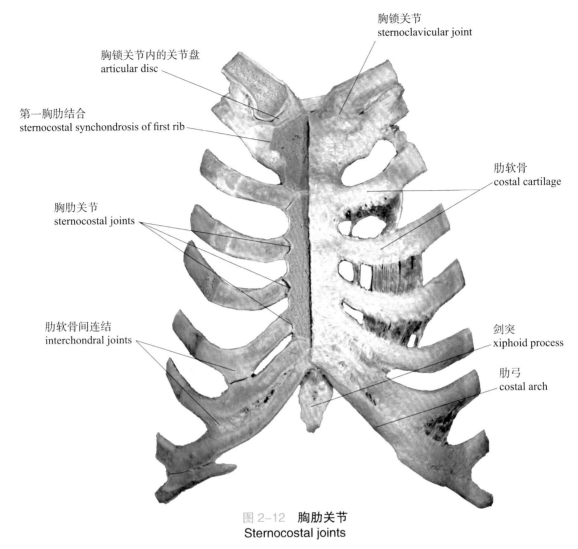

胸锁关节
sternoclavicular joint

胸锁关节内的关节盘
articular disc

第一胸肋结合
sternocostal synchondrosis of first rib

肋软骨
costal cartilage

胸肋关节
sternocostal joints

肋软骨间连结
interchondral joints

剑突
xiphoid process

肋弓
costal arch

图 2-12　胸肋关节
Sternocostal joints

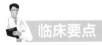 临床要点

脊柱的临床要点

1. 椎间盘结构坚韧，富有弹性，不仅使椎体之间牢固连结，而且起着弹性垫的作用，可缓冲外力对脊柱和颅骨的冲击以保护脊髓和脑。

2. 人体各部的椎间盘厚薄不一，下颈部和上胸部较薄，而上颈部和腰部较厚，故颈部和腰部脊柱的运动幅度较大。

3. 人体各部椎间盘的形态差异与脊柱的生理弯曲有关。颈段和腰段脊柱凸向前方，故其椎间盘前部较后部稍厚，而胸段脊柱凸向后方，故其椎间盘后部较前部稍厚。

4. 过度的负重和劳损可导致纤维环破裂，髓核膨出，形成椎间盘突出症。由于椎间盘的前方有宽而强的前纵韧带，而其后方的后纵韧带窄而弱，故髓核常向后外侧脱出，以致压迫脊髓和脊神经根。

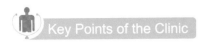 Key Points of the Clinic

Clinical points of the vertebral column

1. The intervertebral discs are tough and elastic, which not only make the vertebral bodies connected firmly, but also

play the role of the elastic pad. It can buffer the impact of external forces on the spine and skull to protect the spinal cord and brain.

2. The thickness of intervertebral discs are different in different parts of the vertebral column. The lower cervical and upper thoracic parts are thinner, and the upper cervical and lumbar parts are thicker. Therefore, the range of movement of the cervical and lumbar parts of spine is wider.

3. The morphological differences of the intervertebral discs in different parts of the spinal column are related to its physiological curvatures. The cervical and lumbar parts convex forwards, so the anterior part of the disc is slightly thicker than the posterior part, while the thoracic part of it convex backwards, so the posterior part of the disc is slightly thicker than the anterior part.

4. The rupture of the annulus fibrosus and the protruding nucleus pulposus can be caused by excessive weight-burden and strain, which leads to the prolapse of intervertebral disc. Because of the anterior longitudinal ligament in front of the intervertebral disc is strong and wide, while the posterior longitudinal ligament behind it is narrow and weak, the nucleus pulposus often prolapses to the posterolateral side, leading to compression of the spinal cord and the roots of spinal nerves.

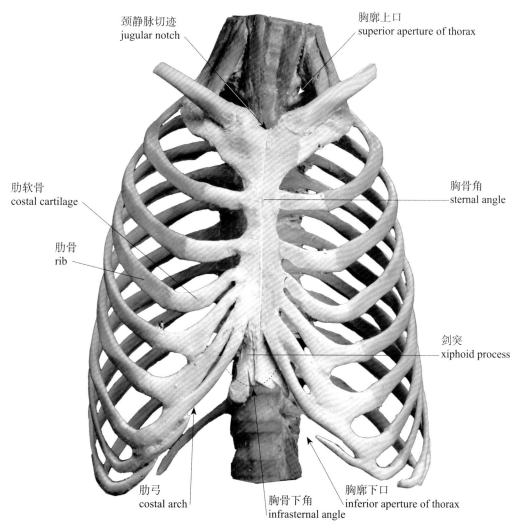

图 2-13 胸廓（前面观）
Thoracic cage (anterior view)

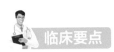

胸廓的临床要点

1. 胸廓参与呼吸运动。胸廓的运动为肋及胸骨的联合运动。肋的运动是以通过肋颈为运动轴的旋转。吸气时，肋向上外举，并使胸骨向前上而扩大胸廓的前后径及横径；呼气时则肋及胸骨下降，从而缩小胸腔。

2. 新生儿胸廓的矢状径较横径稍大，略呈桶状；成年胸廓呈近似圆锥形；女性胸廓较男性者短而圆；老年人胸廓因弹性减退、运动减弱而呈长扁形。

3. 肺及支气管疾病患者胸廓可呈桶状；儿童患佝偻病时胸骨明显凸出，胸廓前后径变大，成为鸡胸。胸廓形态异常，将影响胸腔内心、肺等重要器官的发育和功能。

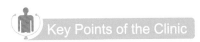

Clinical points of the thorax

1. The thorax is involved in the breathing movement. The motion of the thorax is the associated movement of the ribs and sternum. The movement of the ribs is the rotation that surrounds the axis passing through the rib neck. When inhaling, the ribs are lifted upward and outward, and the sternum is raised forward to enlarge the anterior-posterior diameter and transverse diameter of the thorax; when exhaling, the ribs and sternum are lowered downward in order to reduce the volume of thoracic cavity.

2. The anterior-posterior diameter of the thoracic cage of the newborn is larger than the transverse diameter, so it is slightly barrel-shaped; the adult thoracic cage is approximately conical, the female is shorter and rounder than the male; the elderly one is long and flat because of reducing elasticity and weakening the movement.

3. The diseases of lung and bronchi can make the chest barrel-shaped, children with rickets can make the protrusion of sternum, while the anterior-posterior diameter of the thoracic cage becomes larger, resulting in a malformation of pigeon breast. Abnormal shape of chest will affect the development and functional activity of important organs such as heart, lung and so on.

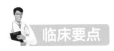

颞下颌关节临床要点

颞下颌关节属于联动关节。张口时，下颌体下降并伴有下颌头和关节盘向前方移动。如果张口过大且关节囊过分松弛，下颌头可滑动至关节结节前方而不能退回关节窝，造成颞下颌关节脱位。故在进行手法复位时，必须先将下颌骨向下拉，使其下颌头低于关节结节，才能再将其回纳至下颌窝内。

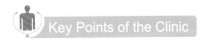

Clinical points of temporomandibular joint

The temporomandibular joint is the associated joint of movement. As the mouth opening, the body of mandible descends while the head of the mandible and the articular disc move forward. If the mouth opens too large and the articular capsule is too loose, the head of mandible can slide to the front of the articular tubercle and not returns back, resulting in dislocation of the temporo mandibular joint. Therefore, during manual reduction, the mandible must be pulled downward to make the head of mandible lower than the articular tubercles, and then it can be returned to the mandibular fossa.

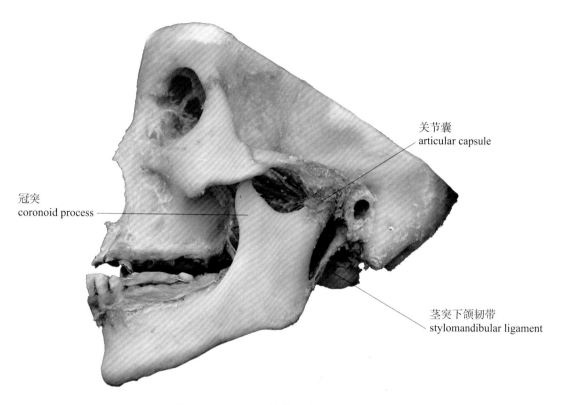

冠突
coronoid process

关节囊
articular capsule

茎突下颌韧带
stylomandibular ligament

图 2-14 颞下颌关节（外侧面观）
Temporomandibular joint (lateral view)

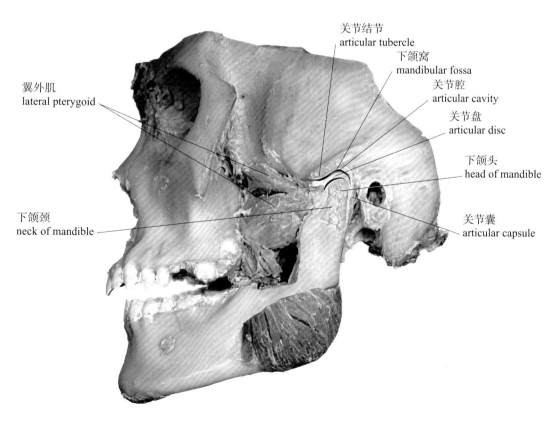

翼外肌
lateral pterygoid

下颌颈
neck of mandible

关节结节
articular tubercle

下颌窝
mandibular fossa

关节腔
articular cavity

关节盘
articular disc

下颌头
head of mandible

关节囊
articular capsule

图 2-15 颞下颌关节（矢状切面）
Temporomandibular joint (sagittal section)

第二节 四肢骨的连结 Section 2 Joints of limbs

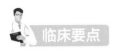 临床要点

肩关节的临床要点

肩周炎又称肩关节周围炎，是一种肩关节囊及其周围韧带、肌腱和滑囊的慢性特异性炎症。好发年龄在 50 岁左右，故有"五十肩"一说。女性发病率略高于男性，多见于体力劳动者。肩周炎的患者，主要表现为日益加重的肩部疼痛及肩关节外展活动受限，其疼痛往往晚上比白天重。该疾病具有一定的自愈性，疼痛逐渐减轻，活动得到改善。

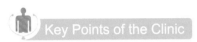 Key Points of the Clinic

Clinical points of shoulder joint

Shoulder periarthritis, also known as periarthritis of shoulder joint, is a chronic and specific inflammation of the articular capsule and its surrounding ligaments, tendons and synovial bursae. The age of onset is about 50 years old, so it is also called as "fifty shoulders". The morbidity in female is slightly higher than that of males, especially in manual workers. The main symptoms of this disease are progressive shoulder pain and limited shoulder abduction. Usually the pain is more serious at night than during the day. The disease has a certain degree of self-healing, pain may be relieved gradually, actirity would be improved.

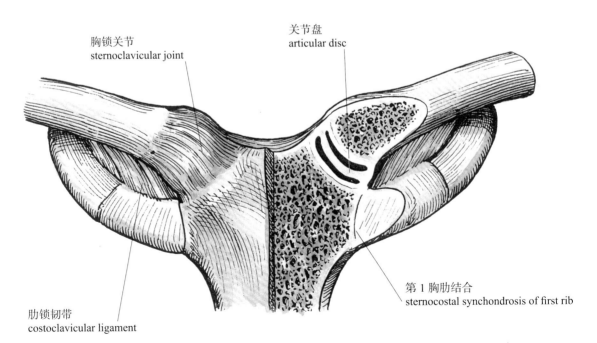

图 2-16 胸锁关节
Sternoclavicular joint

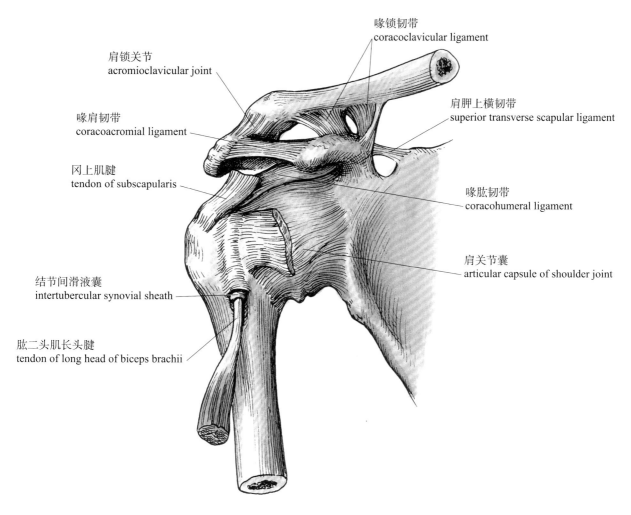

喙锁韧带
coracoclavicular ligament

肩锁关节
acromioclavicular joint

肩胛上横韧带
superior transverse scapular ligament

喙肩韧带
coracoacromial ligament

冈上肌腱
tendon of subscapularis

喙肱韧带
coracohumeral ligament

肩关节囊
articular capsule of shoulder joint

结节间滑液囊
intertubercular synovial sheath

肱二头肌长头腱
tendon of long head of biceps brachii

图 2-17 肩部的关节和韧带
Joints and ligaments of shoulder

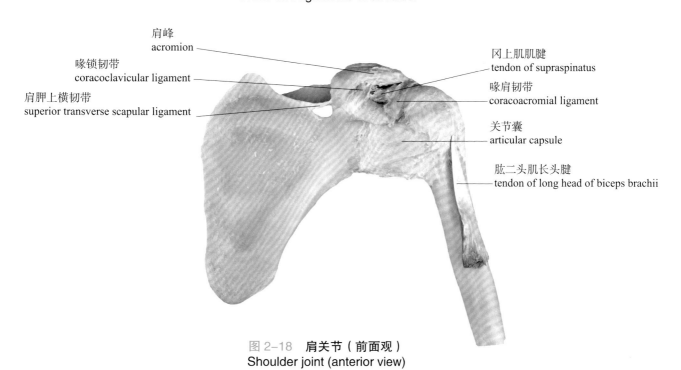

肩峰
acromion

冈上肌肌腱
tendon of supraspinatus

喙锁韧带
coracoclavicular ligament

肩胛上横韧带
superior transverse scapular ligament

喙肩韧带
coracoacromial ligament

关节囊
articular capsule

肱二头肌长头腱
tendon of long head of biceps brachii

图 2-18 肩关节（前面观）
Shoulder joint (anterior view)

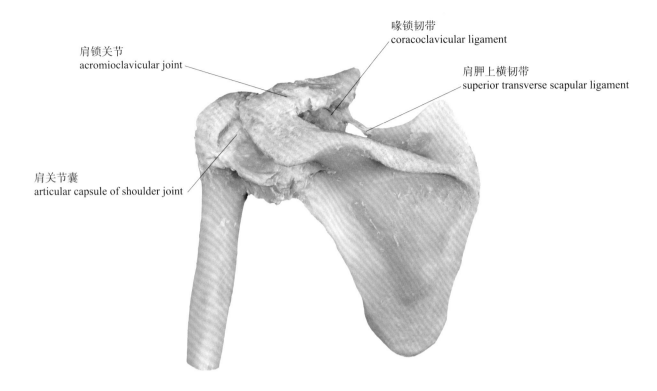

喙锁韧带
coracoclavicular ligament

肩锁关节
acromioclavicular joint

肩胛上横韧带
superior transverse scapular ligament

肩关节囊
articular capsule of shoulder joint

图 2-19 肩关节（后面观）
Shoulder joint (posterior view)

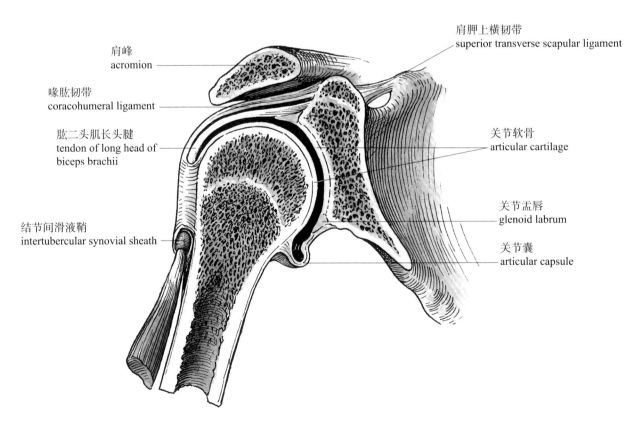

肩峰
acromion

喙肱韧带
coracohumeral ligament

肱二头肌长头腱
tendon of long head of
biceps brachii

结节间滑液鞘
intertubercular synovial sheath

肩胛上横韧带
superior transverse scapular ligament

关节软骨
articular cartilage

关节盂唇
glenoid labrum

关节囊
articular capsule

图 2-20 肩关节（冠状切面，模式图）
Shoulder joint (coronal section, diagram)

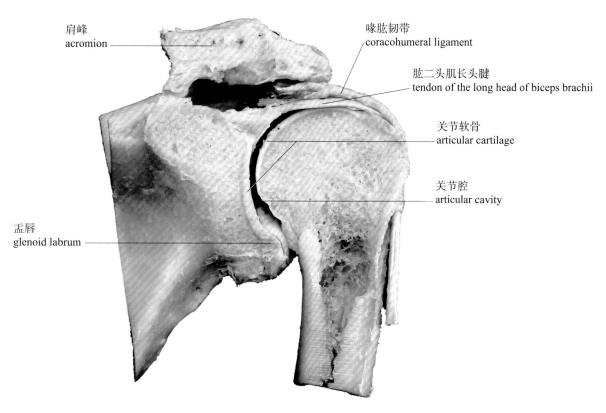

肩峰
acromion

喙肱韧带
coracohumeral ligament

肱二头肌长头腱
tendon of the long head of biceps brachii

关节软骨
articular cartilage

关节腔
articular cavity

盂唇
glenoid labrum

图 2-21　肩关节（冠状切面）
Shoulder joint (coronal section)

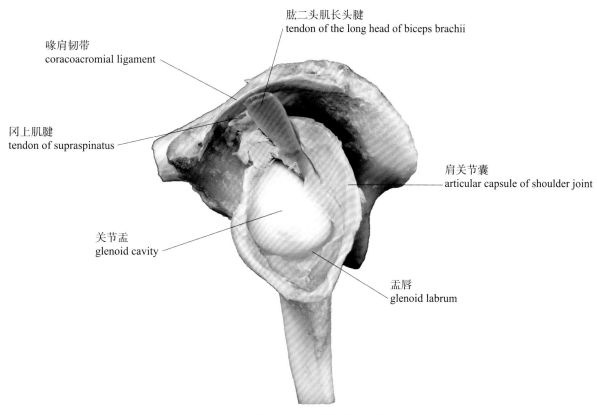

肱二头肌长头腱
tendon of the long head of biceps brachii

喙肩韧带
coracoacromial ligament

冈上肌腱
tendon of supraspinatus

肩关节囊
articular capsule of shoulder joint

关节盂
glenoid cavity

盂唇
glenoid labrum

图 2-22　肩关节（打开）
Shoulder joint (opened)

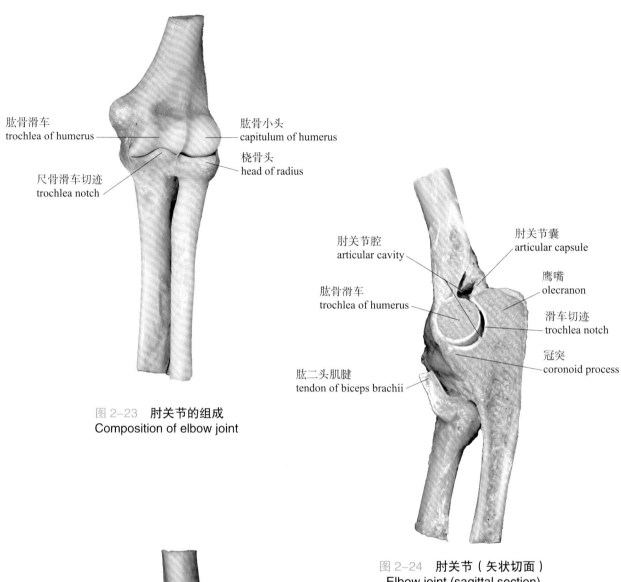

肱骨滑车
trochlea of humerus

肱骨小头
capitulum of humerus

桡骨头
head of radius

尺骨滑车切迹
trochlea notch

肘关节腔
articular cavity

肘关节囊
articular capsule

肱骨滑车
trochlea of humerus

鹰嘴
olecranon

滑车切迹
trochlea notch

冠突
coronoid process

肱二头肌腱
tendon of biceps brachii

图 2-23　肘关节的组成
Composition of elbow joint

图 2-24　肘关节（矢状切面）
Elbow joint (sagittal section)

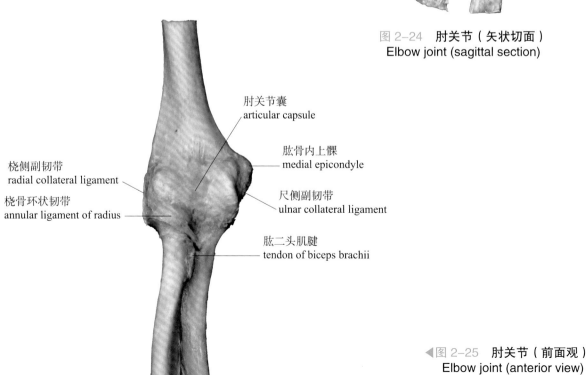

肘关节囊
articular capsule

肱骨内上髁
medial epicondyle

桡侧副韧带
radial collateral ligament

桡骨环状韧带
annular ligament of radius

尺侧副韧带
ulnar collateral ligament

肱二头肌腱
tendon of biceps brachii

◀图 2-25　肘关节（前面观）
Elbow joint (anterior view)

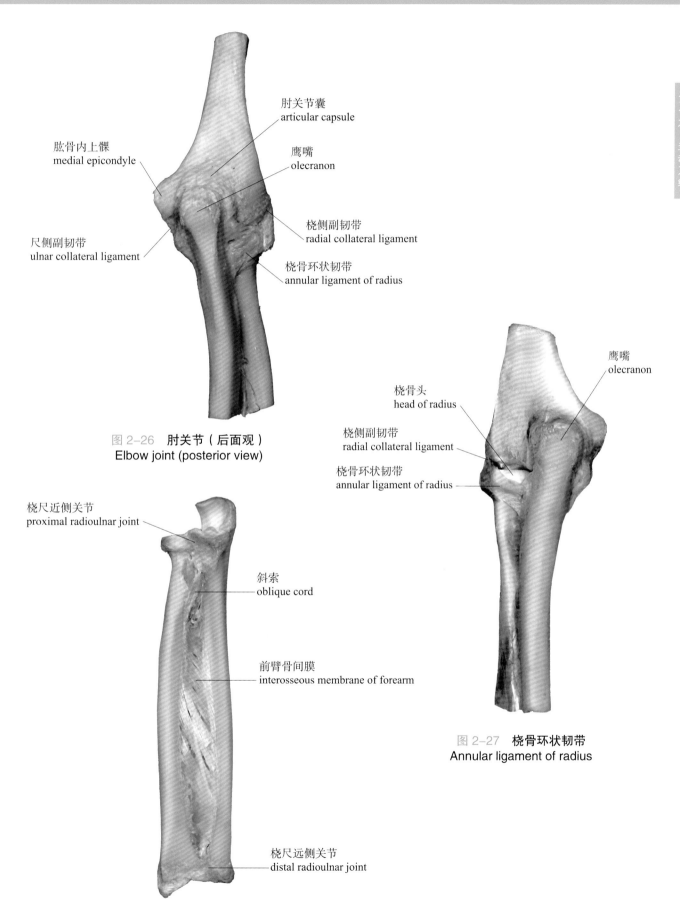

肘关节囊
articular capsule

鹰嘴
olecranon

肱骨内上髁
medial epicondyle

桡侧副韧带
radial collateral ligament

尺侧副韧带
ulnar collateral ligament

桡骨环状韧带
annular ligament of radius

图 2-26　肘关节（后面观）
Elbow joint (posterior view)

鹰嘴
olecranon

桡骨头
head of radius

桡侧副韧带
radial collateral ligament

桡骨环状韧带
annular ligament of radius

图 2-27　桡骨环状韧带
Annular ligament of radius

桡尺近侧关节
proximal radioulnar joint

斜索
oblique cord

前臂骨间膜
interosseous membrane of forearm

桡尺远侧关节
distal radioulnar joint

图 2-28　前臂骨间连结
Joints between ulna and radius

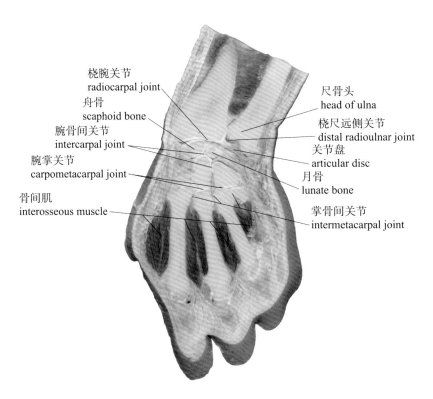

图 2-29　手的关节（冠状面）
Joints of hand (coronal section)

桡腕关节
radiocarpal joint

舟骨
scaphoid bone

腕骨间关节
intercarpal joint

腕掌关节
carpometacarpal joint

骨间肌
interosseous muscle

尺骨头
head of ulna

桡尺远侧关节
distal radioulnar joint

关节盘
articular disc

月骨
lunate bone

掌骨间关节
intermetacarpal joint

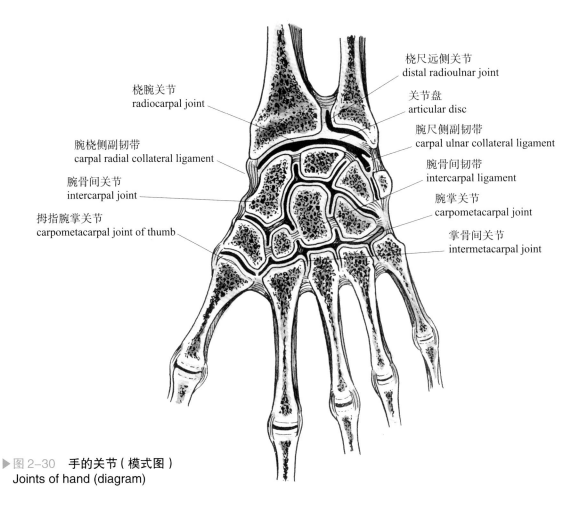

▶图 2-30　手的关节（模式图）
Joints of hand (diagram)

桡腕关节
radiocarpal joint

腕桡侧副韧带
carpal radial collateral ligament

腕骨间关节
intercarpal joint

拇指腕掌关节
carpometacarpal joint of thumb

桡尺远侧关节
distal radioulnar joint

关节盘
articular disc

腕尺侧副韧带
carpal ulnar collateral ligament

腕骨间韧带
intercarpal ligament

腕掌关节
carpometacarpal joint

掌骨间关节
intermetacarpal joint

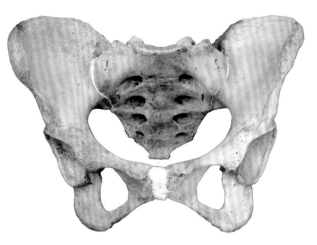

图 2-31 女性骨盆（前面观）
Female pelvis (anterior view)

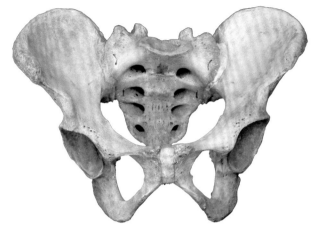

图 2-32 男性骨盆（前面观）
Male pelvis (anterior view)

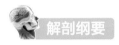

男性和女性骨盆的差异

结构	差异	
	男性	女性
骨盆外形	狭小而高	宽大且矮
骨盆入口	呈心形，前后狭窄	呈圆形或椭圆形，前后宽阔
骨盆出口	狭小	宽大
耻骨下角	较小，为 70° ~ 75°	较大，为 90° ~ 100°
坐骨结节间距	较近	较远

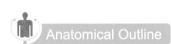

The differences between the male and female pelvis

Structure	Difference	
	male	female
External features	Narrow and high	Wide and low
Inlet of pelvis	Heart-shaped Anterior-posterior short,	Round or oval shape Anterior-posterior long
Outlet of pelvis	Narrow	wide
Subpubic angle	Smaller, 70°-75°	Larger, 90°-100°
Biischial diameter	Shorter	Longer

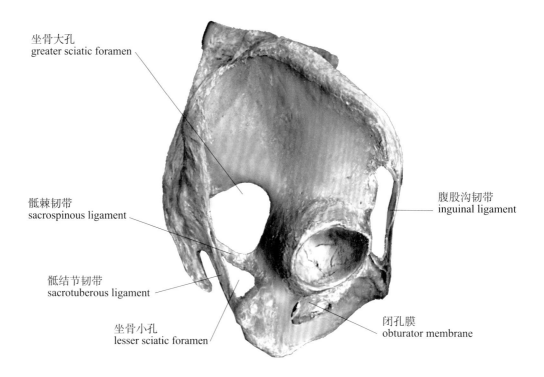

坐骨大孔
greater sciatic foramen

腹股沟韧带
inguinal ligament

骶棘韧带
sacrospinous ligament

骶结节韧带
sacrotuberous ligament

坐骨小孔
lesser sciatic foramen

闭孔膜
obturator membrane

图 2-33 骨盆的韧带（外面观）
Ligaments of pelvis (external view)

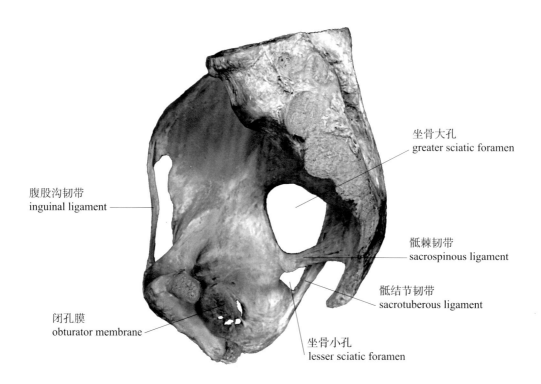

腹股沟韧带
inguinal ligament

坐骨大孔
greater sciatic foramen

骶棘韧带
sacrospinous ligament

骶结节韧带
sacrotuberous ligament

闭孔膜
obturator membrane

坐骨小孔
lesser sciatic foramen

图 2-34 骨盆的韧带（内面观）
Ligaments of pelvis (internal view)

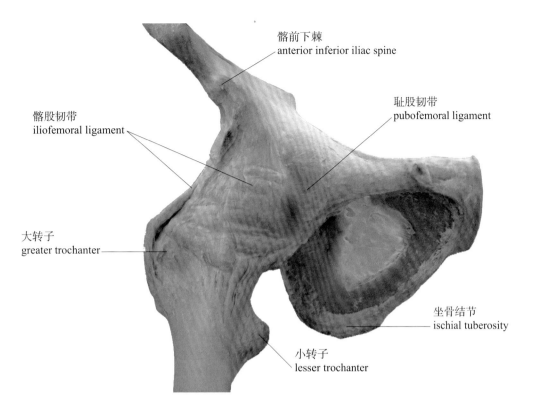

髂前下棘
anterior inferior iliac spine

耻股韧带
pubofemoral ligament

髂股韧带
iliofemoral ligament

大转子
greater trochanter

坐骨结节
ischial tuberosity

小转子
lesser trochanter

图 2-35　髋关节（前面观）
Hip joint (anterior view)

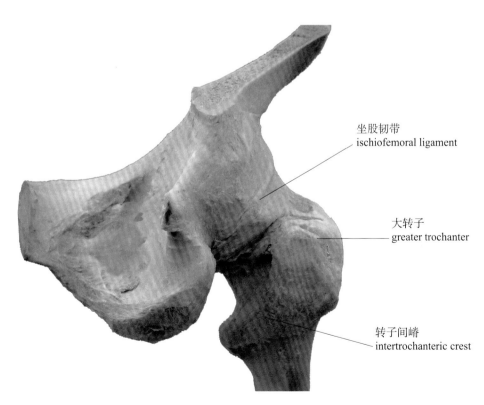

坐股韧带
ischiofemoral ligament

大转子
greater trochanter

转子间嵴
intertrochanteric crest

图 2-36　髋关节（后面观）
Hip joint (posterior view)

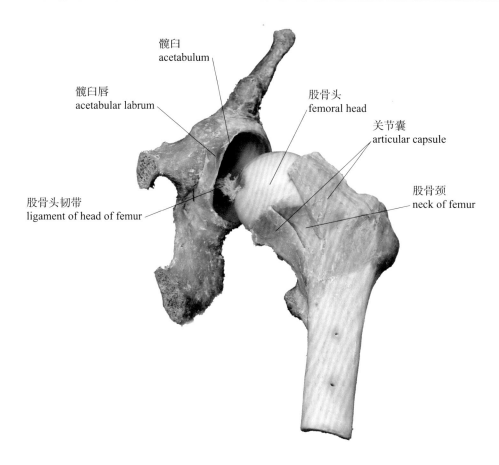

髋臼
acetabulum

髋臼唇
acetabular labrum

股骨头
femoral head

关节囊
articular capsule

股骨头韧带
ligament of head of femur

股骨颈
neck of femur

图 2-37　髋关节（打开）
Hip joint (opened)

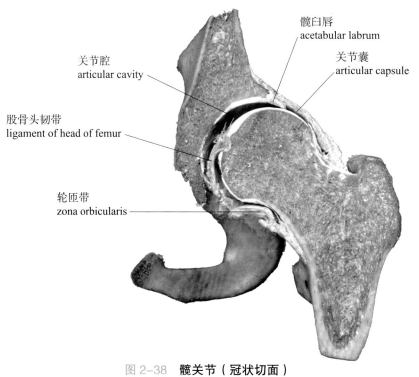

髋臼唇
acetabular labrum

关节囊
articular capsule

关节腔
articular cavity

股骨头韧带
ligament of head of femur

轮匝带
zona orbicularis

图 2-38　髋关节（冠状切面）
Hip joint (coronal section)

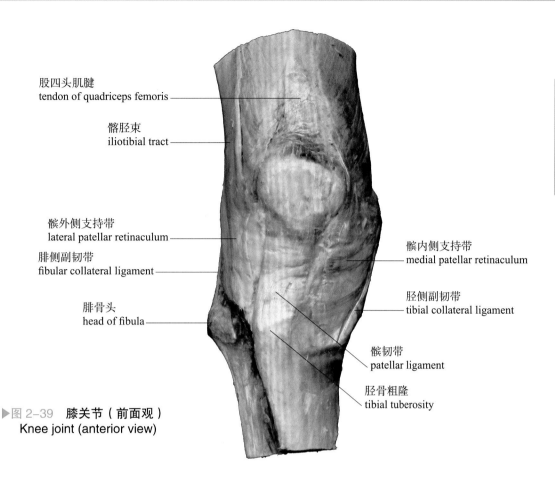

股四头肌腱
tendon of quadriceps femoris

髂胫束
iliotibial tract

髌外侧支持带
lateral patellar retinaculum

腓侧副韧带
fibular collateral ligament

腓骨头
head of fibula

髌内侧支持带
medial patellar retinaculum

胫侧副韧带
tibial collateral ligament

髌韧带
patellar ligament

胫骨粗隆
tibial tuberosity

▶图 2-39 膝关节（前面观）
Knee joint (anterior view)

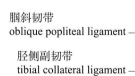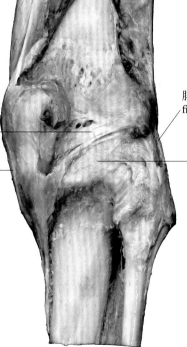

腘斜韧带
oblique popliteal ligament

胫侧副韧带
tibial collateral ligament

腓侧副韧带
fibular collateral ligament

膝关节囊后壁
posterior wall of articular capsule of knee joint

◀图 2-40 膝关节（后面观）
Knee joint (posterior view)

临床要点

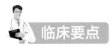

膝关节临床要点

膝关节是人体内最大、结构最复杂的关节。半月板具有一定的弹性，位于股骨下端和胫骨上端之间，使关节面紧密接触，以增加关节的稳定性。同时，半月板还具有一定的活动性，可随膝关节的运动而移动，在膝关节的伸直稳定中起重要的绞索作用。当突然进行有爆发力的运动时，易使半月板损伤或撕裂。

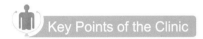

Clinical points of knee joint

The knee joint is the largest and most complex joint of the human body. Because of a certain degree of elasticity, the menisci can make articular surfaces contact closely and increase the stability of the joint which is located between the lower end of the femur and the upper end of the tibia. The menisci also have a certain degree of mobility, they can shift with the movement of the knee joint and play an important noose role in the extending stability of the knee. When the movement of knee is erupting, the injury or tear of menisci can happen easily.

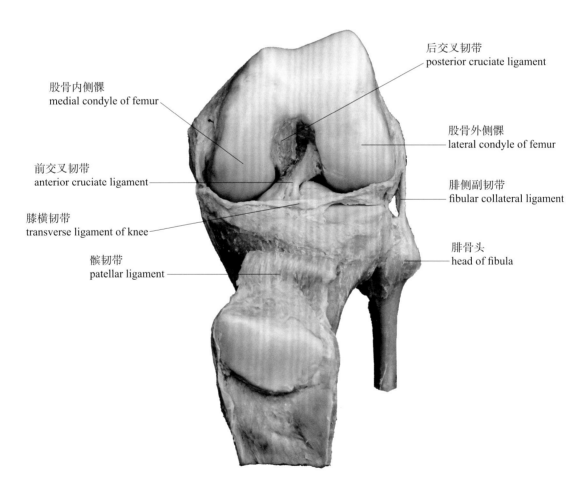

图 2-41　膝关节（前面观，示前交叉韧带）
Knee joint (anterior view, anterior cruciate ligament)

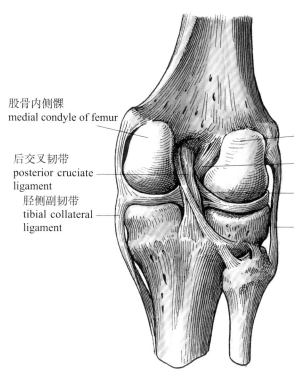

股骨内侧髁
medial condyle of femur

后交叉韧带
posterior cruciate ligament

胫侧副韧带
tibial collateral ligament

股骨外侧髁
lateral condyle of femur

前交叉韧带
anterior cruciate ligament

板股后韧带
posterior meniscofemoral ligament

腓侧副韧带
fibular collateral ligament

图 2-42　膝关节（后面观，模式图）
Knee joint (posterior view, diagram)

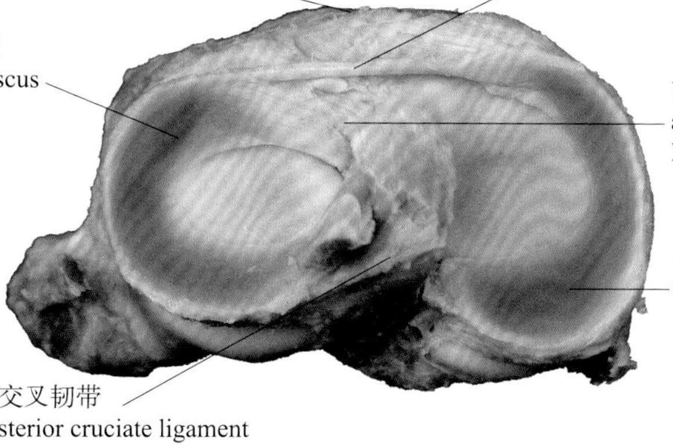

胫骨粗隆
tibial tuberosity

外侧半月板
lateral meniscus

膝横韧带
transverse ligament of knee

前交叉韧带
anterior cruciate ligament

内侧半月板
medial meniscus

后交叉韧带
posterior cruciate ligament

图 2-43　膝关节（上面观，示半月板）
Knee joint (superior view, meniscus)

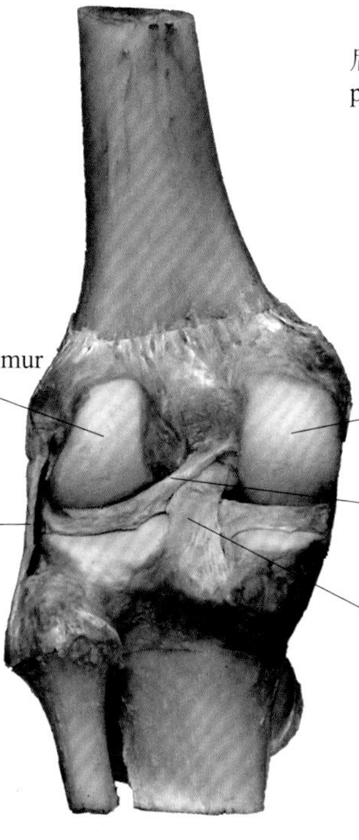

股骨外侧髁
lateral condyle of femur

腓侧副韧带
fibular collateral ligament

股骨内侧髁
medial condyle of femur

板股韧带
meniscofemoral ligament

后交叉韧带
posterior cruciate ligament

图 2-44　膝关节（后面观，示后交叉韧带）
Knee joint (posterior view, posterior cruciate ligament)

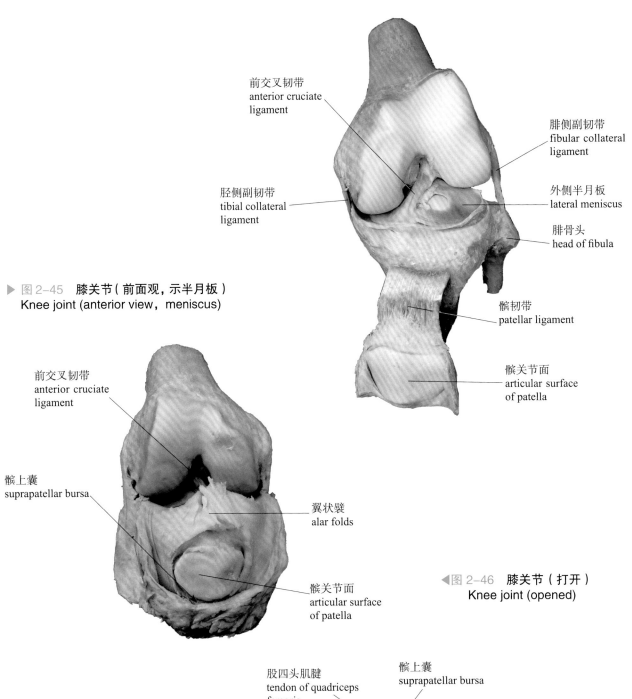

前交叉韧带
anterior cruciate
ligament

腓侧副韧带
fibular collateral
ligament

胫侧副韧带
tibial collateral
ligament

外侧半月板
lateral meniscus

腓骨头
head of fibula

髌韧带
patellar ligament

髌关节面
articular surface
of patella

▶ 图 2-45　膝关节（前面观，示半月板）
Knee joint (anterior view，meniscus)

前交叉韧带
anterior cruciate
ligament

髌上囊
suprapatellar bursa

翼状襞
alar folds

髌关节面
articular surface
of patella

◀图 2-46　膝关节（打开）
Knee joint (opened)

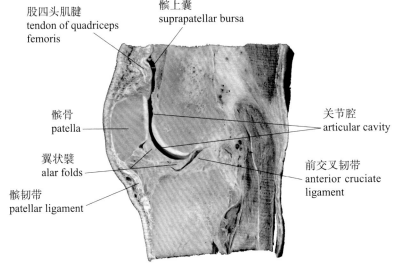

股四头肌腱
tendon of quadriceps
femoris

髌上囊
suprapatellar bursa

髌骨
patella

关节腔
articular cavity

翼状襞
alar folds

前交叉韧带
anterior cruciate
ligament

髌韧带
patellar ligament

▶ 图 2-47　膝关节（矢状切面）
Knee joint (sagittal section)

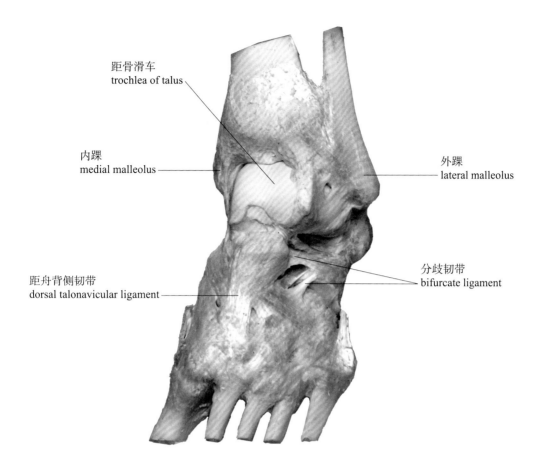

距骨滑车
trochlea of talus

内踝
medial malleolus

外踝
lateral malleolus

分歧韧带
bifurcate ligament

距舟背侧韧带
dorsal talonavicular ligament

图 2-48 踝关节（前面观）
Talocrural joint (anterior view)

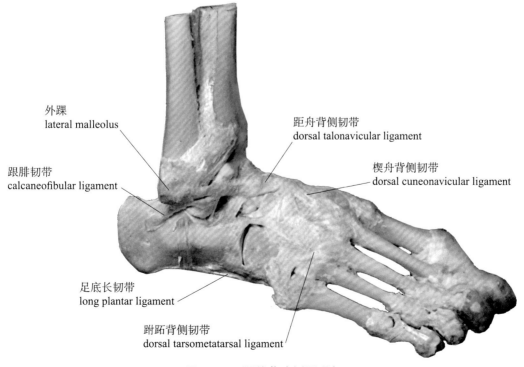

外踝
lateral malleolus

跟腓韧带
calcaneofibular ligament

距舟背侧韧带
dorsal talonavicular ligament

楔舟背侧韧带
dorsal cuneonavicular ligament

足底长韧带
long plantar ligament

跗跖背侧韧带
dorsal tarsometatarsal ligament

图 2-49 踝关节（侧面观）
Talocrural joint (lateral view)

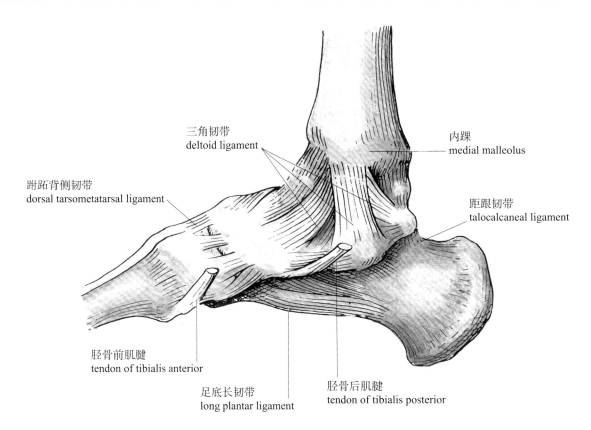

三角韧带
deltoid ligament

内踝
medial malleolus

跗跖背侧韧带
dorsal tarsometatarsal ligament

距跟韧带
talocalcaneal ligament

胫骨前肌腱
tendon of tibialis anterior

足底长韧带
long plantar ligament

胫骨后肌腱
tendon of tibialis posterior

图 2-50 踝和足的韧带（内侧面）
Ligaments of ankle and foot (medial view)

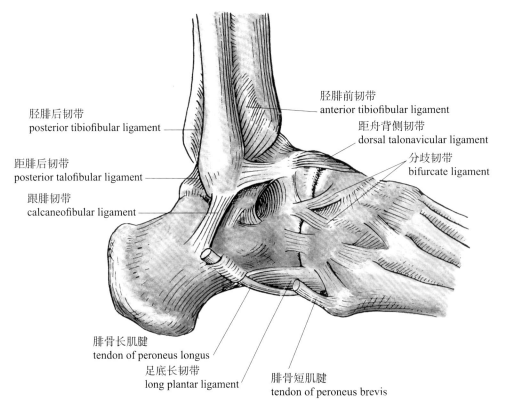

胫腓后韧带
posterior tibiofibular ligament

胫腓前韧带
anterior tibiofibular ligament

距舟背侧韧带
dorsal talonavicular ligament

距腓后韧带
posterior talofibular ligament

分歧韧带
bifurcate ligament

跟腓韧带
calcaneofibular ligament

腓骨长肌腱
tendon of peroneus longus

足底长韧带
long plantar ligament

腓骨短肌腱
tendon of peroneus brevis

图 2-51 踝和足的韧带（外侧面）
Ligaments of ankle and foot (lateral view)

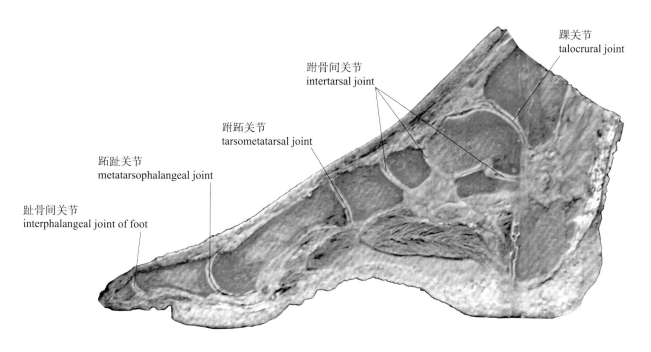

图 2-52　足的关节（矢状面）
Joints of foot (sagittal section)

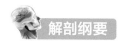

四肢主要关节的小结

关节名称	组成	结构特点	运动
肩关节	关节盂、肱骨头	① 球窝关节，头大盂小，盂周缘有关节唇 ② 关节囊松弛，前、后、上方有韧带和肌腱加强，唯下壁薄弱 ③ 关节囊内有肱二头肌长头腱通过	屈伸、收展、旋转和环转，为全身最灵活的关节
肘关节	肱骨下端，桡、尺骨上端	① 复关节，包含 3 个关节（肱尺、肱桡、桡尺近侧关节），6 个关节面 ② 关节囊前、后壁松弛，两侧有副韧带加强 ③ 桡骨头周围有桡骨环状韧带	蜗状关节为主，可做屈伸运动，桡尺近侧关节参与前臂旋转
桡腕关节	舟、月、三角骨，腕关节面和尺骨下方的关节盘	① 椭圆关节 ② 前、后及两侧均有韧带加强	二轴关节，可做屈伸、收展运动
髋关节	髋臼、股骨头	① 杵臼关节，头大窝深，有髋臼唇 ② 关节囊坚韧，其前、上和后壁均有韧带加强 ③ 股骨颈后面的外 1/3 露于囊外 ④ 关节囊内有股骨头韧带	屈伸、收展、旋转和环转，活动范围小于肩关节
膝关节	股骨下端、胫骨上端和髌骨	① 关节囊宽阔而松弛，囊外有韧带加强 ② 关节囊内有前、后交叉韧带 ③ 关节囊内有内、外侧半月板 ④ 关节囊的滑膜层形成滑膜皱襞（翼状襞）和滑膜囊（髌上囊）	铰链关节，主要为屈伸运动，半屈位时可做轻度旋转运动
踝关节	胫、腓骨下端，距骨滑车	① 滑车关节，距骨滑车前宽后窄，跖屈时稳固性低 ② 关节囊前后松弛，两侧分别有内侧和外侧韧带加强	足背屈和跖屈

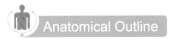 Anatomical Outline

The summary of important joints of limbs

Name	Composition	Structural characteristics	Movement
Shoulder joint	Glenoid cavity and head of the humerus	① Ball and socket joint, head is large but glenoid small, with the glenoid labrum ② Articular capsule is loose, anterior, posterior and superior parts are enhanced by ligaments and tendons, the inferior part is weak only ③ The tendon of long head of biceps passes within it	Flexion and extension, adduction and abduction, rotation and circumduction. It's the most movable joint in the body
Elbow joint	The lower end of humerus the upper end of radius and ulna	① Complex joint, 3 joints (humeroulnar, humeroradial, and proximal radioulnar joints), 6 articular surfaces ② The anterior and posterior wall of capsule is slack, and the collateral ligaments strengthen on both sides ③ The annular ligament of radius encloses the head of the radius	Cochlear joint, flexion and extension mainly, and the proximal radioulnar joint is involved in the rotation of forearm
Radiocarpal joint	Scaphoid, lunate, and triquetral bones; radial carpal articular surface and articular disc	① Ellipsoid joint ② The ligaments reinforce anterior, posterior and both sides of the capsule	Biaxial joints can be flexed and extended
Hip joint	Acetabulum and head of the femur	① Enarthrosis, head is large and socket is deep, with the acetabular labrum ② Articular capsule is tough, and its anterior, posterior and posterior walls are reinforced by ligaments ③ The lateral 1/3 of the neck of the femur behind is exposed outside the capsule ④ Ligament of head of femur is within capsule	Flexion and extension, adduction and abduction, rotation and circumduction Range of motion is smaller than shoulder joint
Knee joint	The lower end of femur, the upper end of tibia, patella	① The articular capsule is broad and loose, with ligaments strengthened outside ② The anterior and posterior cruciate ligaments are within the capsule ③ There are medial and lateral menisci in the articular capsule ④ The synovial layer of capsule forms synovial plica (alar fold) and synovial bursa (suprapatellar bursa)	Hinge joint, mainly flexion and extension, while slight rotation can be done at half flexed position
Ankle joint	The lower end of tibia and fibula, and trochlea of talus	① Trochlear joint, trochlea of talus anterior width and posterior narrowness, low stability with plantarflexed ② The anterior and posterior articular capsule is relaxed, and the medial and lateral ligaments are strengthened on both sides	The dorsal flexion and plantar flexion

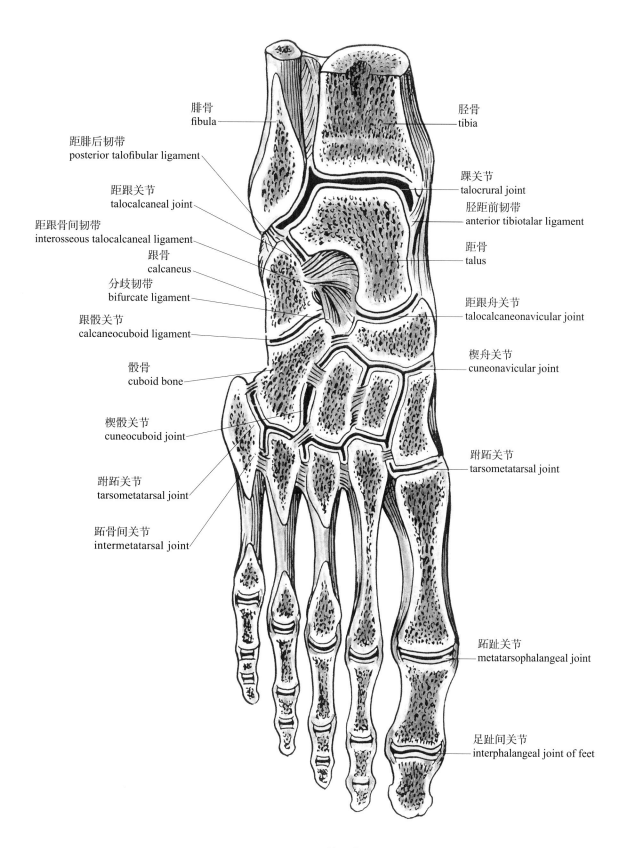

腓骨
fibula

胫骨
tibia

距腓后韧带
posterior talofibular ligament

距跟关节
talocalcaneal joint

距跟骨间韧带
interosseous talocalcaneal ligament

跟骨
calcaneus

分歧韧带
bifurcate ligament

跟骰关节
calcaneocuboid ligament

骰骨
cuboid bone

楔骰关节
cuneocuboid joint

跗跖关节
tarsometatarsal joint

跖骨间关节
intermetatarsal joint

踝关节
talocrural joint

胫距前韧带
anterior tibiotalar ligament

距骨
talus

距跟舟关节
talocalcaneonavicular joint

楔舟关节
cuneonavicular joint

跗跖关节
tarsometatarsal joint

跖趾关节
metatarsophalangeal joint

足趾间关节
interphalangeal joint of feet

图 2-53　足的关节（背侧面观）
Joints of foot (dorsal view)

第三章 肌学
Chapter 3 Myology

第一节 肌学总论 Section 1 Introduction of myology

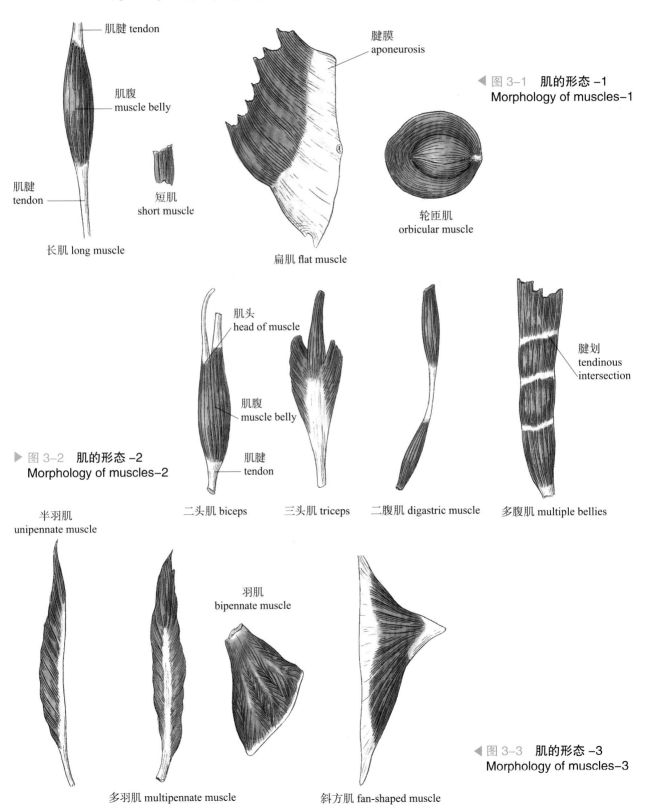

◀ 图 3-1 肌的形态 -1
Morphology of muscles-1

肌腱 tendon

肌腹
muscle belly

肌腱
tendon

短肌
short muscle

长肌 long muscle

腱膜
aponeurosis

轮匝肌
orbicular muscle

扁肌 flat muscle

▶ 图 3-2 肌的形态 -2
Morphology of muscles-2

肌头
head of muscle

肌腹
muscle belly

肌腱
tendon

腱划
tendinous
intersection

半羽肌
unipennate muscle

二头肌 biceps   三头肌 triceps   二腹肌 digastric muscle   多腹肌 multiple bellies

羽肌
bipennate muscle

◀ 图 3-3 肌的形态 -3
Morphology of muscles-3

多羽肌 multipennate muscle   斜方肌 fan-shaped muscle

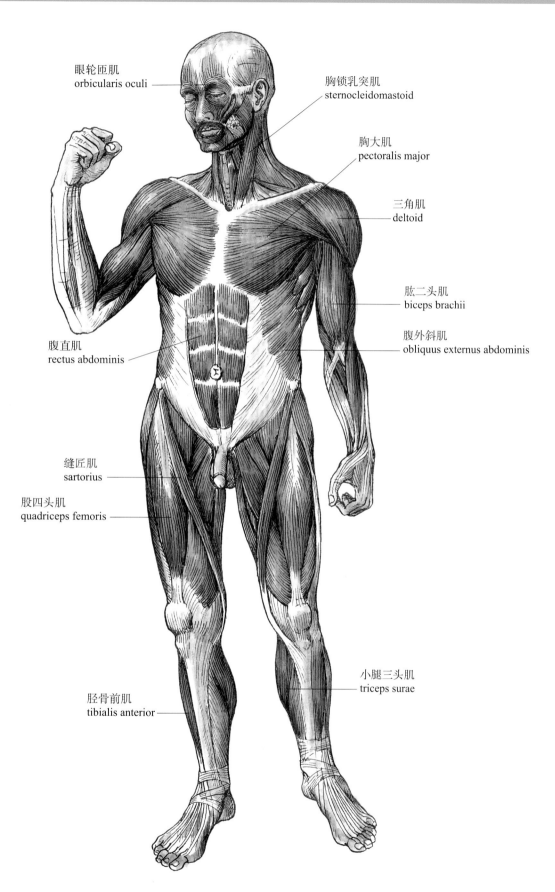

眼轮匝肌
orbicularis oculi

胸锁乳突肌
sternocleidomastoid

胸大肌
pectoralis major

三角肌
deltoid

肱二头肌
biceps brachii

腹外斜肌
obliquus externus abdominis

腹直肌
rectus abdominis

缝匠肌
sartorius

股四头肌
quadriceps femoris

小腿三头肌
triceps surae

胫骨前肌
tibialis anterior

图 3-4　全身肌肉（前面观）
Muscles of body (anterior view)

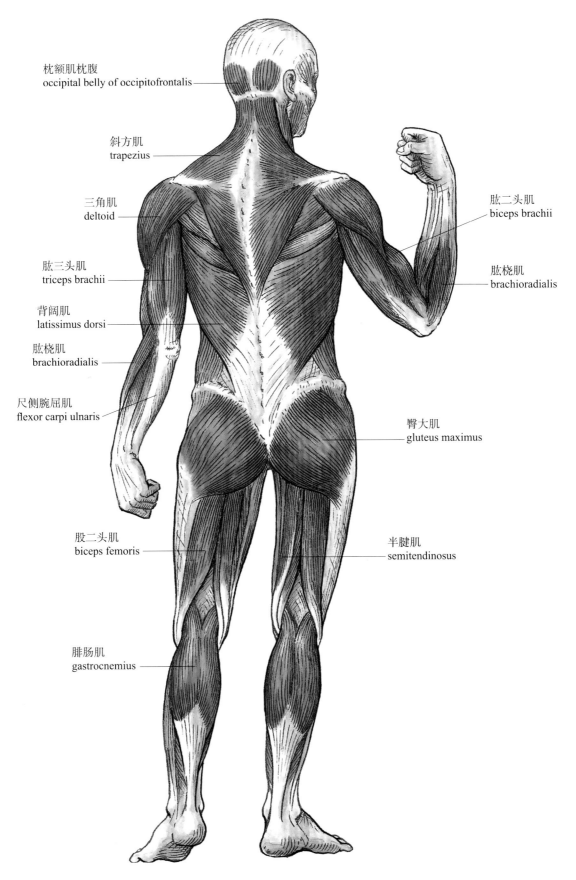

枕额肌枕腹
occipital belly of occipitofrontalis

斜方肌
trapezius

三角肌
deltoid

肱三头肌
triceps brachii

背阔肌
latissimus dorsi

肱桡肌
brachioradialis

尺侧腕屈肌
flexor carpi ulnaris

股二头肌
biceps femoris

腓肠肌
gastrocnemius

肱二头肌
biceps brachii

肱桡肌
brachioradialis

臀大肌
gluteus maximus

半腱肌
semitendinosus

图 3-5　全身肌肉（后面观）
Muscles of body (posterior view)

第二节 头肌与颈肌 Section 2 Muscles of head and neck

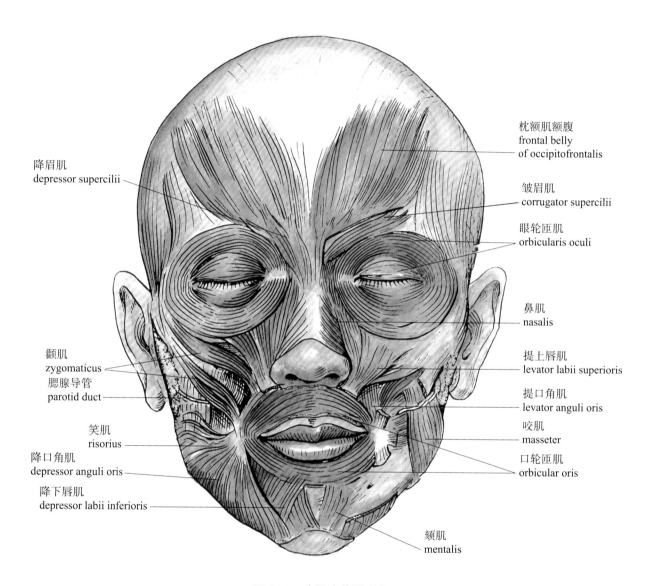

图 3-6 头肌（前面观）
Muscles of head (anterior view)

降眉肌
depressor supercilii

枕额肌额腹
frontal belly
of occipitofrontalis

皱眉肌
corrugator supercilii

眼轮匝肌
orbicularis oculi

鼻肌
nasalis

提上唇肌
levator labii superioris

提口角肌
levator anguli oris

咬肌
masseter

口轮匝肌
orbicular oris

颏肌
mentalis

颧肌
zygomaticus

腮腺导管
parotid duct

笑肌
risorius

降口角肌
depressor anguli oris

降下唇肌
depressor labii inferioris

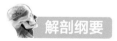 解剖纲要

头部肌肉 ┬ 面肌
　　　　　└ 咀嚼肌：咬肌、颞肌、翼内肌和翼外肌

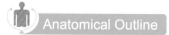 Anatomical Outline

Muscles of head ┬ Facial muscles
　　　　　　　　└ Masticatory muscles: masseter, temporalis, medial and lateral pterygoid muscles

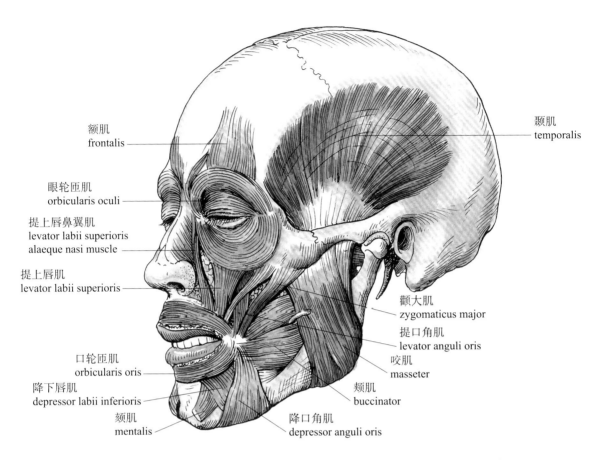

额肌
frontalis

颞肌
temporalis

眼轮匝肌
orbicularis oculi

提上唇鼻翼肌
levator labii superioris
alaeque nasi muscle

提上唇肌
levator labii superioris

颧大肌
zygomaticus major

提口角肌
levator anguli oris

咬肌
masseter

口轮匝肌
orbicularis oris

颊肌
buccinator

降下唇肌
depressor labii inferioris

颏肌
mentalis

降口角肌
depressor anguli oris

图 3-7 头肌（侧面观）
Muscles of head (lateral view)

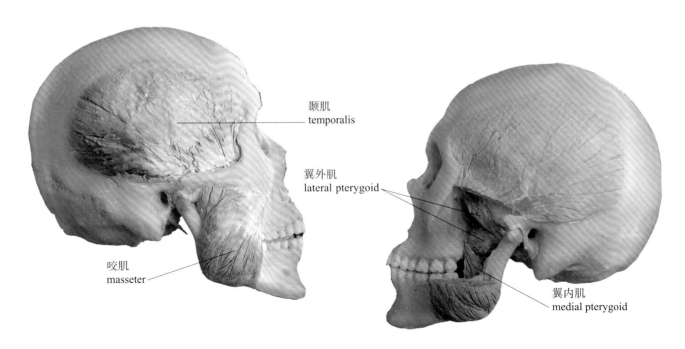

颞肌
temporalis

翼外肌
lateral pterygoid

咬肌
masseter

翼内肌
medial pterygoid

图 3-8 咀嚼肌（浅层）
Masticatory muscles (superficial layer)

图 3-9 咀嚼肌（深层）
Masticatory muscles (deep layer)

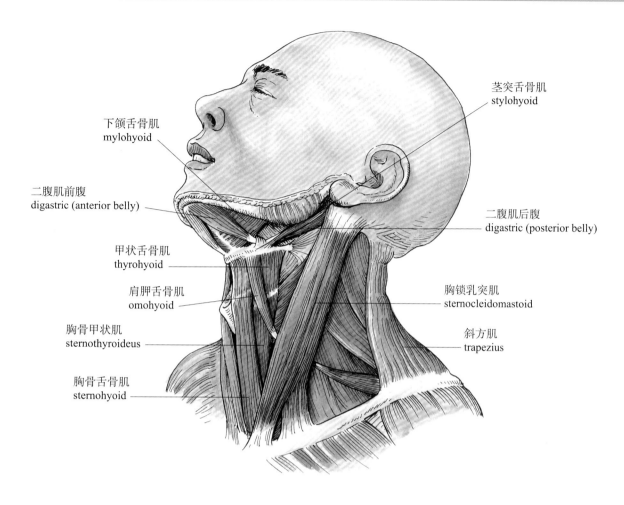

茎突舌骨肌
stylohyoid

下颌舌骨肌
mylohyoid

二腹肌前腹
digastric (anterior belly)

二腹肌后腹
digastric (posterior belly)

甲状舌骨肌
thyrohyoid

肩胛舌骨肌
omohyoid

胸锁乳突肌
sternocleidomastoid

胸骨甲状肌
sternothyroideus

斜方肌
trapezius

胸骨舌骨肌
sternohyoid

图 3-10　颈肌（浅层）
Muscles of neck (superficial layer)

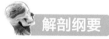 解剖纲要

颈部肌肉
- 浅层：颈阔肌、胸锁乳突肌
- 中层
  - 舌骨上肌群：下颌舌骨肌、颏舌骨肌、二腹肌、茎突舌骨肌
  - 舌骨下肌群：胸骨舌骨肌、肩胛舌骨肌、胸骨甲状肌、甲状舌骨肌
- 深层
  - 外侧肌群：前斜角肌、中斜角肌、后斜角肌
  - 内侧肌群：颈长肌、头长肌

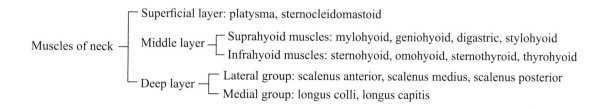 Anatomical Outline

Muscles of neck
- Superficial layer: platysma, sternocleidomastoid
- Middle layer
  - Suprahyoid muscles: mylohyoid, geniohyoid, digastric, stylohyoid
  - Infrahyoid muscles: sternohyoid, omohyoid, sternothyroid, thyrohyoid
- Deep layer
  - Lateral group: scalenus anterior, scalenus medius, scalenus posterior
  - Medial group: longus colli, longus capitis

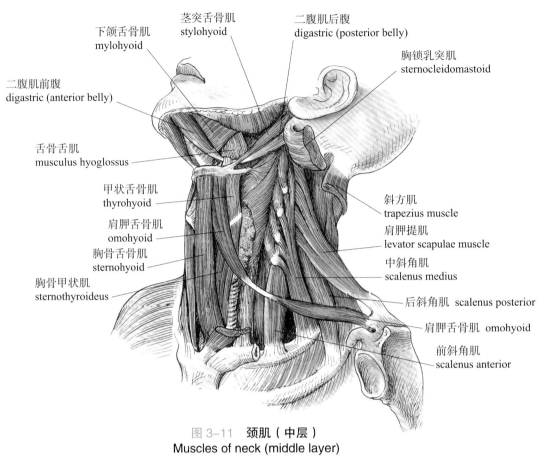

下颌舌骨肌
mylohyoid

茎突舌骨肌
stylohyoid

二腹肌后腹
digastric (posterior belly)

胸锁乳突肌
sternocleidomastoid

二腹肌前腹
digastric (anterior belly)

舌骨舌肌
musculus hyoglossus

甲状舌骨肌
thyrohyoid

肩胛舌骨肌
omohyoid

胸骨舌骨肌
sternohyoid

胸骨甲状肌
sternothyroideus

斜方肌
trapezius muscle

肩胛提肌
levator scapulae muscle

中斜角肌
scalenus medius

后斜角肌 scalenus posterior

肩胛舌骨肌 omohyoid

前斜角肌
scalenus anterior

图 3-11 颈肌（中层）
Muscles of neck (middle layer)

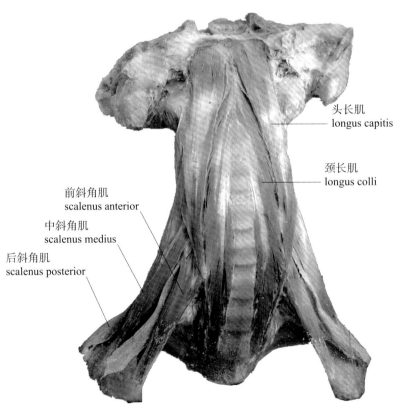

头长肌
longus capitis

颈长肌
longus colli

前斜角肌
scalenus anterior

中斜角肌
scalenus medius

后斜角肌
scalenus posterior

图 3-12 颈肌（深层）
Muscles of neck (deep layer)

第一篇　运动系统　Part 1 Locomotor System

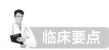
临床要点

先天性肌性斜颈：一侧胸锁乳突肌收缩使头偏向同侧，脸朝向对侧。如一侧胸锁乳突肌挛缩则引起头颈歪斜，如临床常见的斜颈畸形——先天性肌性斜颈。

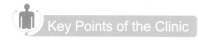
Key Points of the Clinic

Congenital myogenic torticollis: When one side of the sternocleidomastoid is contracting, the head leans to the same side and the face rotates to the opposite side. If one side of sternocleidomastoid contracture will cause head and neck deviation, such as congenital muscular torticollis, a common clinical torticollis.

第三节　躯干肌　Section 3　Muscles of trunk

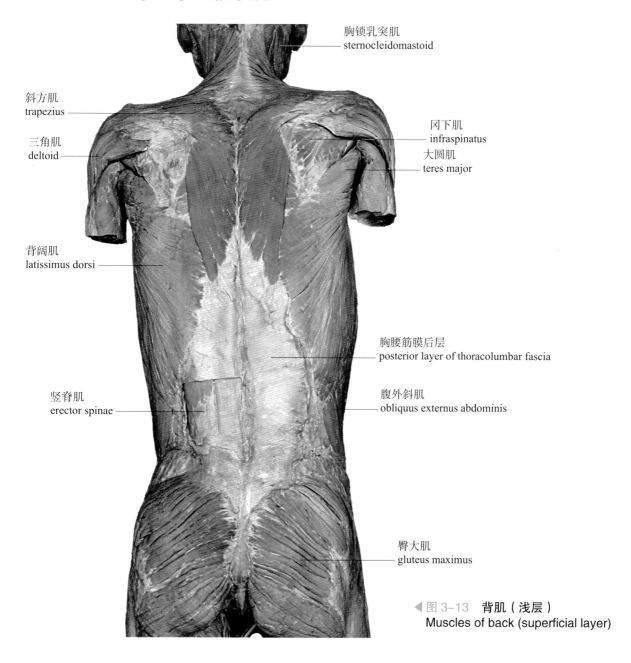

胸锁乳突肌 sternocleidomastoid
斜方肌 trapezius
三角肌 deltoid
冈下肌 infraspinatus
大圆肌 teres major
背阔肌 latissimus dorsi
胸腰筋膜后层 posterior layer of thoracolumbar fascia
竖脊肌 erector spinae
腹外斜肌 obliquus externus abdominis
臀大肌 gluteus maximus

◀ 图 3-13　背肌（浅层）
Muscles of back (superficial layer)

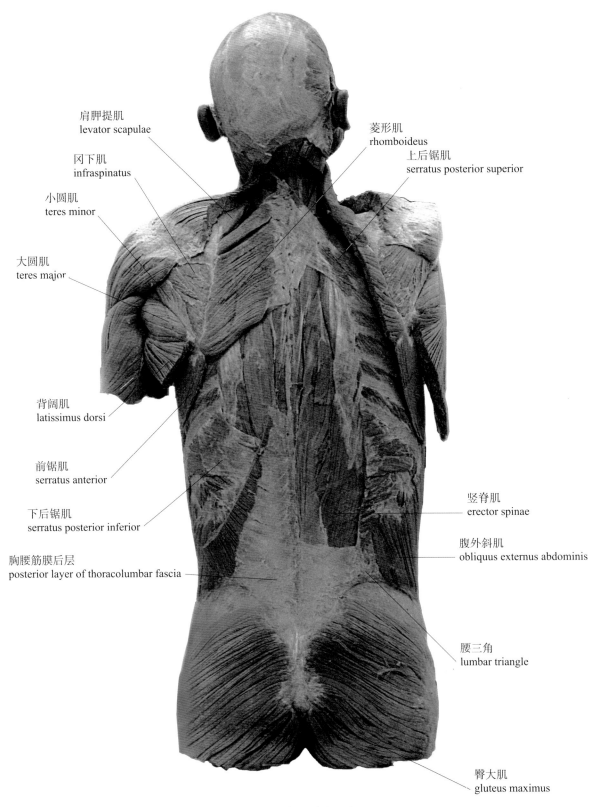

肩胛提肌
levator scapulae

冈下肌
infraspinatus

小圆肌
teres minor

大圆肌
teres major

背阔肌
latissimus dorsi

前锯肌
serratus anterior

下后锯肌
serratus posterior inferior

胸腰筋膜后层
posterior layer of thoracolumbar fascia

菱形肌
rhomboideus

上后锯肌
serratus posterior superior

竖脊肌
erector spinae

腹外斜肌
obliquus externus abdominis

腰三角
lumbar triangle

臀大肌
gluteus maximus

图 3-14 背肌（中层）
Muscles of back (middle layer)

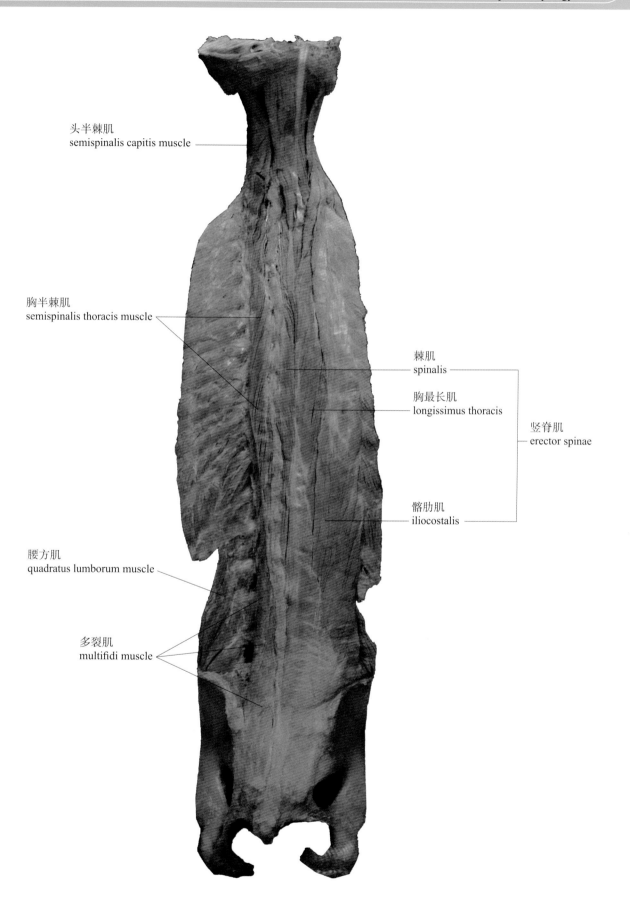

头半棘肌
semispinalis capitis muscle

胸半棘肌
semispinalis thoracis muscle

棘肌
spinalis

胸最长肌
longissimus thoracis

竖脊肌
erector spinae

髂肋肌
iliocostalis

腰方肌
quadratus lumborum muscle

多裂肌
multifidi muscle

图 3-15 背肌（深层）
Muscles of back (deep layer)

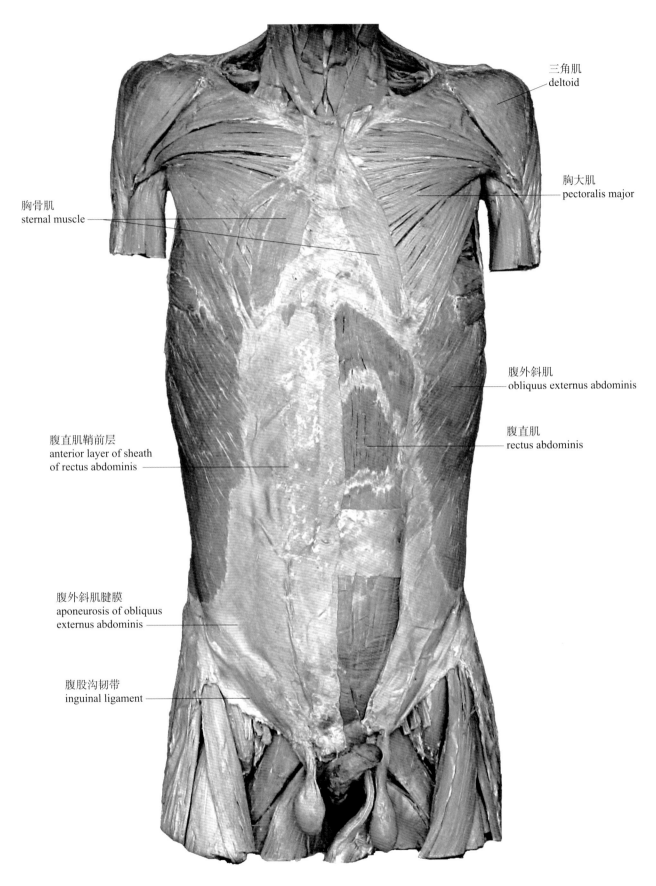

三角肌
deltoid

胸大肌
pectoralis major

胸骨肌
sternal muscle

腹外斜肌
obliquus externus abdominis

腹直肌
rectus abdominis

腹直肌鞘前层
anterior layer of sheath
of rectus abdominis

腹外斜肌腱膜
aponeurosis of obliquus
externus abdominis

腹股沟韧带
inguinal ligament

图 3-16 胸腹肌（浅层）
Muscles of thorax and abdomen (superficial layer)

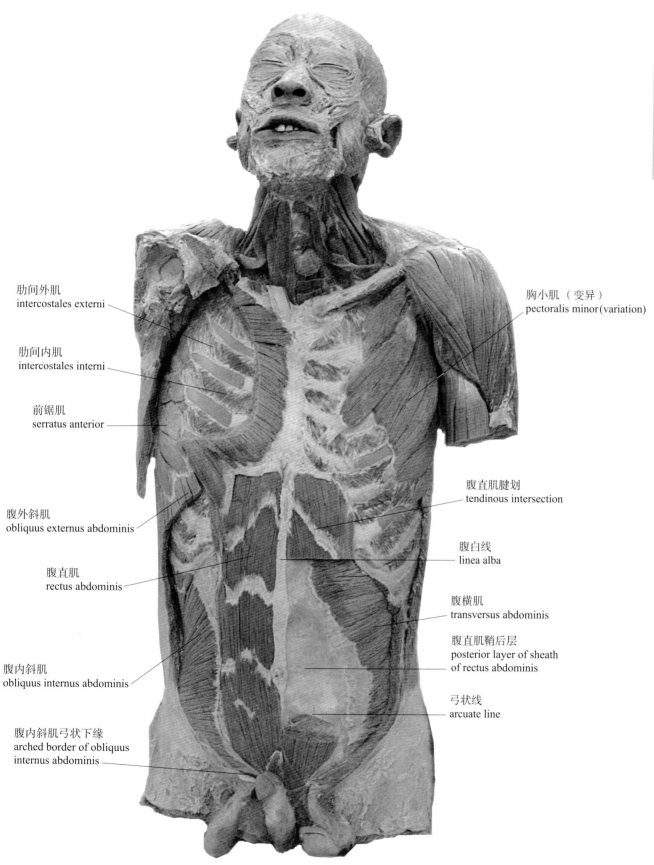

肋间外肌
intercostales externi

肋间内肌
intercostales interni

前锯肌
serratus anterior

腹外斜肌
obliquus externus abdominis

腹直肌
rectus abdominis

腹内斜肌
obliquus internus abdominis

腹内斜肌弓状下缘
arched border of obliquus
internus abdominis

胸小肌（变异）
pectoralis minor(variation)

腹直肌腱划
tendinous intersection

腹白线
linea alba

腹横肌
transversus abdominis

腹直肌鞘后层
posterior layer of sheath
of rectus abdominis

弓状线
arcuate line

图 3-17 胸腹肌（深层）
Muscles of thorax and abdomen (deep layer)

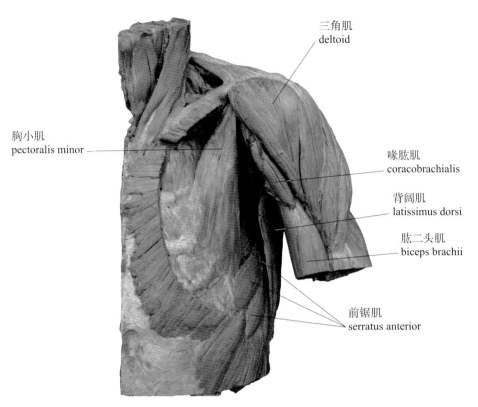

三角肌
deltoid

胸小肌
pectoralis minor

喙肱肌
coracobrachialis

背阔肌
latissimus dorsi

肱二头肌
biceps brachii

前锯肌
serratus anterior

图 3-18 **胸小肌**
Pectoralis minor

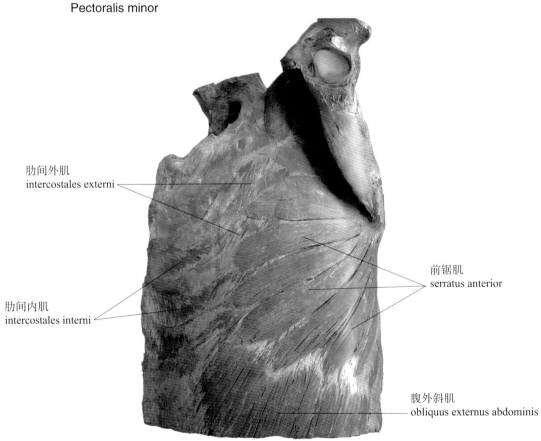

肋间外肌
intercostales externi

前锯肌
serratus anterior

肋间内肌
intercostales interni

腹外斜肌
obliquus externus abdominis

图 3-19 **前锯肌**
Serratus anterior

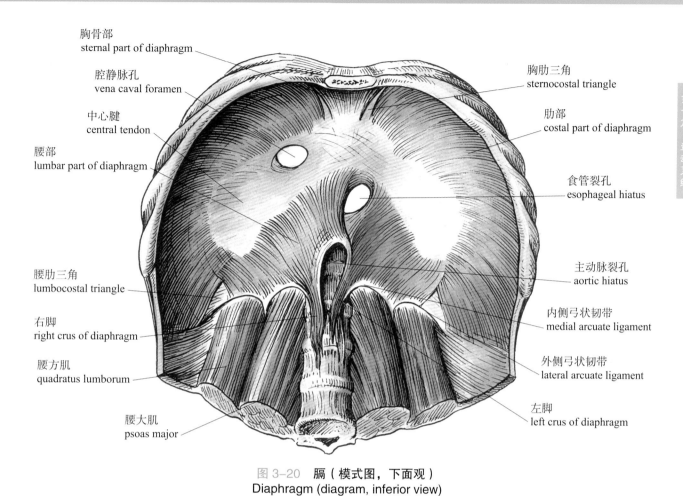

胸骨部
sternal part of diaphragm

腔静脉孔
vena caval foramen

中心腱
central tendon

腰部
lumbar part of diaphragm

腰肋三角
lumbocostal triangle

右脚
right crus of diaphragm

腰方肌
quadratus lumborum

腰大肌
psoas major

胸肋三角
sternocostal triangle

肋部
costal part of diaphragm

食管裂孔
esophageal hiatus

主动脉裂孔
aortic hiatus

内侧弓状韧带
medial arcuate ligament

外侧弓状韧带
lateral arcuate ligament

左脚
left crus of diaphragm

图 3-20　膈（模式图，下面观）
Diaphragm (diagram, inferior view)

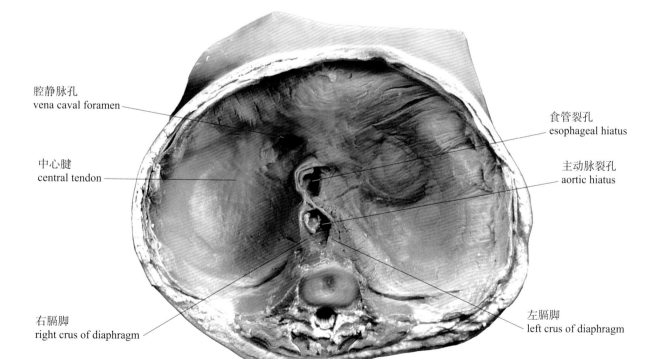

腔静脉孔
vena caval foramen

中心腱
central tendon

右膈脚
right crus of diaphragm

食管裂孔
esophageal hiatus

主动脉裂孔
aortic hiatus

左膈脚
left crus of diaphragm

图 3-21　膈（下面观）
Diaphragm (inferior view)

主要背部肌肉

名称	起点	止点	主要作用	神经支配
斜方肌	上项线、枕外隆凸、项韧带和全部胸椎棘突	锁骨外侧 1/3、肩峰、肩胛冈	拉肩胛骨向脊柱靠拢；提肩胛骨；降肩胛骨	副神经
背阔肌	下 6 个胸椎棘突、全部腰椎棘突及髂嵴后部	肱骨小结节嵴	使肩关节后伸、内收和旋内	胸背神经
竖脊肌	骶骨背面、髂嵴后部和腰椎棘突	肋骨、椎骨及颞骨乳突等	一侧收缩使脊柱侧屈；两侧同时收缩使脊柱后伸和仰头	脊神经后支

Main muscles of back

Name	Origin	Insertion	Actions	Nerve
Trapezius	Superior nuchal line, external occipital protuberance, ligamentum nuchae, the spinous processes of all thoracic vertebrae	Lateral 1/3 of the clavicle, acromion and the spine of scapula	Draws scapula closer to the spinal column, raises and descends scapula	Accessory nerve
Latissimus dorsi	Spinous processes of the lower six thoracic, whole lumbar and sacral vertebrae, and iliac crest	Crest of the lesser tubercle	Allows the shoulder jcint to extend, to adduct and to rotate medially	Thoracodorsal nerve
Erector spinae	The back of sacrum, ilium and spinous processes of lumbar vertebrae	Ribs, vertebrae and mastoid process of the temporal bone	Bends and rotates the vertebral column toward the opposite side when acting on one side, when acting on both sides, they extend the vertebral column	Posterior branches of spinal nerves

主要胸部肌肉

名称	起点	止点	主要作用	神经支配
胸大肌	锁骨内侧 2/3 段、胸骨前面、第 1～6 肋软骨前面	肱骨大结节嵴	使肩关节内收、旋内和前屈	胸内、外侧神经
胸小肌	第 3～5 肋骨前面	肩胛骨喙突	拉肩胛骨向前下方	胸内侧神经
前锯肌	上 8 或 9 个肋骨外面	肩胛骨内侧缘和下角	拉肩胛骨向前并紧贴胸廓	胸长神经

Main muscles of thorax

Name	Origin	Insertion	Actions	Nerve
Pectoral major	Medial 2/3 of the clavicle, anterior surface of the sternum and anterior surfaces of the the 1st to 6th costal cartilage	Crest of the greater tubercle	Allows the shoulder joint to adduct, to rotate medially and to flex	Lateral and medial pectoral nerves
Pectoral minor	Anterior surfaces of the 3rd to 5th ribs	Coracoid process of the scapula	Pulls the scapula forward and downward	Medial nerve
Serratus anterior	External surfaces of the upper 8 or 9 ribs	Medial border and inferior angle of the scapula	Pulls the scapula forward and keeps it close to the thoracic cage	Long thoracic nerve

膈肌和腹部肌肉

名称	起点	止点	主要作用	神经支配
膈	剑突后面、下 6 对肋内面和上 2~3 腰椎体	中心腱	助呼吸；增加腹压	膈神经
腹外斜肌	下 8 位肋骨外面	髂嵴前部、腹股沟韧带、白线	保护腹腔脏器，维持和增加腹压；降肋助呼气；使脊柱前屈、侧屈和旋转	第 5~11 肋间神经、肋下神经、髂腹下神经和髂腹股沟神经
腹内斜肌	胸腰筋膜、髂嵴和腹股沟韧带外侧半	白线		
腹横肌	下 6 对肋软骨内面、胸腰筋膜、髂嵴和腹股沟韧带外侧 1/3	白线		
腹直肌	耻骨联合、耻骨嵴	胸骨剑突、第 5~7 肋软骨前面		第 5~11 肋间神经、肋下神经
腰方肌	髂嵴后侧	第 12 肋内侧半，上 4 腰椎横突	固定和降 12 肋，使脊柱侧屈	腰神经前支

Main muscles of thorax

Name	Origin	Insertion	Actions	Nerve
Diaphragm	Posterior aspect of the xiphoid process, internal surfaces of the lower six ribs and the bodies of the upper 2 or 3 lumbar vertebrae	Central tendon	Helps breathing, increase abdominal pressure	Phrenic nerve
Obliquus externus abdominis	External surfaces of the lower eight ribs	Anterior part of the iliac crest, inguinal ligament and linea alba	Protects the abdominal organs, maintains and increases intraabdominal pressure, falling ribs to help exhale, allows the vertebral column to flex forward, to flex lateral and to rotate	The 5th to 11th intercostal nerves, subcostal nerve, iliohypogastric nerve, and ilioinguinal nerve
Obliquus internus abdominis	Thoracolumbar fascia, iliac crest and later half of the inguinal ligament	Linea alba		
Transversus abdominis	Inner surfaces of the lower 6 ribs, thoracolumbar fascia and lateral 1/3 of the inguinal ligament	Linea alba		
Rectus abdominis	Pubic symphysis and pubic crest	Xiphoid process of the sternum, anterior surfaces of the 5th to 7th costal cartilages		The 5th to 11th intercostal nerves, subcostal nerve
Quadratus lumborum	Posterior part of the iliac crest	Medial half of the 12th rib, transverse processes of the upper four lumbar vertebrae	Fixes and reduces the 12th rib, allows the vertebral column to flex lateral	Anterior branches of lumbar nerves

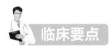

临床要点

腹肌、腹股沟管的临床要点

1. 腹股沟管是一条肌间裂隙，男性的精索以及女性的子宫圆韧带通过该管。管的内口称腹股沟管深环，外口称腹股沟管浅环。

2. 腹股沟三角位于腹前壁下部，由腹直肌外侧缘、腹股沟韧带和腹壁下动脉围成。

3. 腹股沟管和腹股沟三角均为腹壁下部的薄弱区，在病理情况下，可致腹腔内容物由此区突出而形成疝。若经腹股沟管深环突出，称斜疝；若从腹股沟三角处膨出，则称直疝。

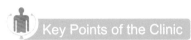

Key Points of the Clinic

Key points of the clinic on the muscles of abdomen and inguinal canal

1. The inguinal canal is an intermuscular fissure through which passes the spermatic cord in male and the round ligament of the uterus in female. The internal aperture of the canal is called deep inguinal ring, and the external aperture of the canal is called superficial inguinal ring.

2. The inguinal triangle lies in the lower part of the anterior abdominal wall. The triangle is bounded by the lateral border of rectus abdominis, the inguinal ligament and the inferior epigastric artery.

3. The inguinal canal and the inguinal triangle are all the weaknesses in the lower part of the anterior abdominal wall. A hernia involves the protrusion of a viscus through these areas in case of pathology. If the viscus protrudes through the deep inguinal ring it is called an indirect inguinal hernia; whereas the protrusion of viscus through the inguinal triangle, is called a direct inguinal hernia.

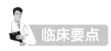

临床要点

膈的临床要点

1. 膈分为 3 部：胸骨部、肋部和腰部。胸骨部起自剑突后面；肋部起自下 6 对肋；腰部以左、右两个膈脚起自上 2 ～ 3 腰椎。

2. 膈肌三部起点之间通常留有一些三角区域：胸肋三角位于胸骨部和肋部起点之间；腰肋三角位于肋部和腰部之间。腹部脏器可能经由这些区域突入胸腔形成膈疝。

3. 膈上有三个孔或裂：主动脉裂孔（通过主动脉和胸导管）、食管裂孔（通过食管和迷走神经）和腔静脉孔（通过下腔静脉）。

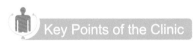

Key Points of the Clinic

Key points of the clinic on the diaphragm

1. The diaphragm can be divided into three parts: sternal, costal and lumbar parts. The sternal part arises from the posterior aspect of the xiphoid process; the costal part arises from the internal surfaces of the lower six ribs; the lumbar part arises from the upper 2-3 lumbar vertebral bodies with right and left crura of diaphragm.

2. There are usually triangular areas between the origin of three parts of the diaphragm: the sternocostal triangles lie between the origin of the sternal part and costal part; the lumbocostal triangles lie between the costal part and lumbar part. The abdominal organs may herniate through these areas into the thorax, this is called diaphragmatic hernia.

3. There are three large foramen or hiatuses on the diaphragm: the aortic hiatus (transmits the aorta and thoracic duct), the esophageal hiatus (transmits the esophagus and vagus nerve), the vena caval foramen (transmits the inferior vena cava).

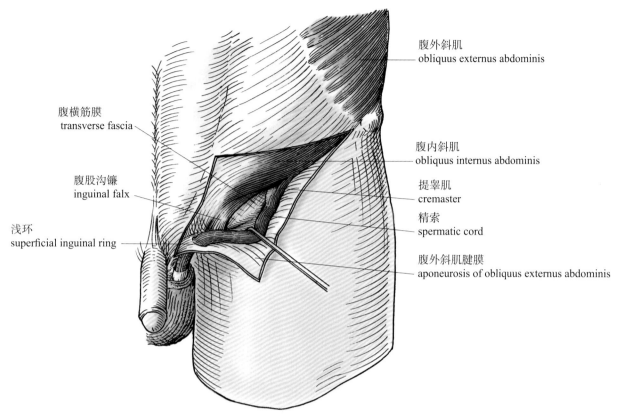

腹外斜肌
obliquus externus abdominis

腹横筋膜
transverse fascia

腹内斜肌
obliquus internus abdominis

腹股沟镰
inguinal falx

提睾肌
cremaster

精索
spermatic cord

浅环
superficial inguinal ring

腹外斜肌腱膜
aponeurosis of obliquus externus abdominis

图 3-22　腹股沟管（前面观）
Inguinal canal (anterior view)

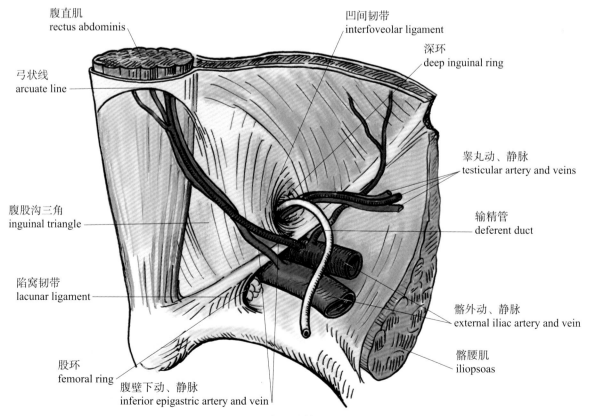

腹直肌
rectus abdominis

凹间韧带
interfoveolar ligament

深环
deep inguinal ring

弓状线
arcuate line

睾丸动、静脉
testicular artery and veins

腹股沟三角
inguinal triangle

输精管
deferent duct

陷窝韧带
lacunar ligament

髂外动、静脉
external iliac artery and vein

髂腰肌
iliopsoas

股环
femoral ring

腹壁下动、静脉
inferior epigastric artery and vein

图 3-23　腹股沟管（后面观）
Inguinal canal (posterior view)

第四节　上肢肌　Section 4　Muscles of upper limb

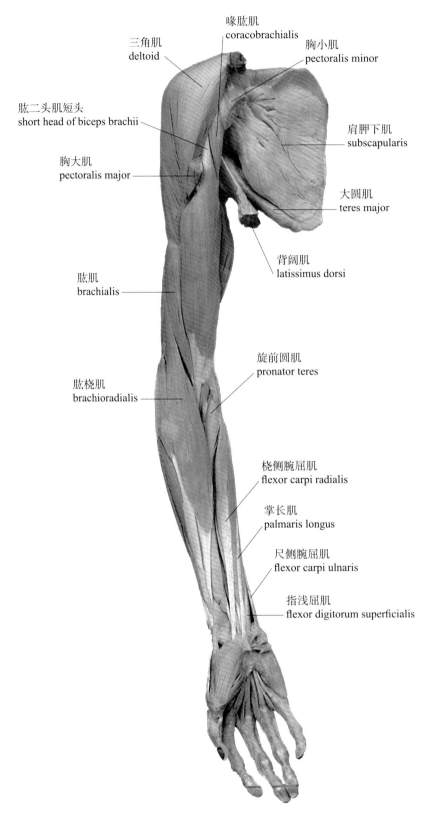

喙肱肌
coracobrachialis

三角肌
deltoid

胸小肌
pectoralis minor

肱二头肌短头
short head of biceps brachii

肩胛下肌
subscapularis

胸大肌
pectoralis major

大圆肌
teres major

背阔肌
latissimus dorsi

肱肌
brachialis

旋前圆肌
pronator teres

肱桡肌
brachioradialis

桡侧腕屈肌
flexor carpi radialis

掌长肌
palmaris longus

尺侧腕屈肌
flexor carpi ulnaris

指浅屈肌
flexor digitorum superficialis

图 3-24　上肢肌（前面观，浅层）
Muscles of upper limb (anterior view, superficial layer)

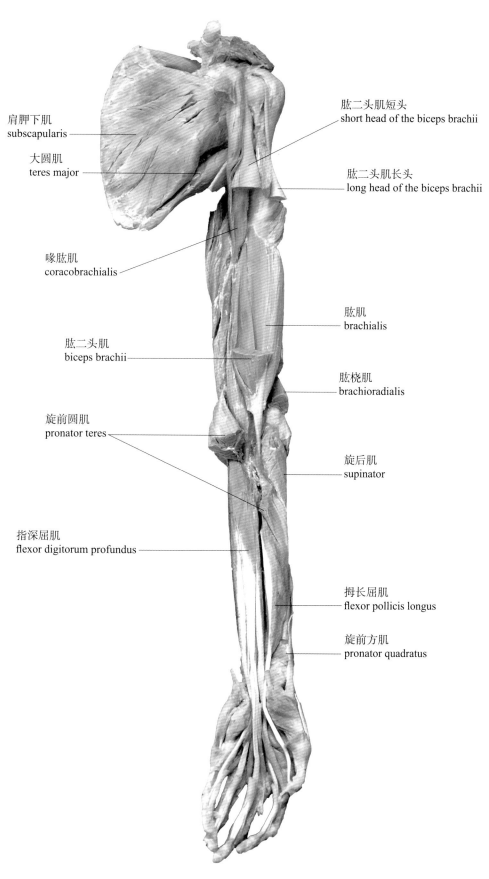

肩胛下肌
subscapularis

大圆肌
teres major

喙肱肌
coracobrachialis

肱二头肌
biceps brachii

旋前圆肌
pronator teres

指深屈肌
flexor digitorum profundus

肱二头肌短头
short head of the biceps brachii

肱二头肌长头
long head of the biceps brachii

肱肌
brachialis

肱桡肌
brachioradialis

旋后肌
supinator

拇长屈肌
flexor pollicis longus

旋前方肌
pronator quadratus

图 3-25　上肢肌（前面观，深层）
Muscles of upper limb (anterior view, deep layer)

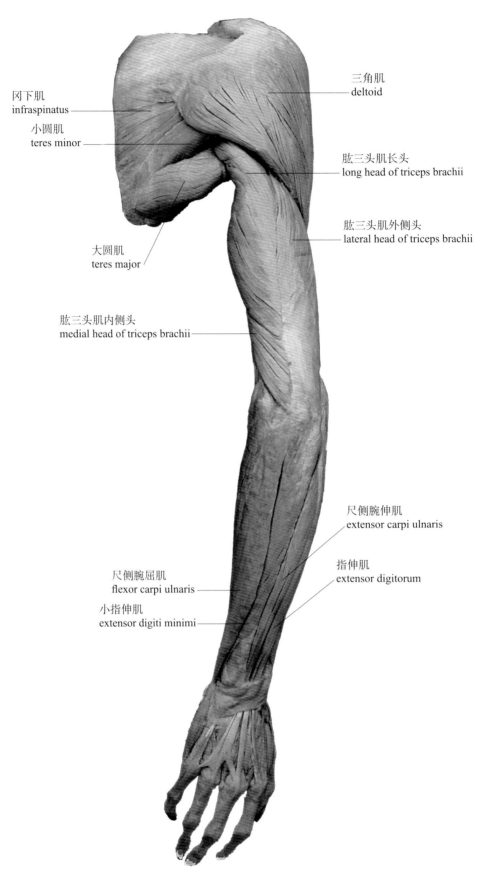

冈下肌
infraspinatus

小圆肌
teres minor

大圆肌
teres major

肱三头肌内侧头
medial head of triceps brachii

尺侧腕屈肌
flexor carpi ulnaris

小指伸肌
extensor digiti minimi

三角肌
deltoid

肱三头肌长头
long head of triceps brachii

肱三头肌外侧头
lateral head of triceps brachii

尺侧腕伸肌
extensor carpi ulnaris

指伸肌
extensor digitorum

图 3-26　上肢肌（后面观）
Muscles of upper limb (posterior view)

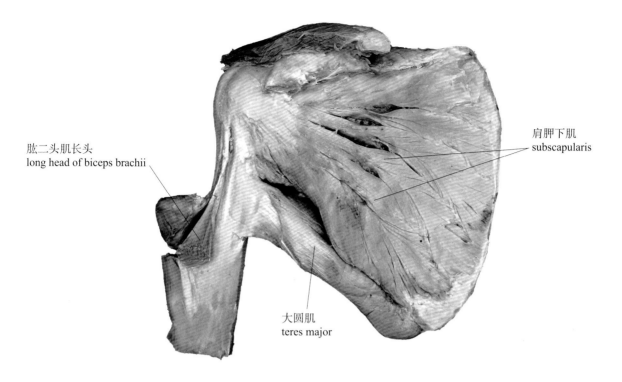

肱二头肌长头
long head of biceps brachii

肩胛下肌
subscapularis

大圆肌
teres major

图 3-27　肩肌（前面观）
Muscles of shoulder (anterior view)

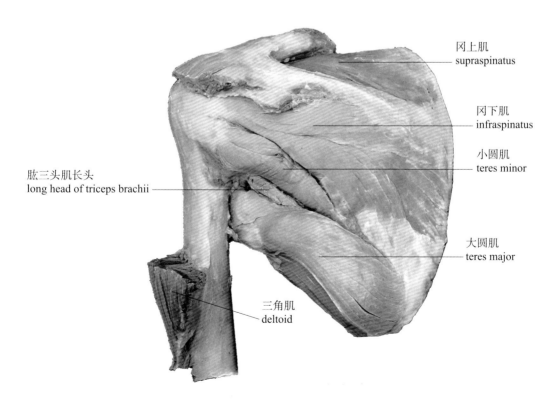

冈上肌
supraspinatus

冈下肌
infraspinatus

小圆肌
teres minor

大圆肌
teres major

肱三头肌长头
long head of triceps brachii

三角肌
deltoid

图 3-28　肩肌（后面观）
Muscles of shoulder (posterior view)

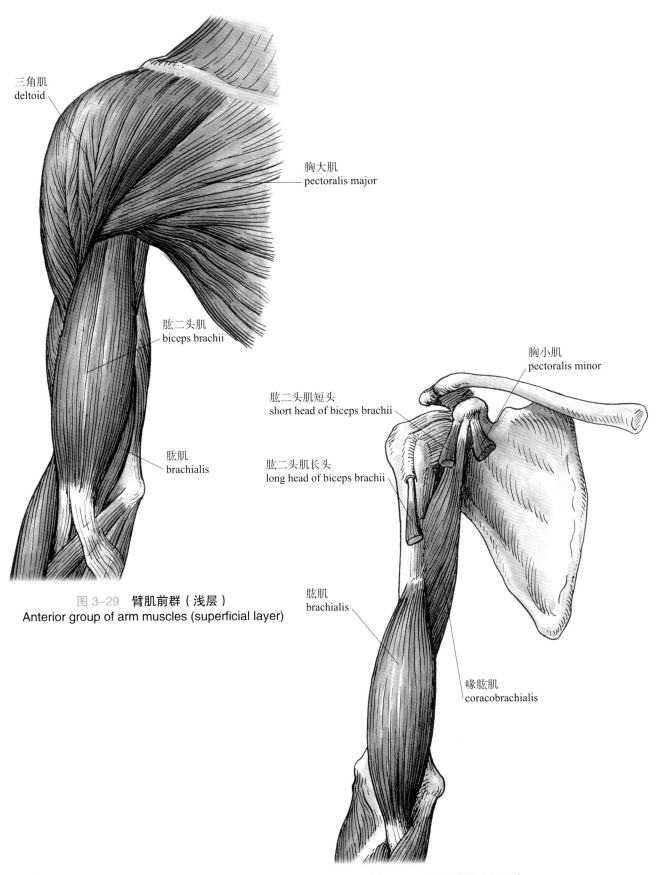

三角肌
deltoid

胸大肌
pectoralis major

肱二头肌
biceps brachii

肱肌
brachialis

图 3-29 臂肌前群（浅层）
Anterior group of arm muscles (superficial layer)

胸小肌
pectoralis minor

肱二头肌短头
short head of biceps brachii

肱二头肌长头
long head of biceps brachii

肱肌
brachialis

喙肱肌
coracobrachialis

图 3-30 臂肌前群（深层）
Anterior group of arm muscles (deep layer)

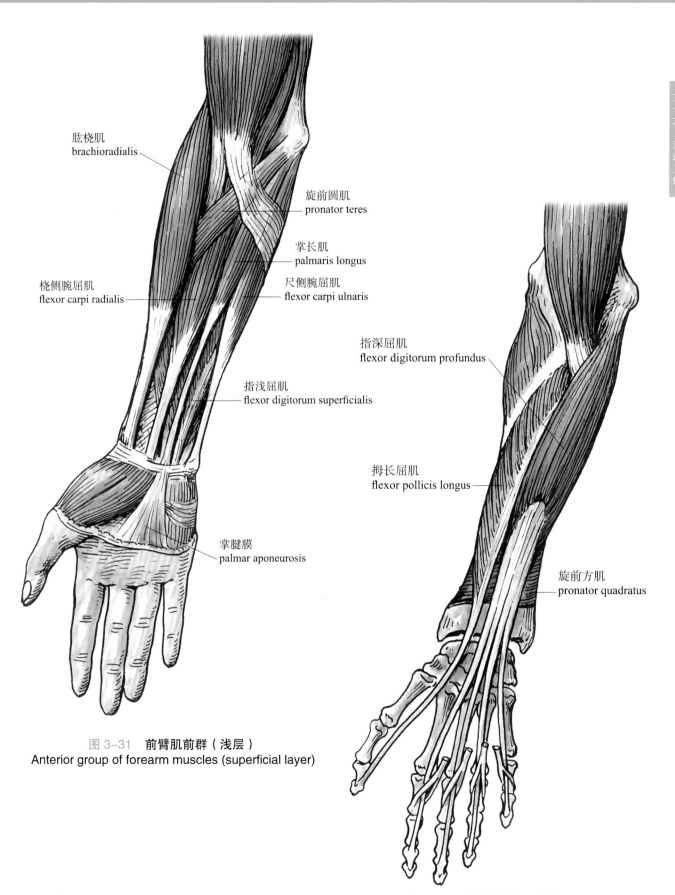

肱桡肌
brachioradialis

旋前圆肌
pronator teres

掌长肌
palmaris longus

桡侧腕屈肌
flexor carpi radialis

尺侧腕屈肌
flexor carpi ulnaris

指深屈肌
flexor digitorum profundus

指浅屈肌
flexor digitorum superficialis

拇长屈肌
flexor pollicis longus

掌腱膜
palmar aponeurosis

旋前方肌
pronator quadratus

图 3-31　前臂肌前群（浅层）
Anterior group of forearm muscles (superficial layer)

图 3-32　前臂肌前群（深层）
Anterior group of forearm muscles (deep layer)

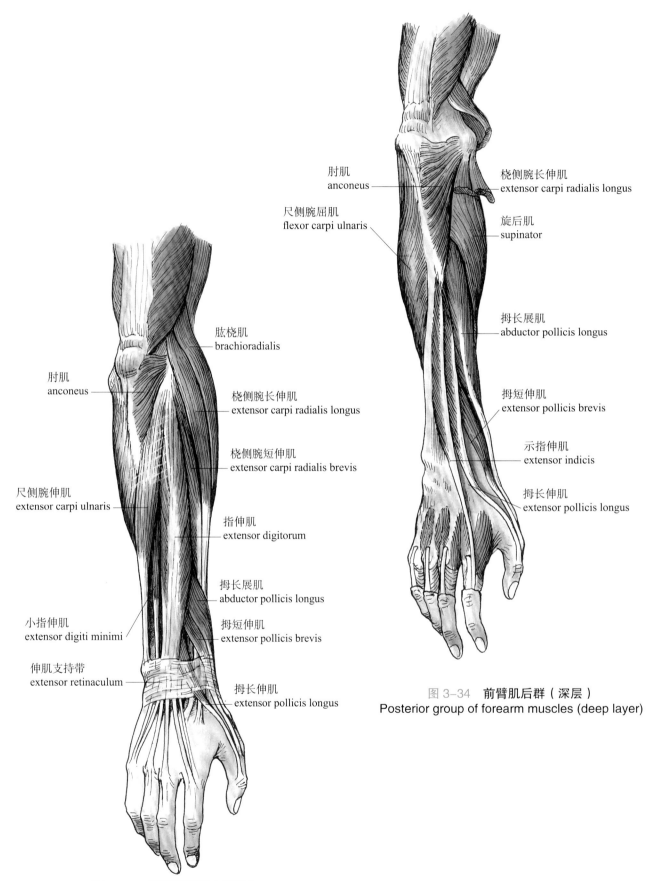

肘肌
anconeus

尺侧腕屈肌
flexor carpi ulnaris

桡侧腕长伸肌
extensor carpi radialis longus

旋后肌
supinator

拇长展肌
abductor pollicis longus

拇短伸肌
extensor pollicis brevis

示指伸肌
extensor indicis

拇长伸肌
extensor pollicis longus

肱桡肌
brachioradialis

肘肌
anconeus

桡侧腕长伸肌
extensor carpi radialis longus

桡侧腕短伸肌
extensor carpi radialis brevis

尺侧腕伸肌
extensor carpi ulnaris

指伸肌
extensor digitorum

拇长展肌
abductor pollicis longus

小指伸肌
extensor digiti minimi

拇短伸肌
extensor pollicis brevis

伸肌支持带
extensor retinaculum

拇长伸肌
extensor pollicis longus

图 3-34　前臂肌后群（深层）
Posterior group of forearm muscles (deep layer)

图 3-33　前臂肌后群（浅层）
Posterior group of forearm muscles (superficial layer)

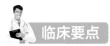
临床要点

参与前臂旋转的肌肉

旋前：旋前圆肌、旋前方肌。

旋后：旋后肌、肱二头肌（前臂旋前时，使其旋后）。

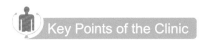
Key Points of the Clinic

Muscles involved in forearm rotation

Pronation: pronator teres, pronator quadratus.

Supination: supinator, biceps brachii (when the forearm pronates, biceps brachii supinate forearm).

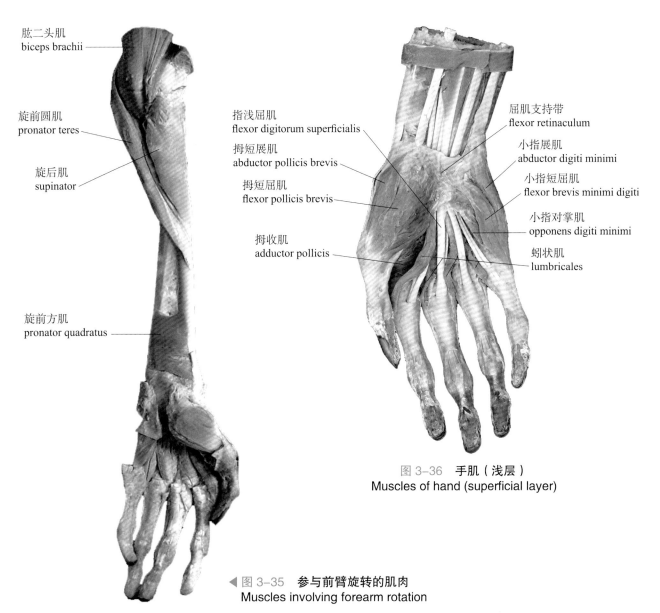

肱二头肌
biceps brachii

旋前圆肌
pronator teres

旋后肌
supinator

旋前方肌
pronator quadratus

指浅屈肌
flexor digitorum superficialis

拇短展肌
abductor pollicis brevis

拇短屈肌
flexor pollicis brevis

拇收肌
adductor pollicis

屈肌支持带
flexor retinaculum

小指展肌
abductor digiti minimi

小指短屈肌
flexor brevis minimi digiti

小指对掌肌
opponens digiti minimi

蚓状肌
lumbricales

图 3-36 手肌（浅层）
Muscles of hand (superficial layer)

◀ 图 3-35 参与前臂旋转的肌肉
Muscles involving forearm rotation

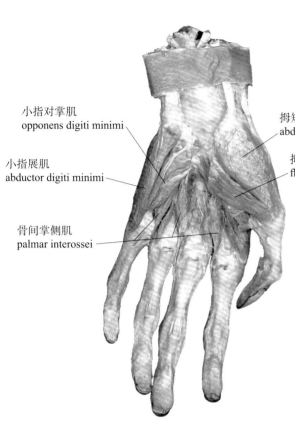

小指对掌肌
opponens digiti minimi

拇短展肌
abductor pollicis brevis

小指展肌
abductor digiti minimi

拇短屈肌
flexor pollicis brevis

骨间掌侧肌
palmar interossei

◀ 图 3-37　手肌（深层）
Muscles of hand (deep layer)

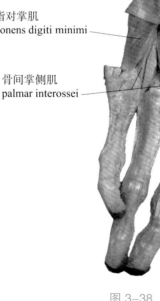

拇对掌肌
opponens pollicis

小指对掌肌
opponens digiti minimi

骨间掌侧肌
palmar interossei

图 3-38　骨间掌侧肌
Palmar interossei

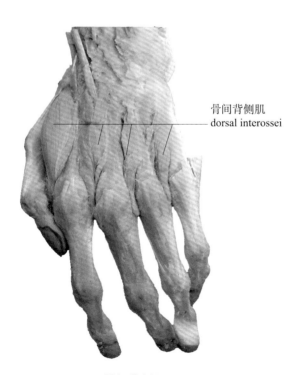

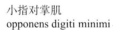

骨间背侧肌
dorsal interossei

图 3-39　骨间背侧肌
Dorsal interossei

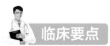 临床要点

"网球肘"

前臂浅层伸肌大都起自肱骨外上髁及其附近的深筋膜，在经常做前臂旋后和伸腕等动作时，会造成肱骨外上髁附近筋膜损伤，称为肱骨外上髁综合征，也称"网球肘"，常见于网球运动员。查体时，可见患者的肱骨外上髁附近有明显压痛，手背屈时疼痛加重。

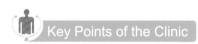 Key Points of the Clinic

"Tennis elbow"

Most of the superficial extensors of the forearm originate from the lateral epicondyle of the humerus and the deep fascia nearby. Frequent action of supination and wrist extension can cause fascia injury near the lateral epicondyle of the humerus, which is called the lateral epicondyle syndrome, also known as the "tennis elbow", which is more common in tennis players. Generally, the patient has obvious tenderness near the lateral epicondyle of the humerus at the time of physical examination, and the pain would be aggravated when the hand is flexed dorsally.

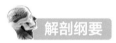 解剖纲要

上肢主要肌

名称	起点	止点	作用	神经支配
三角肌	锁骨外 1/3、肩峰、肩胛冈	肱骨三角肌粗隆	肩关节外展、前屈或后伸	腋神经
肱二头肌	长头：盂上结节 短头：喙突	桡骨粗隆	屈肩、屈肘、前臂旋后	肌皮神经
肱三头肌	长头：盂下结节 外侧头：桡神经沟上方 内侧头：桡神经沟下方	尺骨鹰嘴	伸肘、肩关节后伸	桡神经

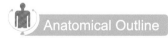 Anatomical Outline

Main muscles of upper limb

Muscle	Origin	Insertion	Action	Innervation
Deltoid	Lateral one-third of clavicle, acromion, and spine of scapula	Deltoid tuberosity of humerus	Abducts, flexes or extends shoulder joint	Axillary nerve
Biceps brachii	Long head: supraglenoid tuberosity Short head: coracoid process	Radial tuberosity	Flexes shoulder and elbow joint, supinates forearm	Musculocutaneous nerve
Triceps brachii	Long head: infraglenoid tuberosity Lateral head: above the sulcus for radial nerver Medial head: below the sulcus for radial nerve	Olecranon of ulna	Extends elbow and shoulder joint	Radial nerve

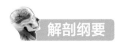 解剖纲要

参与上肢关节运动的主要肌肉

关节	运动方式	主要肌肉
肩关节	屈	胸大肌、三角肌（前部肌束）、肱二头肌长头
	伸	三角肌（后部肌束）、背阔肌、肱三头肌长头
	内收	胸大肌、大圆肌、肩胛下肌、肱三头肌长头、背阔肌
	外展	三角肌、岗上肌
	旋内	胸大肌、三角肌（前部肌束）、大圆肌、肩胛下肌、背阔肌
	旋外	三角肌（后部肌束）、岗下肌、小圆肌
肘关节	屈	肱二头肌、肱肌、肱桡肌、旋前圆肌、桡侧腕屈肌、尺侧腕屈肌
	伸	肱三头肌
桡尺连结	旋前	旋前圆肌、旋前方肌
	旋后	旋后肌、肱二头肌
桡腕关节	屈	桡侧腕屈肌、尺侧腕屈肌、指浅屈肌、指深屈肌
	伸	桡侧腕长伸肌、桡侧腕短伸肌、指伸肌、尺侧腕伸肌
	内收	尺侧腕屈肌、尺侧腕伸肌
	外展	桡侧腕屈肌、桡侧腕长伸肌、桡侧腕短伸肌

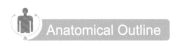 Anatomical Outline

The muscles involve in upper limb joint movement

Joint	Movement	Main muscles
Shoulder	Flexion	Pectoralis major, deltoid (anterior fibres) and long head of biceps brachii
	Extension	Deltoid (posterior fibres), latissimus dorsi and long head of triceps brachii
	Adduction	Pectoralis major, teres major, subscapularis, long head of triceps brachii and latissimus dorsi
	Abduction	Deltoid and supraspinatus
	Medial rotation	Pectoralis major, deltoid (anterior fibres), teres major, subscapularis and latissimus dorsi
	Lateral rotation	Deltoid (posterior fibres), infraspinatus and teres minor
Elbow	Flexion	Biceps brachii, brachialis, brachioradialis, pronator teres, flexor carpi radialis and flexor carpi ulnaris
	Extension	Triceps brachii
Radioulnar syndesmosis	Pronation	Pronator teres and pronator quadratus
	Supination	Supinator and biceps brachii
Radiocarpal joint	Flexion	Flexor carpi radialis, flexor carpi ulnaris, superficial digital flexor and deep digital flexor
	Extension	Extensor carpi radialis longus, Extensor carpi radialis brevis, extensor digitorum communis and extensor carpi ulnaris
	Adduction	Flexor carpi ulnaris and extensor carpi ulnaris
	Abduction	Flexor carpi radialis, extensor carpi radialis longus and extensor carpi radialis brevis

第五节 下肢肌 Section 5 Muscles of lower limb

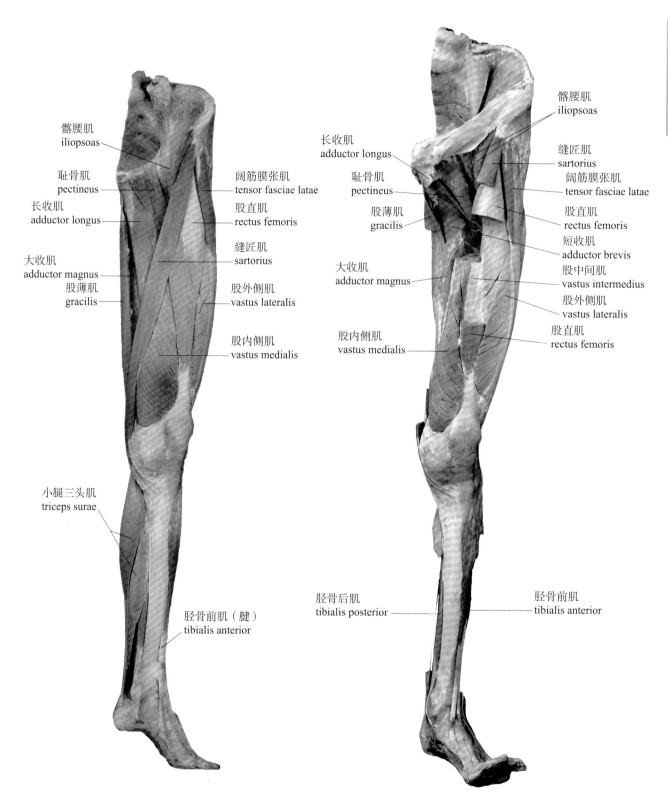

髂腰肌
iliopsoas

耻骨肌
pectineus

长收肌
adductor longus

大收肌
adductor magnus

股薄肌
gracilis

阔筋膜张肌
tensor fasciae latae

股直肌
rectus femoris

缝匠肌
sartorius

股外侧肌
vastus lateralis

股内侧肌
vastus medialis

小腿三头肌
triceps surae

胫骨前肌（腱）
tibialis anterior

长收肌
adductor longus

耻骨肌
pectineus

股薄肌
gracilis

大收肌
adductor magnus

股内侧肌
vastus medialis

髂腰肌
iliopsoas

缝匠肌
sartorius

阔筋膜张肌
tensor fasciae latae

股直肌
rectus femoris

短收肌
adductor brevis

股中间肌
vastus intermedius

股外侧肌
vastus lateralis

股直肌
rectus femoris

胫骨后肌
tibialis posterior

胫骨前肌
tibialis anterior

图 3-40 下肢肌（前面观，浅层）
Muscles of lower limb (anterior view, superficial layer)

图 3-41 下肢肌（前面观，深层）
Muscles of lower limb (anterior view, deep layer)

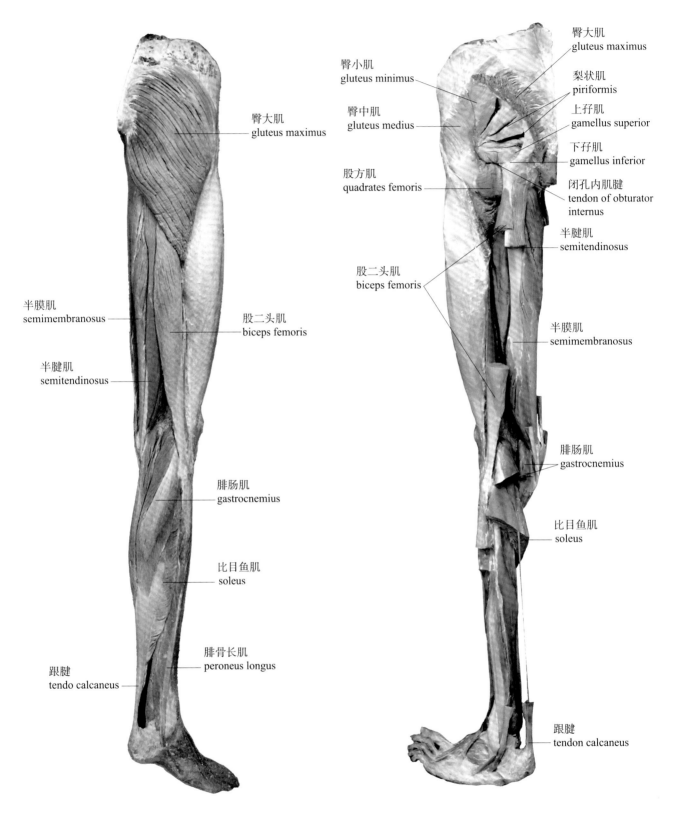

臀大肌
gluteus maximus

半膜肌
semimembranosus

半腱肌
semitendinosus

股二头肌
biceps femoris

腓肠肌
gastrocnemius

比目鱼肌
soleus

腓骨长肌
peroneus longus

跟腱
tendo calcaneus

臀小肌
gluteus minimus

臀中肌
gluteus medius

股方肌
quadrates femoris

股二头肌
biceps femoris

臀大肌
gluteus maximus

梨状肌
piriformis

上孖肌
gamellus superior

下孖肌
gamellus inferior

闭孔内肌腱
tendon of obturator internus

半腱肌
semitendinosus

半膜肌
semimembranosus

腓肠肌
gastrocnemius

比目鱼肌
soleus

跟腱
tendon calcaneus

图 3-42　下肢肌（后面观，浅层）
Muscles of lower limb (posterior view, superficial layer)

图 3-43　下肢肌（后面观，深层）
Muscles of lower limb (posterior view, deep layer)

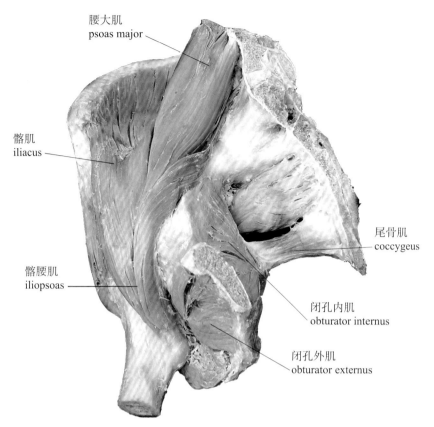

腰大肌
psoas major

髂肌
iliacus

髂腰肌
iliopsoas

尾骨肌
coccygeus

闭孔内肌
obturator internus

闭孔外肌
obturator externus

图 3-44 髋肌（前面观）
Muscles of hip (anterior view)

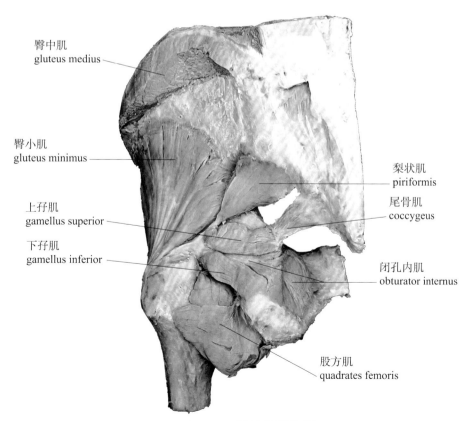

臀中肌
gluteus medius

臀小肌
gluteus minimus

上孖肌
gamellus superior

下孖肌
gamellus inferior

梨状肌
piriformis

尾骨肌
coccygeus

闭孔内肌
obturator internus

股方肌
quadrates femoris

图 3-45 髋肌（后面观）
Muscles of hip (posterior view)

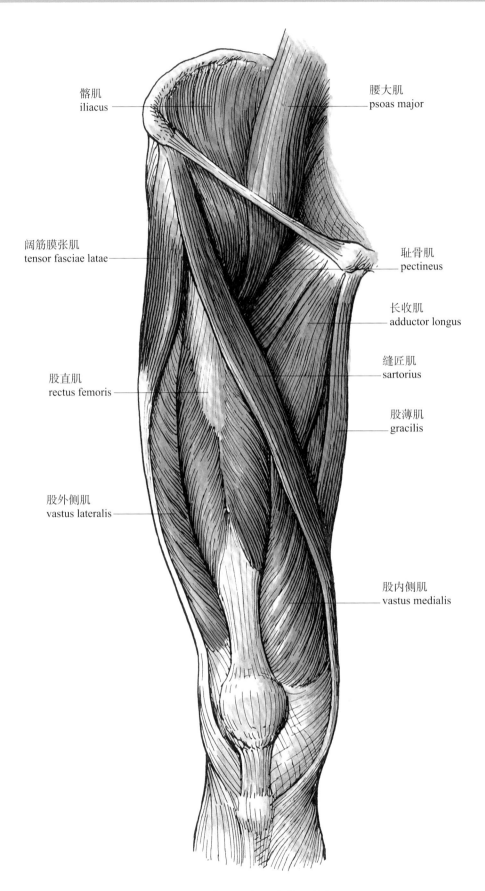

髂肌
iliacus

腰大肌
psoas major

阔筋膜张肌
tensor fasciae latae

耻骨肌
pectineus

长收肌
adductor longus

缝匠肌
sartorius

股直肌
rectus femoris

股薄肌
gracilis

股外侧肌
vastus lateralis

股内侧肌
vastus medialis

图 3-46 大腿肌浅层（前面观）
Superficial layer muscles of thigh (anterior view)

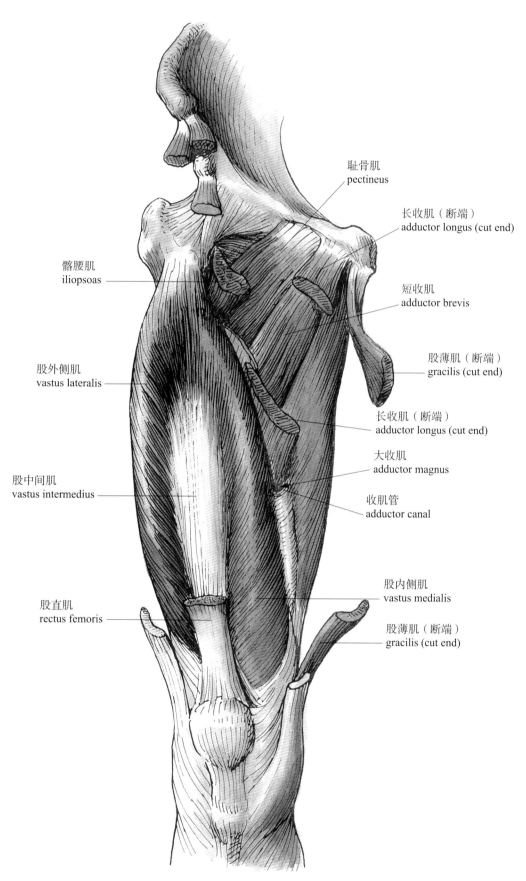

耻骨肌
pectineus

长收肌（断端）
adductor longus (cut end)

髂腰肌
iliopsoas

短收肌
adductor brevis

股薄肌（断端）
gracilis (cut end)

股外侧肌
vastus lateralis

长收肌（断端）
adductor longus (cut end)

大收肌
adductor magnus

收肌管
adductor canal

股中间肌
vastus intermedius

股内侧肌
vastus medialis

股直肌
rectus femoris

股薄肌（断端）
gracilis (cut end)

图 3-47　大腿肌深层（前面观）
Deep layer muscles of thigh (anterior view)

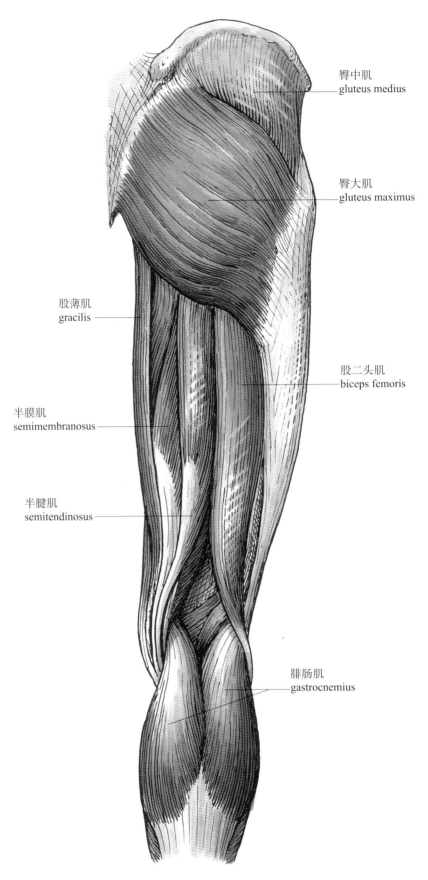

臀中肌
gluteus medius

臀大肌
gluteus maximus

股薄肌
gracilis

股二头肌
biceps femoris

半膜肌
semimembranosus

半腱肌
semitendinosus

腓肠肌
gastrocnemius

图 3-48 大腿肌（后面观）
Muscles of thigh (posterior view)

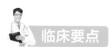

临床要点

阔筋膜张肌

　　阔筋膜张肌位置表浅，有恒定的血供及神经分布，切取后对髋关节的功能影响不大，所以经常用作临床肌皮瓣或髂胫束瓣供体。

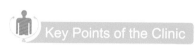

The tensor fasciae latae

　　The tensor fasciae latae is located superficially and it has a constant blood supply and nerve distribution. There is little effect on the function of hip joint after cutting, so it is often used as a myocutaneous flap donor or an iliotibial tract flap donor.

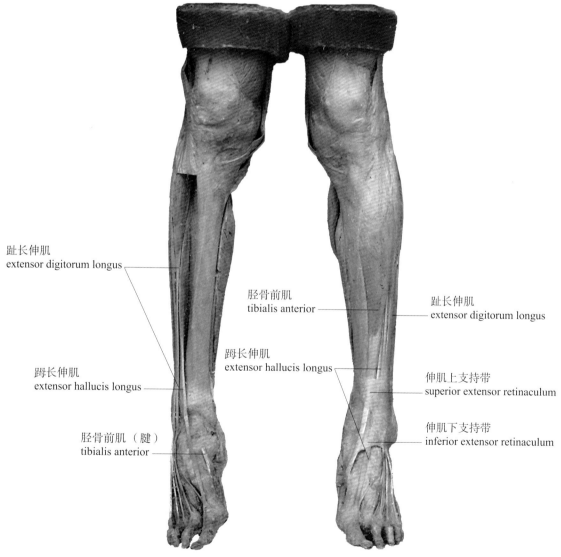

趾长伸肌
extensor digitorum longus

胫骨前肌
tibialis anterior

趾长伸肌
extensor digitorum longus

𧿹长伸肌
extensor hallucis longus

伸肌上支持带
superior extensor retinaculum

𧿹长伸肌
extensor hallucis longus

伸肌下支持带
inferior extensor retinaculum

胫骨前肌（腱）
tibialis anterior

图 3-49　小腿肌（前面观）
Muscles of leg (anterior view)

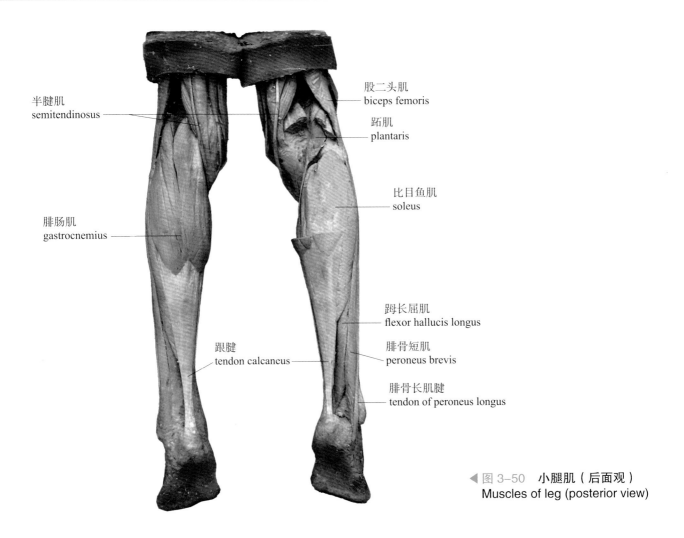

半腱肌
semitendinosus

股二头肌
biceps femoris

跖肌
plantaris

比目鱼肌
soleus

腓肠肌
gastrocnemius

姆长屈肌
flexor hallucis longus

腓骨短肌
peroneus brevis

跟腱
tendon calcaneus

腓骨长肌腱
tendon of peroneus longus

◀ 图 3-50　小腿肌（后面观）
Muscles of leg (posterior view)

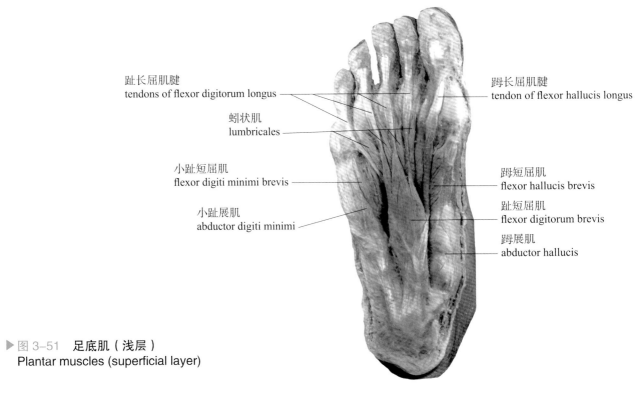

趾长屈肌腱
tendons of flexor digitorum longus

姆长屈肌腱
tendon of flexor hallucis longus

蚓状肌
lumbricales

小趾短屈肌
flexor digiti minimi brevis

姆短屈肌
flexor hallucis brevis

小趾展肌
abductor digiti minimi

趾短屈肌
flexor digitorum brevis

姆展肌
abductor hallucis

▶ 图 3-51　足底肌（浅层）
Plantar muscles (superficial layer)

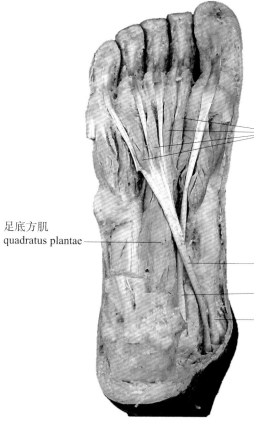

蚓状肌
lumbricales

足底方肌
quadratus plantae

趾长屈肌腱
tendon of flexor digitorum longus

蹄长屈肌腱
tendon of flexor hallucis longus

胫骨后肌腱
tendon of tibialis posterior

图 3-52 足底肌（中层）
Plantar muscles (middle layer)

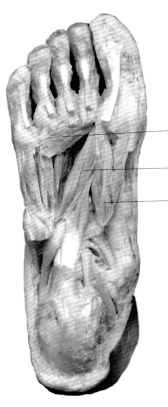

蹄收肌横头
cross head of adductor hallucis

蹄收肌斜头
oblique head of adductor hallucis

蹄短屈肌
flexor hallucis brevis

图 3-53 足底肌（深层）
Plantar muscles (deep layer)

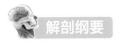 解剖纲要

下肢主要肌

名称	起点	止点	作用	神经支配
髂腰肌	腰大肌：腰椎横突 髂肌：髂窝	股骨小转子	屈髋并旋外	腰丛
臀大肌	髂骨翼和骶骨的背面	臀肌粗隆及髂胫束	伸髋并旋外	臀下神经
股四头肌	髂前下棘、股骨粗线及前面	胫骨粗隆	屈髋并伸膝	股神经
缝匠肌	髂前上棘	胫骨上端内侧面	屈髋、屈膝 屈膝时使小腿旋内	股神经
股二头肌	长头：坐骨结节 短头：股骨粗线	腓骨头	伸髋、屈膝	坐骨神经
小腿三头肌	腓肠肌：股骨内、外侧髁 比目鱼肌：胫、腓骨上端后面	以跟腱止于跟骨结节	屈膝，使足跖屈	胫神经

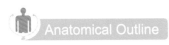 Anatomical Outline

Main muscles of lower limb

Muscle	Origin	Insertion	Action	Innervation
Iliopsoas	Psoas major：transverse processes of all lumbar vertebrae Iliacus：iliac fossa	Lesser trochanter of femur	Flexes and rotates thigh laterally at the hip joint	Lumbar plexus
Gluteus maximus	Ala of ilium and dorsal surface of the sacrum	Gluteal tuberosity and iliotibial tract	Extends and rotates thigh laterally at the hip joint	Inferior gluteal nerve
Quadriceps femoris	Anterior inferior iliac spine, linea aspera and anterior surface of femur	Tibial tuberosity	Flexes hip joint; extends knee joint	Femoral nerve
Sartorius	Anterior superior iliac spine	Medial surface of upper end of tibia	Flexes hip and knee joints; rotates leg medially at knee joint when flexes knee joint	Femoral nerve
Biceps femoris	Long head: ischial tuberosity Short head: linea aspera of femur	Head of fibula	Extends hip joint, flexes knee joint	Sciatic nerve
Triceps surae	Gastrocnemius: lateral and medial condyle of femur Soleus: posterior surface of upper end of fibula and tibia	Calcaneal tuberosity by calcaneal tendon	Plantar flexes foot at ankle, flexes knee joint	Tibial nerve

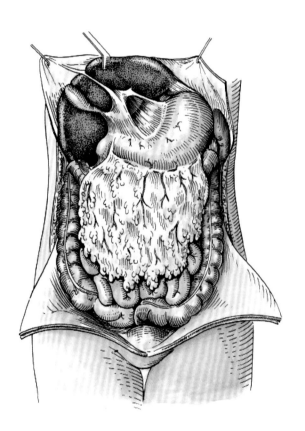

第二篇
内脏学

Part 2 Splanchnology

第四章 消化系统
Chapter 4 Alimentary system

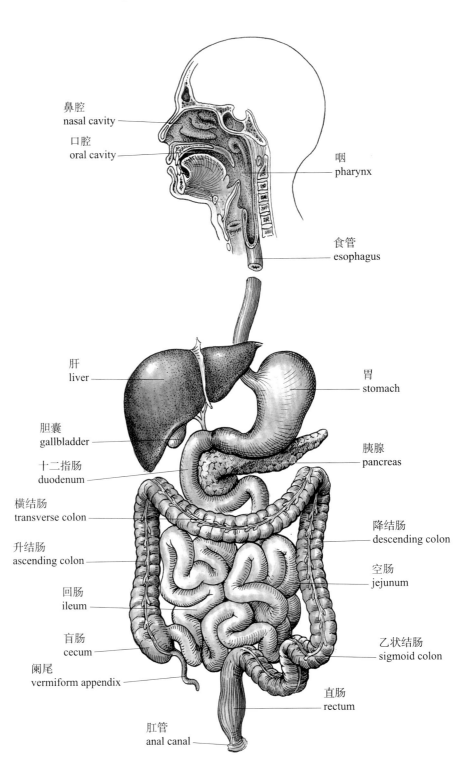

鼻腔
nasal cavity

口腔
oral cavity

咽
pharynx

食管
esophagus

肝
liver

胃
stomach

胆囊
gallbladder

胰腺
pancreas

十二指肠
duodenum

横结肠
transverse colon

降结肠
descending colon

升结肠
ascending colon

空肠
jejunum

回肠
ileum

盲肠
cecum

乙状结肠
sigmoid colon

阑尾
vermiform appendix

直肠
rectum

肛管
anal canal

图 4-1 消化系统概观（模式图）
Overview of alimentary system (diagram)

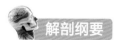

消化系统组成

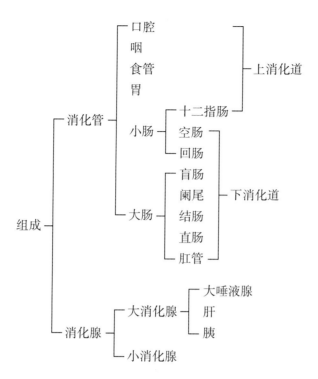

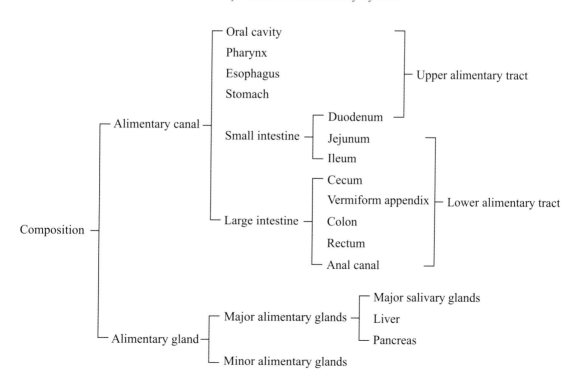

Composition of alimentary system

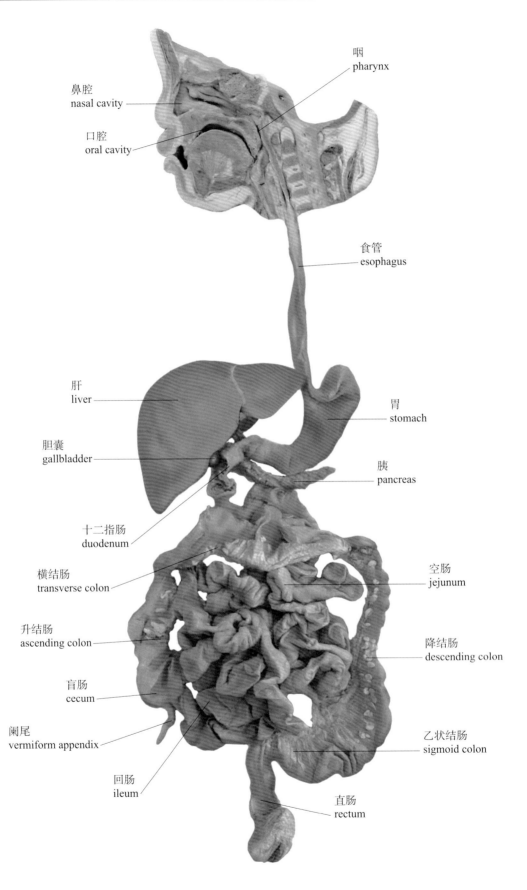

鼻腔
nasal cavity

口腔
oral cavity

咽
pharynx

食管
esophagus

肝
liver

胃
stomach

胆囊
gallbladder

胰
pancreas

十二指肠
duodenum

横结肠
transverse colon

空肠
jejunum

升结肠
ascending colon

降结肠
descending colon

盲肠
cecum

阑尾
vermiform appendix

乙状结肠
sigmoid colon

回肠
ileum

直肠
rectum

图 4-2　消化系统概观
Overview of alimentary system

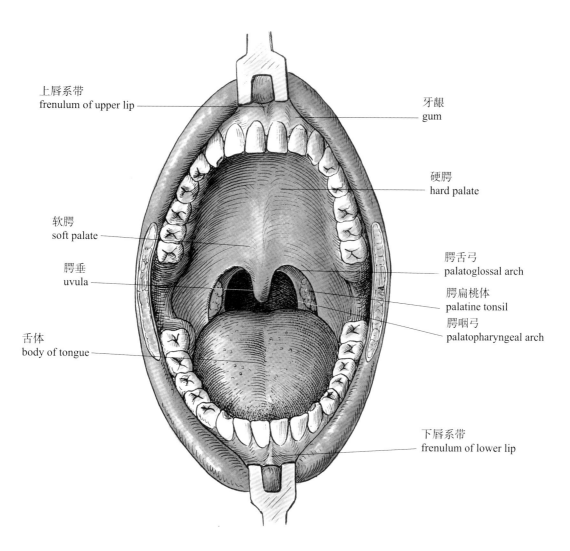

图 4-3 口腔
Oral cavity

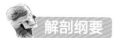

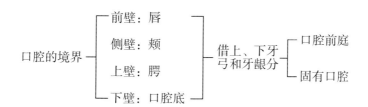

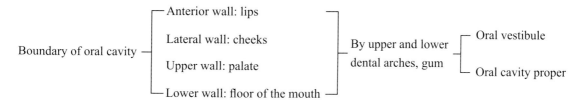

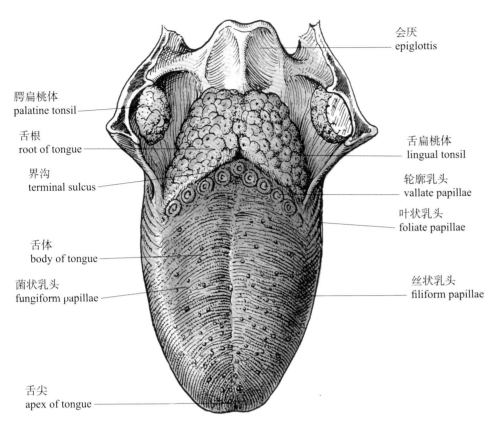

会厌
epiglottis

腭扁桃体
palatine tonsil

舌根
root of tongue

界沟
terminal sulcus

舌体
body of tongue

菌状乳头
fungiform papillae

舌尖
apex of tongue

舌扁桃体
lingual tonsil

轮廓乳头
vallate papillae

叶状乳头
foliate papillae

丝状乳头
filiform papillae

图 4-4　舌（背面观，模式图）
Tongue (dorsal view, diagram)

舌根
root of tongue

轮廓乳头
vallate papillae

菌状乳头
fungiform papillae

舌体
body of tongue

舌尖
apex of tongue

舌扁桃体
lingual tonsil

界沟
terminal sulcus

叶状乳头
foliate papillae

丝状乳头
filiform papillae

图 4-5　舌（背面观）
Tongue (dorsal view)

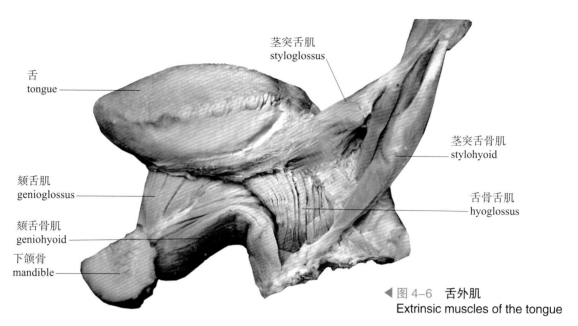

茎突舌肌
styloglossus

舌
tongue

茎突舌骨肌
stylohyoid

颏舌肌
genioglossus

舌骨舌肌
hyoglossus

颏舌骨肌
geniohyoid

下颌骨
mandible

◀ 图 4-6　舌外肌
Extrinsic muscles of the tongue

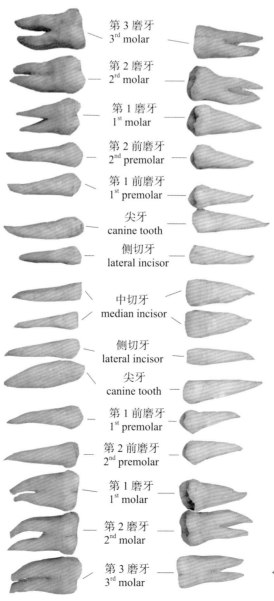

第 3 磨牙
3rd molar

第 2 磨牙
2nd molar

第 1 磨牙
1st molar

第 2 前磨牙
2nd premolar

第 1 前磨牙
1st premolar

尖牙
canine tooth

侧切牙
lateral incisor

中切牙
median incisor

侧切牙
lateral incisor

尖牙
canine tooth

第 1 前磨牙
1st premolar

第 2 前磨牙
2nd premolar

第 1 磨牙
1st molar

第 2 磨牙
2nd molar

第 3 磨牙
3rd molar

◀ 图 4-7　游离恒牙
Dissociative permanent teeth

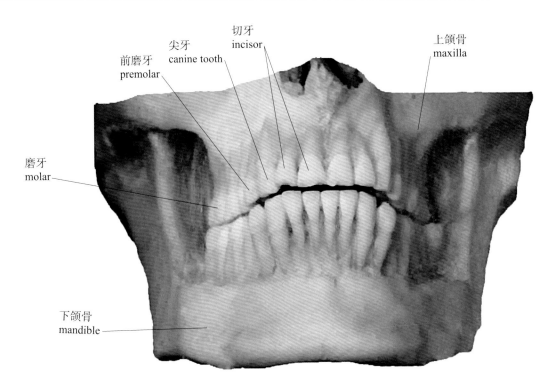

前磨牙 premolar
尖牙 canine tooth
切牙 incisor
上颌骨 maxilla
磨牙 molar
下颌骨 mandible

图 4-8　原位恒牙
Permanent teeth in situ

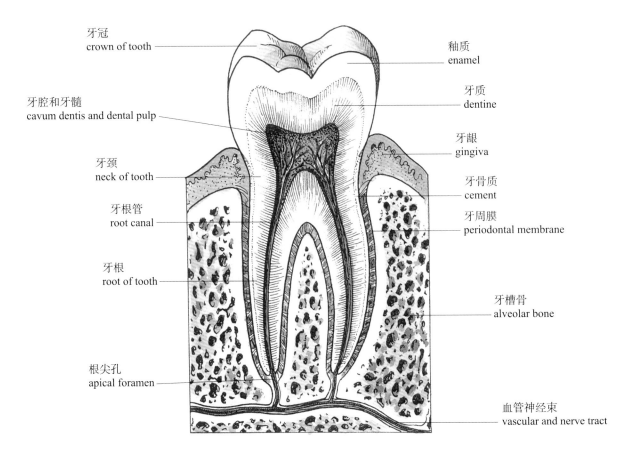

牙冠 crown of tooth
釉质 enamel
牙腔和牙髓 cavum dentis and dental pulp
牙质 dentine
牙颈 neck of tooth
牙龈 gingiva
牙根管 root canal
牙骨质 cement
牙周膜 periodontal membrane
牙根 root of tooth
牙槽骨 alveolar bone
根尖孔 apical foramen
血管神经束 vascular and nerve tract

图 4-9　牙的构造
Structure of the tooth

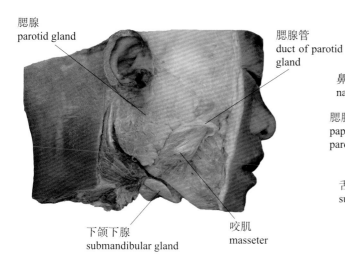

图 4-10 唾液腺（腮腺和下颌下腺）
Salivary glands (parotid gland and submandibular gland)

图 4-11 唾液腺（下颌下腺和舌下腺）
Salivary glands (submandibular gland and sublingual gland)

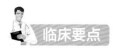 临床要点

大唾液腺位置和开口部位

名称	位置	开口部位
腮腺	浅部位于耳垂下方，咬肌后 1/3 浅面；深部位于下颌后窝内	腮腺管乳头（平对上颌第二磨牙牙冠的颊黏膜）
下颌下腺	下颌体内面的下颌下腺窝内	舌下阜
舌下腺	舌下襞深面	大导管：舌下阜 小导管：舌下襞黏膜表面

Key Points of the Clinic

Location and opening of major salivary glands

Gland	Location	Opening
Parotid gland	Superficial part is located below the auricular lobule, superficial surface of posterior one-third of masseter muscle; deep part lies in mandibular posterior fossa	Parotid papilla (buccal mucosa opposite the maxillary second molar crown)
Submandibular gland	Submandibular fossa on the medial surface of the body of the mandible	Sublingual caruncle
Sublingual gland	Under the sublingual fold	Major sublingual duct: sublingual caruncle minor sublingual dusct: mucosa of ublingual fold

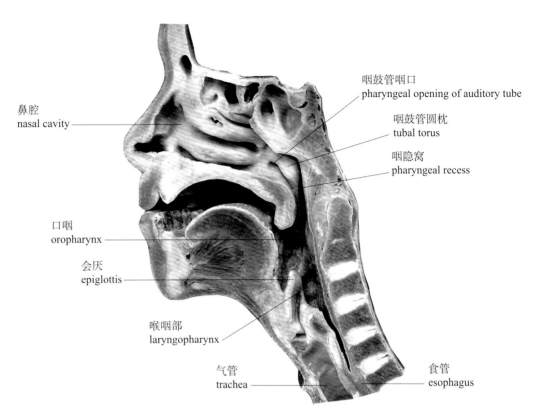

鼻腔
nasal cavity

咽鼓管咽口
pharyngeal opening of auditory tube

咽鼓管圆枕
tubal torus

咽隐窝
pharyngeal recess

口咽
oropharynx

会厌
epiglottis

喉咽部
laryngopharynx

气管
trachea

食管
esophagus

图 4-12　鼻腔、口腔、喉腔和咽（正中矢状切面）
Nasal cavity, oral cavity, laryngeal cavity and pharynx (median sagittal section)

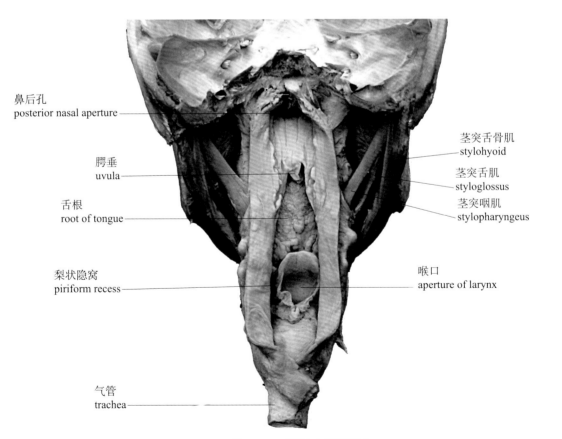

鼻后孔
posterior nasal aperture

腭垂
uvula

舌根
root of tongue

梨状隐窝
piriform recess

气管
trachea

茎突舌骨肌
stylohyoid

茎突舌肌
styloglossus

茎突咽肌
stylopharyngeus

喉口
aperture of larynx

图 4-13　咽腔（后面观）
Pharyngeal cavity (posterior aspect)

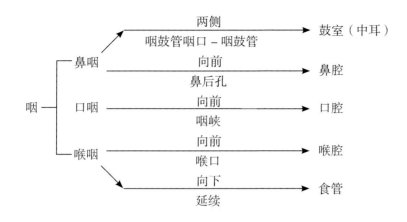

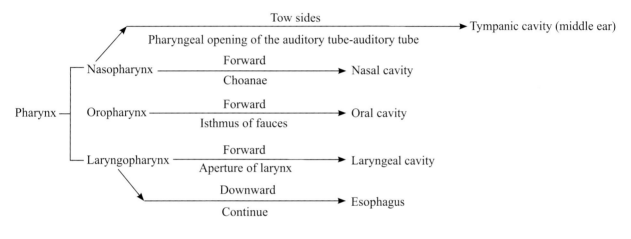

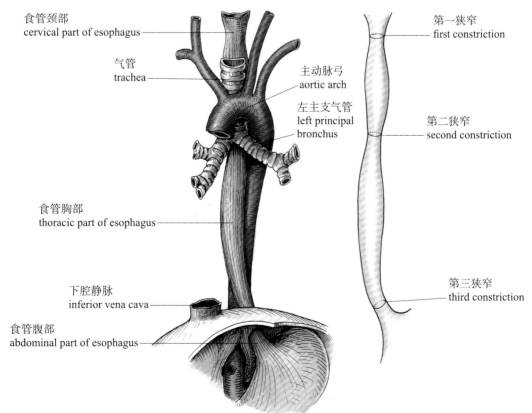

图 4-14 食管
Esophagus

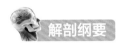 解剖纲要

食管的狭窄部位与意义

狭窄	部位	相当的椎体水平	距中切牙距离（cm）	意义
第一狭窄	起始处	第6颈椎体下缘	15	异物易滞留和食管癌的好发部位
第二狭窄	与左主支气管交叉处	第4、5胸椎体之间	25	
第三狭窄	穿食管裂孔处	第10胸椎	40	

食管分部：颈部、胸部和腹部。

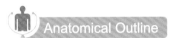 Anatomical Outline

Esophageal constriction and its location and significance

Stricture	Location	Comparable vertebral body level	Distance from the incisor teeth (cm)	Significance
First constricture	Commencement	Lower border of the sixth cervical vertebral body	15	Foreign matter retention and the most common site of esophageal cancer
Second constricture	To cross anteriorly by left principal bronchus	Between fourth and fifth thoracic vertebral body	25	
Third constricture	To pass through esophageal hiatus	Tenth thoracic vertebra	40	

Parts of esophagus: cervical portion, thoracic portion and abdominal portion

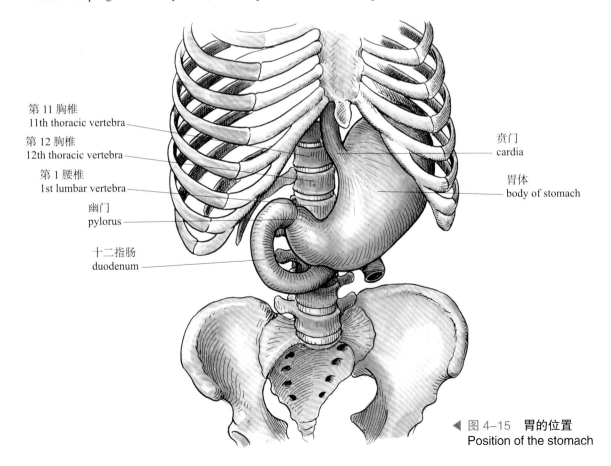

第 11 胸椎
11th thoracic vertebra

第 12 胸椎
12th thoracic vertebra

第 1 腰椎
1st lumbar vertebra

幽门
pylorus

十二指肠
duodenum

贲门
cardia

胃体
body of stomach

◀ 图 4–15　**胃的位置**
Position of the stomach

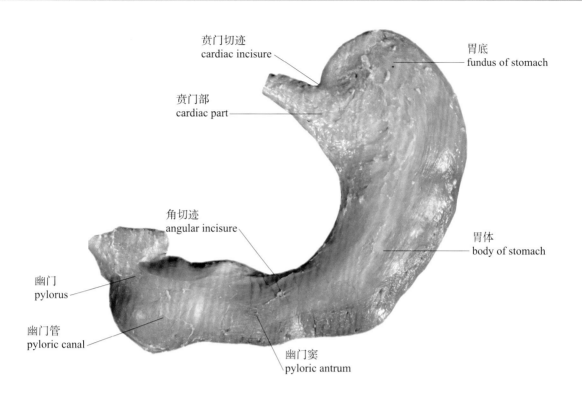

贲门切迹
cardiac incisure

胃底
fundus of stomach

贲门部
cardiac part

角切迹
angular incisure

胃体
body of stomach

幽门
pylorus

幽门管
pyloric canal

幽门窦
pyloric antrum

图 4-16 胃的形态和分部
Shape and parts of the stomach

解剖纲要

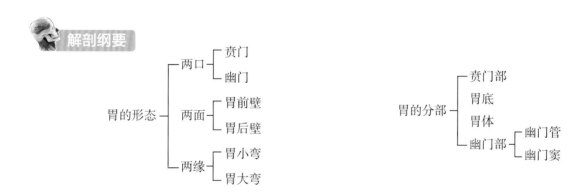

Anatomical Outline

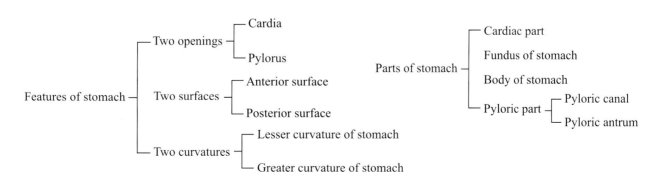

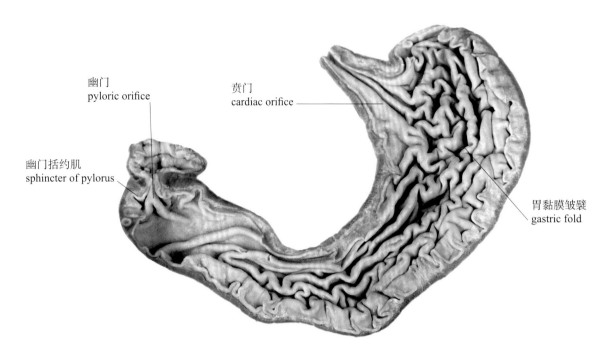

幽门
pyloric orifice

贲门
cardiac orifice

幽门括约肌
sphincter of pylorus

胃黏膜皱襞
gastric fold

图 4-17 **胃黏膜**
Mucous membrane of the stomach

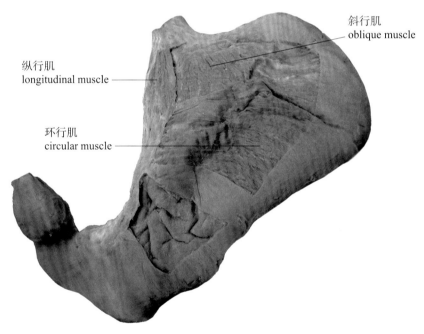

斜行肌
oblique muscle

纵行肌
longitudinal muscle

环行肌
circular muscle

图 4-18 **胃肌**
Muscles of the stomach

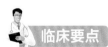 **临床要点**

　　幽门部在临床上常称作"胃窦"，幽门部包括幽门窦和幽门管两部分，幽门窦通常位于胃的最低部，胃溃疡和胃癌多发生于胃的幽门窦近胃小弯处。

　　十二指肠：紧贴腹后壁，整体呈"C"形，环抱胰头，分为上部、降部、水平部和升部。其中，上部临床上称为十二指肠球部，十二指肠溃疡多发于此。

十二指肠升部与空肠转折形成十二指肠空肠曲，该曲的上后壁有十二指肠悬肌连于右膈脚上，十二指肠悬肌与包绕其下段的腹膜皱襞共同构成十二指肠悬韧带，又称 Treitz 韧带，是确定空肠起始部的重要标志。

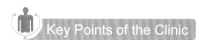

Key Points of the Clinic

The pyloric part is often called "gastric antrum" in clinic. The pyloric part is divided into two parts: pyloric antrum and pyloric canal. The pyloric antrum is usually located at the lowest part of the stomach. Gastric ulcer and gastric cancer often occur near the small curvature of the pyloric antrum.

Duodenum is attached to the posterior abdominal wall closely, and forms an elongated 'C'. The head of the pancreas lies within the concavity of the duodenum. The duodenum is divided into superior, descending, horizontal and ascending parts. Clinically, the superior part is referred to as the duodenal bulb, where duodenal ulcer often occur.

Ascending part turns sharply at the duodenojejunal flexure to become continuous with the jejunum. The suspensory muscle of duodenum is connected to the right crus on the superior posterior wall of the flexure. The suspensory muscle of duodenum and a double fold of peritoneum that wraps the former lower section constitutes of the suspensory ligament of the duodenum (or ligament of Treitz). It is an important sign to determine the beginning of the jejunum.

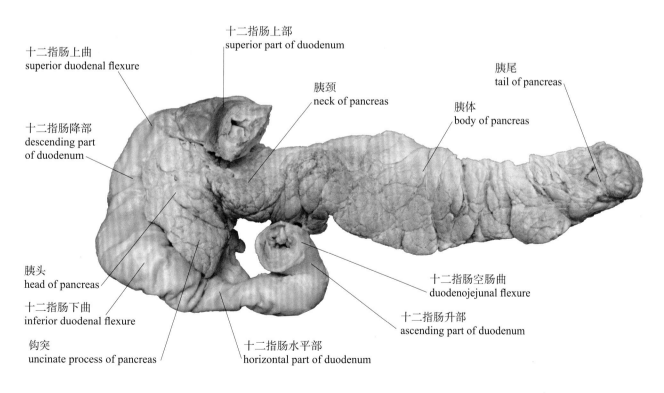

图 4-19　十二指肠和胰
Duodenum and pancreas

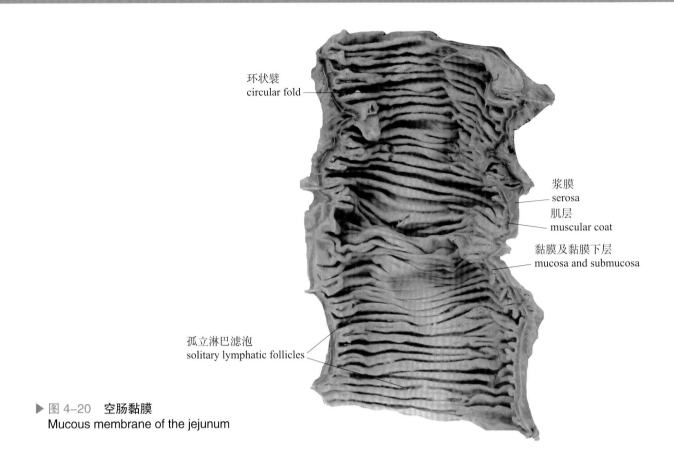

环状襞
circular fold

浆膜
serosa

肌层
muscular coat

黏膜及黏膜下层
mucosa and submucosa

孤立淋巴滤泡
solitary lymphatic follicles

▶ 图 4-20　空肠黏膜
Mucous membrane of the jejunum

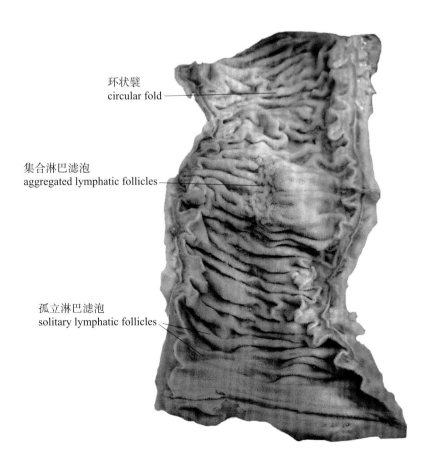

环状襞
circular fold

集合淋巴滤泡
aggregated lymphatic follicles

孤立淋巴滤泡
solitary lymphatic follicles

◀ 图 4-21　回肠黏膜
Mucous membrane of the ileum

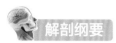 解剖纲要

空肠、回肠的区别

类别	空肠	回肠
位置	左腰区、脐区	脐区、右髂区、下腹区
长度	近侧 2/5	远侧 3/5
外观	粗、粉红、血管多	细、粉灰、血管少
淋巴滤泡	孤立	集合和孤立
血管弓	级数较少	级数较多

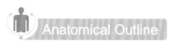 Anatomical Outline

The difference between jejunum and ileum

Items	Jejunum	Ileum
Position	Left lumbar region, umbilical region	Umbilical region, right iliac region, hypogastric region
Length	Proximal two-fifths	Distal three-fifths
Appearance	Thick, pink, more vascular	Thin, pink gray, less vascular
Lymph follicle	Solitary	Aggregated and solitary
Vascular arches	The series is less	The series is more

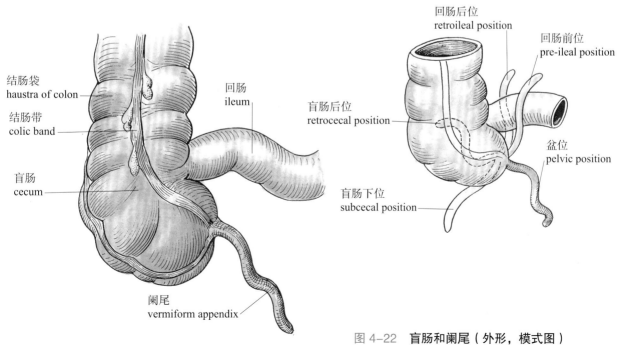

图 4-22 盲肠和阑尾（外形，模式图）
Cecum and vermiform appendix (external features, diagram)

Part 2 Splanchnology 第二篇 内脏学

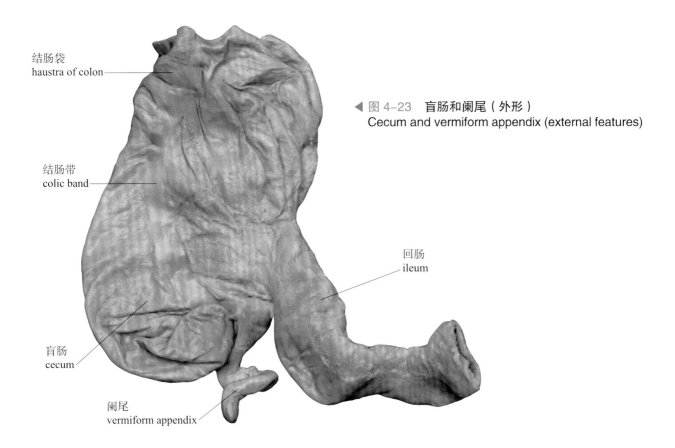

结肠袋
haustra of colon

结肠带
colic band

回肠
ileum

盲肠
cecum

阑尾
vermiform appendix

◀ 图 4-23 盲肠和阑尾（外形）
Cecum and vermiform appendix (external features)

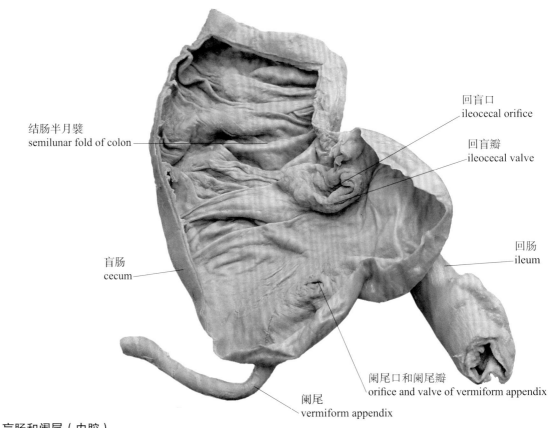

结肠半月襞
semilunar fold of colon

回盲口
ileocecal orifice

回盲瓣
ileocecal valve

回肠
ileum

盲肠
cecum

阑尾口和阑尾瓣
orifice and valve of vermiform appendix

阑尾
vermiform appendix

图 4-24 盲肠和阑尾（内腔）
▶ Cecum and vermiform appendix (internal lumen)

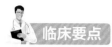

临床要点

　　阑尾根部的体表投影（McBurney 点）：右髂前上棘与脐连线的中、外 1/3 交点处。阑尾尖端为游离盲端，移动性大。3 条结肠带均在阑尾根部集中，故沿结肠带向下追踪，是手术中寻找阑尾的可靠方法。因阑尾位置的不同，阑尾炎症状和体征有一定的差异，因此 McBurney 点仅可作为诊断时的参考，右下腹的局限性、固定的压痛点常更有临床诊断意义。

Key Points of the Clinic

　　The surface projection of the root of the vermiform appendix (McBurney's point): It's the junction of the lateral and the middle one third of the line joining the umbilicus and the right anterior superior iliac spine. The tip of the vermiform appendix is a free blind end with great mobility. All three colic bands converge at the root of the vermiform appendix, making it a reliable method of tracking down the colonic bands, in order to find the vermiform appendix during surgery. The difference in the position of the vermiform appendix would pertain to different symptoms and signs of appendicitis. Therefore, the McBurney's point just provides a reference, that is a limited and fixed tenderness point in the right lower abdomen, which usually is greater significance for the diagnosis.

Part 2 Splanchnology　第二篇　内脏学

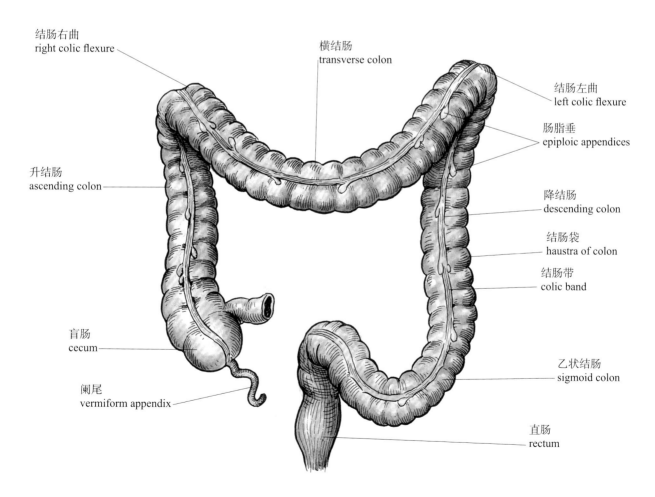

结肠右曲
right colic flexure

横结肠
transverse colon

结肠左曲
left colic flexure

肠脂垂
epiploic appendices

升结肠
ascending colon

降结肠
descending colon

结肠袋
haustra of colon

结肠带
colic band

盲肠
cecum

阑尾
vermiform appendix

乙状结肠
sigmoid colon

直肠
rectum

图 4-25　**大肠**
Large intestine

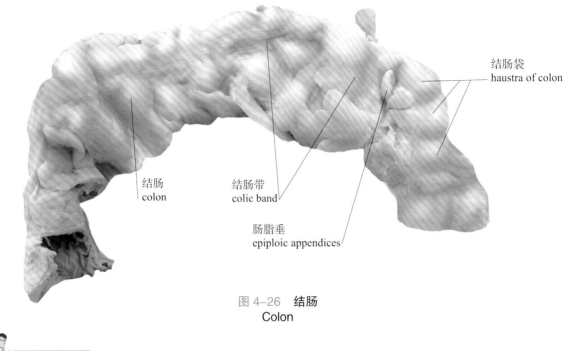

结肠袋
haustra of colon

结肠
colon

结肠带
colic band

肠脂垂
epiploic appendices

图 4-26　结肠
Colon

临床要点

结肠和盲肠特征性结构：结肠带、结肠袋和肠脂垂，是腹部手术中鉴别大、小肠的主要依据。

Key Points of the Clinic

The characteristic structure of colon and cecum: colic band, haustra of colon and epiploic appendice, which are main evidences for identification of large and small intestine in abdominal surgery.

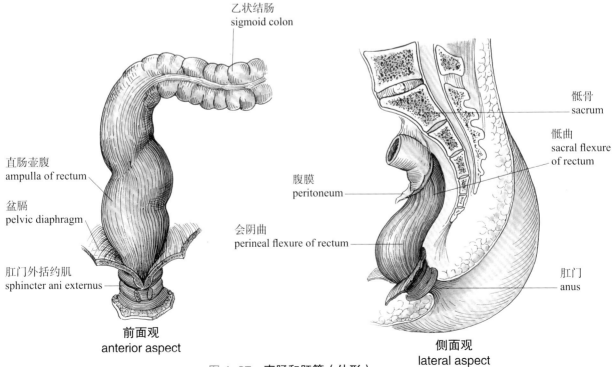

乙状结肠
sigmoid colon

直肠壶腹
ampulla of rectum

盆膈
pelvic diaphragm

肛门外括约肌
sphincter ani externus

骶骨
sacrum

骶曲
sacral flexure of rectum

腹膜
peritoneum

会阴曲
perineal flexure of rectum

肛门
anus

前面观
anterior aspect

侧面观
lateral aspect

图 4-27　直肠和肛管（外形）
Rectum and anal canal (external features)

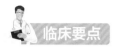 临床要点

直肠弯曲及其临床意义

直肠在矢状面上形成 2 个弯曲，上段形成凸向后的弯曲称直肠骶曲，下段形成凸向前的弯曲称直肠会阴曲。直肠在冠状面上形成 3 个弯曲，但不恒定，一般中间较大的凸向左侧，上、下 2 个凸向右侧。临床进行直肠镜、乙状结肠镜检查时，应注意弯曲，以免损伤肠壁。

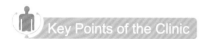 Key Points of the Clinic

Rectal bending and its clinical significance

The rectum forms 2 flexures on the sagittal plane. The upper part forms a flexure convex backward called sacral flexure, and the lower part forms a flexure convex forward called perineal flexure. Rectum forms 3 flexures on coronal plane, but not constant, general middle bigger convex to the left; the upper and lower two convex to the right. In clinical proctoscopy and sigmoidoscopy, attention should be paid to flexures so as not to damage the intestinal wall.

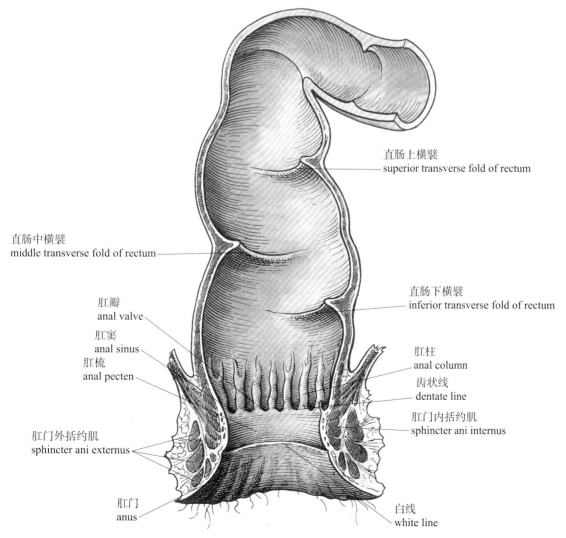

图 4-28 直肠和肛管（内腔，模式图）
Rectum and anal canal (internal lumen, diagram)

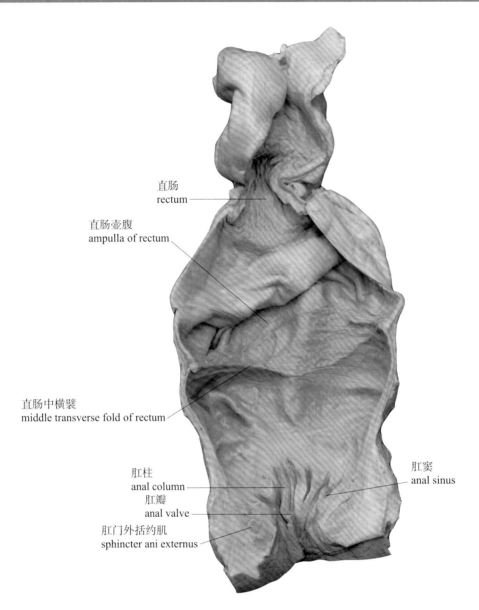

直肠
rectum

直肠壶腹
ampulla of rectum

直肠中横襞
middle transverse fold of rectum

肛窦
anal sinus

肛柱
anal column
肛瓣
anal valve
肛门外括约肌
sphincter ani externus

图 4-29　直肠和肛管（内腔）
Rectum and anal canal (internal lumen)

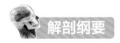 解剖纲要

肛管齿状线上、下部的比较

内容	齿状线以上	齿状线以下
覆盖上皮	单层柱状上皮	复层扁平上皮
动脉来源	直肠上、下动脉	肛动脉
静脉回流	直肠上静脉—肠系膜下静脉—脾静脉—肝门静脉	肛门静脉—阴部内静脉—髂内静脉—髂总静脉—下腔静脉
淋巴引流	肠系膜下淋巴结和髂内淋巴结	腹股沟浅淋巴结
神经分布	内脏神经	躯体神经

Anatomical Outline

Comparison of the structures in anal canal above and below the dentate line

Contents	Above the dentate line	Below the dentate line
Epithelium	simple columnar epithelium	stratified squamous epithelium
Arterial supply	superior and inferior rectal artery	anal artery
Venous return	superior rectal veins—inferior mesenteric vein—splenic vein—hepatic portal vein	anal vein—internal pudendal vein—internal iliac vein—common iliac vein—inferior vena cava
Lymphatic drainage	inferior mesenteric lymph node, internal iliac lymph node	superficial inguinal lymph node
Nerve innervation	visceral nerves	somatic nerves

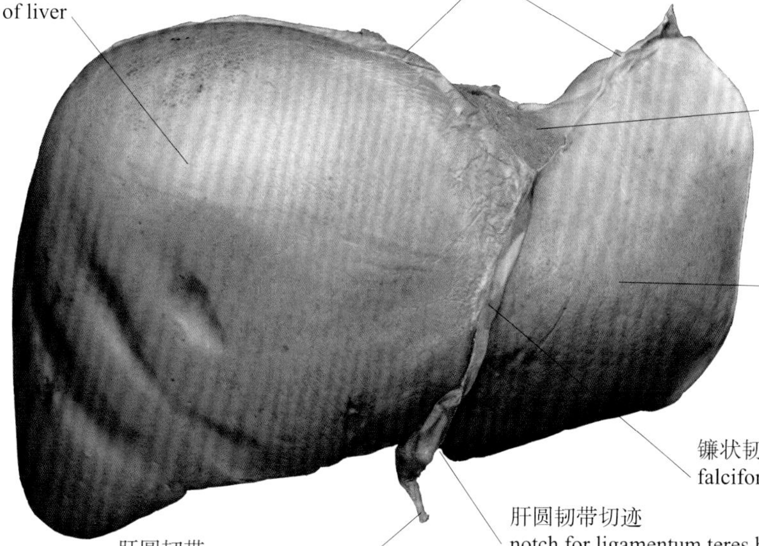

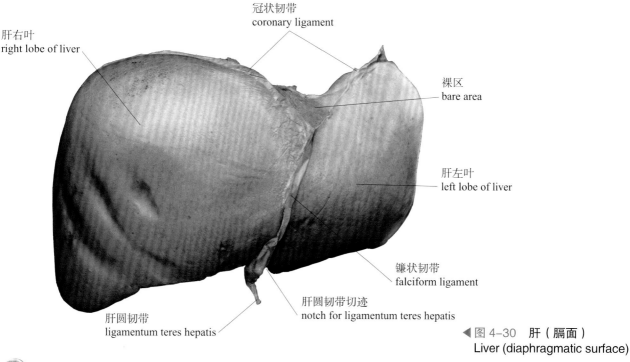

图 4–30 肝（膈面）
Liver (diaphragmatic surface)

解剖纲要

肝的位置与形态

肝大部分位于右季肋区和腹上区，小部分位于左季肋区。

肝包括上、下两面，前、后、左、右四缘。肝上面膨隆，与膈肌毗邻，称为膈面 , 可见镰状韧带和冠状韧带。镰状韧带将肝分为左、右叶。膈面后部无腹膜覆盖处为裸区。肝下面为脏面，与腹腔脏器毗邻，凹凸不平，中部有“H”形沟，由左侧的肝圆韧带裂与静脉韧带裂、右侧的胆囊窝与腔静脉沟和中间横行的肝门构成。出入肝门的结构被结缔组织包绕称为肝蒂，内含左、右肝管，肝固有动脉，肝门静脉，神经和淋巴管。“H”形沟将肝分为肝左叶、肝右叶、方叶和尾状叶。

肝前缘可见胆囊切迹和肝圆韧带切迹，肝后缘和右缘圆钝，肝左缘锐利。

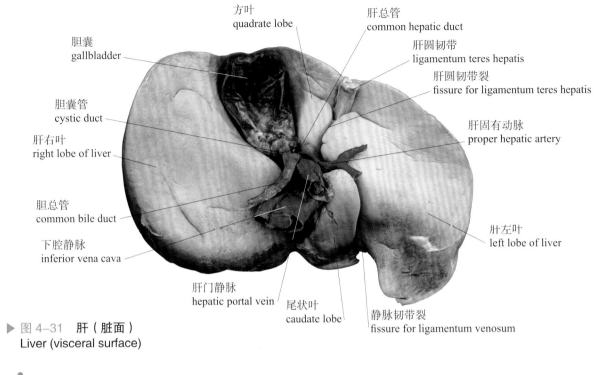

▶ 图 4-31 肝（脏面）
Liver (visceral surface)

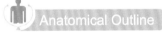

Location and features of liver

The liver mostly lies in the right hypochondriac region and epigastric region, and partly in the left hypochondriac region.

Liver includes superior and inferior surfaces, anterior, posterior, left and right borders. The superior surface is enlarged and lies immediately below the diaphragm, known as the diaphragmatic surface. There are falciform ligament and coronal ligament on it. The falciform ligament divides the liver into left and right lobes. There is a bare area, with no peritoneum covering at the posterior part of the diaphragmatic surface. The inferior uneven aspect of the liver is the visceral surface, adjacent to the abdominal organs, the middle has an "H" sulcus, by the left side of fissure for ligamentum teres hepatis and fissure for ligamentum venosum, the right side of the fossa of the gallbladder and the sulcus for vena cava, and the middle transverse porta hepatis. The structures passing through the porta hepatis is surrounded by connective tissue called the hepatic pedicle, containing the left and right hepatic ducts, the proper hepatic artery, the hepatic portal vein, the nerve, and the lymphatic vessels. "H" sulcus divides the liver into left, right, quadrate and caudate lobes.

Gallbladder notch and ligamentum teres hepatis are found in the anterior border of the liver; the posterior and right border of the liver is round and obtuse; the left border of the liver is sharp.

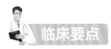

1. 肝的膈面前部被肋所掩盖，仅在腹上区的左、右肋弓之间，有一小部分露于剑突下，直接与腹前壁相接触。当腹上区和右季肋区遭到暴力冲击或肋骨骨折时，肝可能被损伤而破裂。

2.肝上界与膈穹窿一致,肝下界右侧与右肋弓一致;中部位于剑突下约3cm处;左侧被肋弓掩盖。故在体检时,在右肋弓下不能触到肝。但3岁以下的健康幼儿,由于腹腔容积较小,而肝的体积相对较大,肝前缘常低于右肋弓下1.5~2.0cm,7岁以后,在右肋弓下不能触到肝,若能触及,则应考虑为病理性肝肿大。

Key Points of the Clinic

1. The anterior part of hepatic diaphragmatic surface is covered by ribs. Only between the left and right costal arches of the epigastrium, a small part is exposed under the xiphoid process and directly contacts the anterior abdominal wall. When the right hypochondrium and epigastrium are violently impacted or damaged by rib fractures, the liver may be damaged and ruptured.

2. The hepatic superior border is consistent with the diaphragm dome. The right side of the hepatic inferior border is consistent with the right costal arch; middle part lies about 3cm below the xiphoid process; left side is covered by the costal arch. Therefore, the liver cannot be palpable under the right costal arch during the physical examination. However, concerning healthy children under 3 years of age, because the volume of the abdominal cavity is smaller and the volume of the liver is relatively larger, the anterior border of the liver is often 1.5 to 2.0 cm below the right costal arch. After 7 years of age, it cannot be palpable under the right costal arch. If it can be palpable, it should be considered as pathological hepatomegaly.

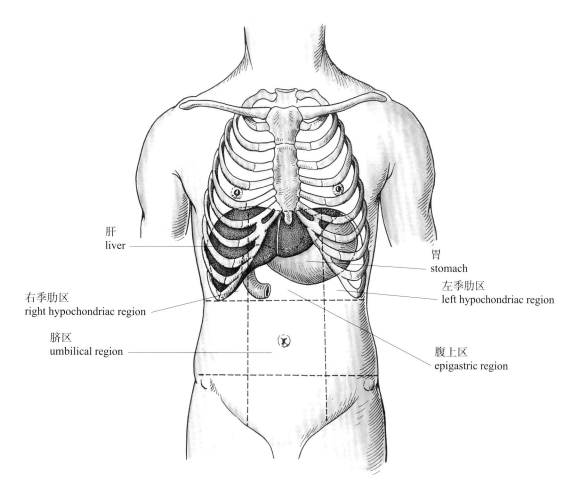

图 4-32　胃和肝的位置
Position of the stomach and liver

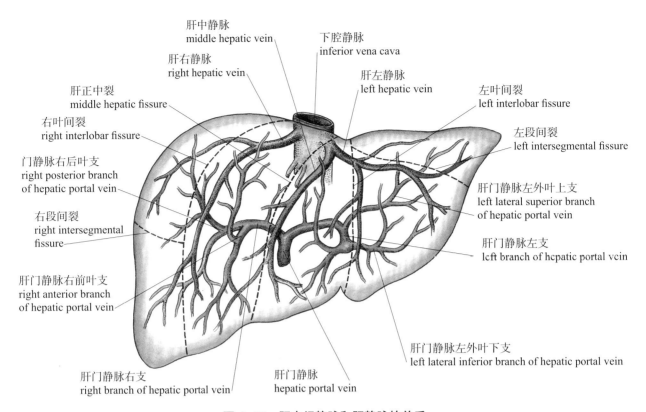

肝中静脉
middle hepatic vein

下腔静脉
inferior vena cava

肝右静脉
right hepatic vein

肝左静脉
left hepatic vein

左叶间裂
left interlobar fissure

肝正中裂
middle hepatic fissure

左段间裂
left intersegmental fissure

右叶间裂
right interlobar fissure

门静脉右后叶支
right posterior branch
of hepatic portal vein

肝门静脉左外叶上支
left lateral superior branch
of hepatic portal vein

右段间裂
right intersegmental
fissure

肝门静脉左支
left branch of hepatic portal vein

肝门静脉右前叶支
right anterior branch
of hepatic portal vein

肝门静脉左外叶下支
left lateral inferior branch of hepatic portal vein

肝门静脉右支
right branch of hepatic portal vein

肝门静脉
hepatic portal vein

图 4-33　肝内门静脉和肝静脉的关系
Relation between intrahepatic portal veins and hepatic veins

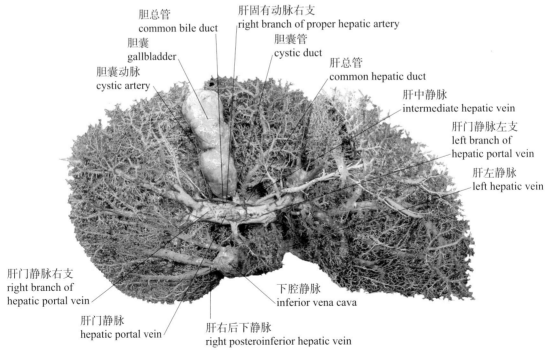

胆总管
common bile duct

肝固有动脉右支
right branch of proper hepatic artery

胆囊
gallbladder

胆囊管
cystic duct

肝总管
common hepatic duct

胆囊动脉
cystic artery

肝中静脉
intermediate hepatic vein

肝门静脉左支
left branch of
hepatic portal vein

肝左静脉
left hepatic vein

肝门静脉右支
right branch of
hepatic portal vein

下腔静脉
inferior vena cava

肝门静脉
hepatic portal vein

肝右后下静脉
right posteroinferior hepatic vein

图 4-34　肝铸型（下面观）
Cast of liver (inferior view)

红色：肝固有动脉及其分支
Red: proper hepatic artery and branches

绿色：肝管、胆管和胆囊
Green: hepatic duct, bile duct and gallbladder

橙色：肝静脉系统
Orange: hepatic vein system

蓝色：肝门静脉系统
Blue: hepatic portal venous system

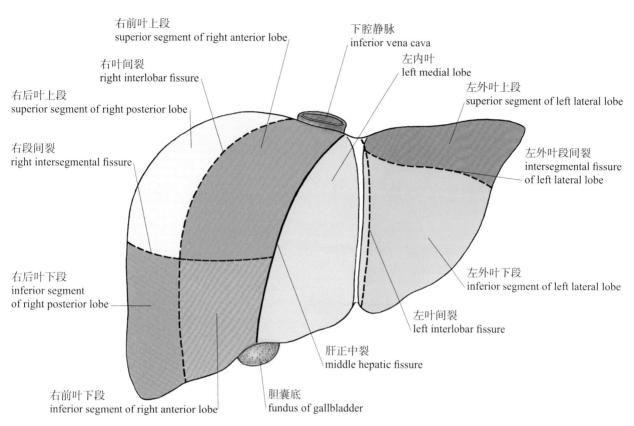

右前叶上段
superior segment of right anterior lobe

右叶间裂
right interlobar fissure

右后叶上段
superior segment of right posterior lobe

右段间裂
right intersegmental fissure

下腔静脉
inferior vena cava

左内叶
left medial lobe

左外叶上段
superior segment of left lateral lobe

左外叶段间裂
intersegmental fissure of left lateral lobe

左外叶下段
inferior segment of left lateral lobe

左叶间裂
left interlobar fissure

右后叶下段
inferior segment of right posterior lobe

肝正中裂
middle hepatic fissure

胆囊底
fundus of gallbladder

右前叶下段
inferior segment of right anterior lobe

图 4-35 肝叶与肝段（前面观）
Hepatic lobes and hepatic segments (anterior view)

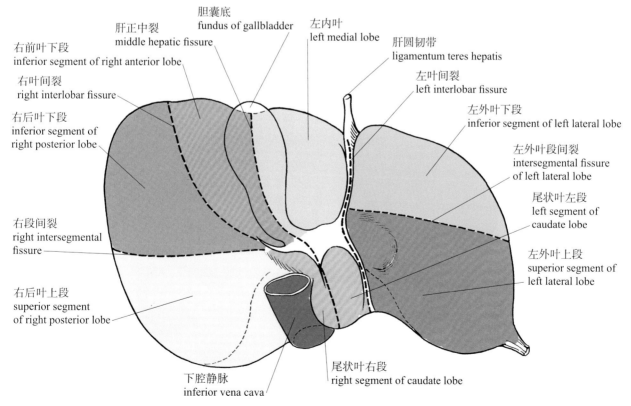

肝正中裂
middle hepatic fissure

胆囊底
fundus of gallbladder

左内叶
left medial lobe

肝圆韧带
ligamentum teres hepatis

右前叶下段
inferior segment of right anterior lobe

右叶间裂
right interlobar fissure

右后叶下段
inferior segment of right posterior lobe

左叶间裂
left interlobar fissure

左外叶下段
inferior segment of left lateral lobe

左外叶段间裂
intersegmental fissure of left lateral lobe

尾状叶左段
left segment of caudate lobe

左外叶上段
superior segment of left lateral lobe

右段间裂
right intersegmental fissure

右后叶上段
superior segment of right posterior lobe

下腔静脉
inferior vena cava

尾状叶右段
right segment of caudate lobe

图 4-36 肝叶与肝段（下面观）
Hepatic lobes and hepatic segments (inferior view)

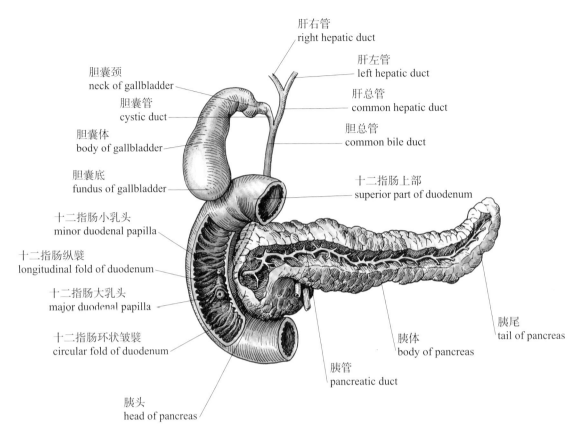

图 4-37　胆囊、输胆管道和胰腺
Gallbladder, biliary ducts and pancreas

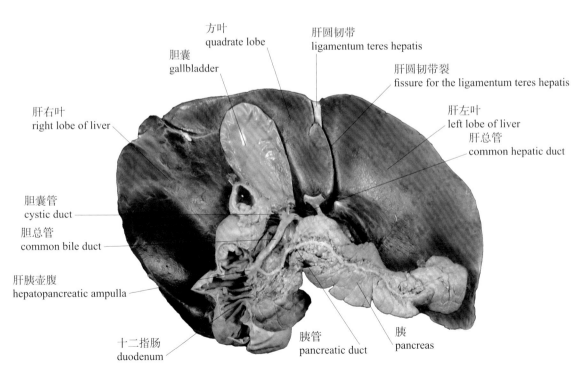

图 4-38　肝外胆道
Extrahepatic biliary tract

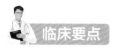

临床上可根据叶、段的区分对肝脏疾病进行较为精确的定位诊断，也可施行肝叶、肝段切除。

胆囊分底、体、颈、管 4 部分。

肝外胆道：胆总管由肝总管和胆囊管汇合而成，在肝十二指肠韧带内下行，在十二指肠后内侧壁内与胰管处汇合，形成肝胰壶腹（或称 Vater 壶腹），开口于十二指肠大乳头。

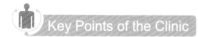

According to the division of lobes and segments in clinical, the liver disease can be accurately located and diagnosed, and the liver lobes or segments can be resected.

The gallbladder is described as having a fundus, body, neck and cystic duct.

Extrahepatic biliary tract: The common bile duct is formed by the junction of the cystic duct and common hepatic ducts. It descends into the hepatoduodenal ligament, and converges with the pancreatic duct in the posterior medial wall of the duodenum. It forms the hepatopancreatic ampulla (or Vater ampulla), opening into the major duodenal papilla.

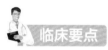

胆囊底的体表投影：右锁骨中线与右肋弓交点附近。胆囊发炎时，该处可有压痛。

The surface projection of the fundus of gallbladder: the crossing of right midclavicular line and the right costal arch. When the gallbladder is inflamed, there may be tenderness.

第五章　呼吸系统
Chapter 5 Respiratory system

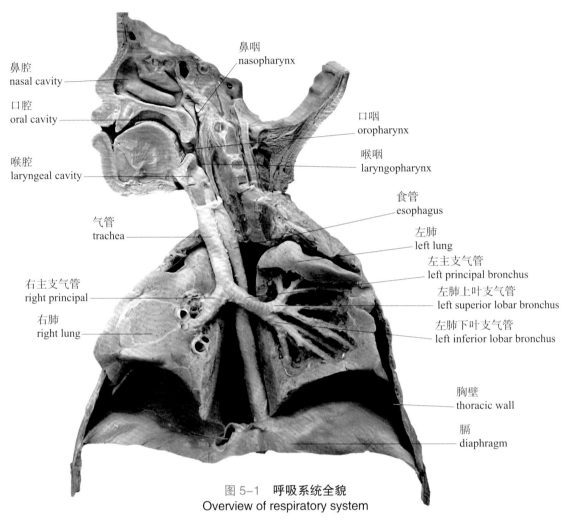

鼻咽
nasopharynx

鼻腔
nasal cavity

口腔
oral cavity

口咽
oropharynx

喉咽
laryngopharynx

喉腔
laryngeal cavity

食管
esophagus

气管
trachea

左肺
left lung

左主支气管
left principal bronchus

右主支气管
right principal

左肺上叶支气管
left superior lobar bronchus

右肺
right lung

左肺下叶支气管
left inferior lobar bronchus

胸壁
thoracic wall

膈
diaphragm

图 5-1　呼吸系统全貌
Overview of respiratory system

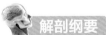解剖纲要

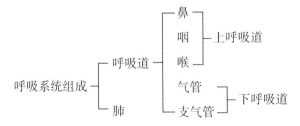

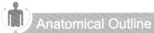Anatomical Outline

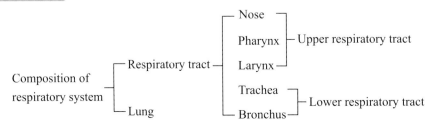

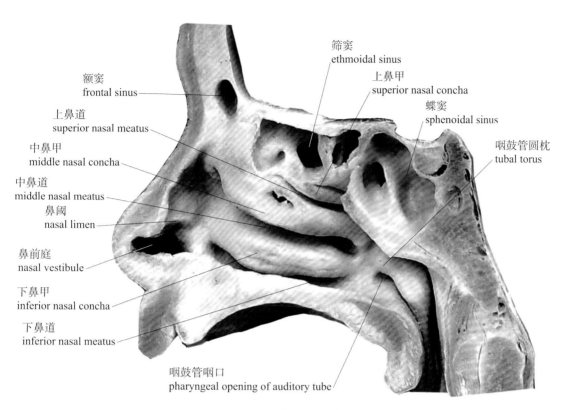

图 5-2　鼻腔外侧壁
Lateral wall of nasal cavity

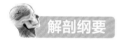解剖纲要

　　喉主要由喉软骨和喉肌构成，它既是呼吸的管道，又是发音的器官，借喉口通喉咽。成年人的喉在第 3~6 颈椎前方。

　　喉软骨是喉的支架，包括甲状软骨、环状软骨、会厌软骨和成对的杓状软骨。

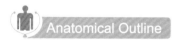Anatomical Outline

　　The larynx is mainly composed of laryngeal cartilages and laryngeal muscles. It is both a respiratory tract and a vocal organ, communicating with laryngopharynx by aperture of larynx. The adult's larynx lies anterior to 3th-6th cervical vertebrae.

　　Laryngeal cartilages are the framework of the larynx, which include thyroid cartilage, cricoid cartilage, epiglottic cartilage and paired arytenoid cartilages.

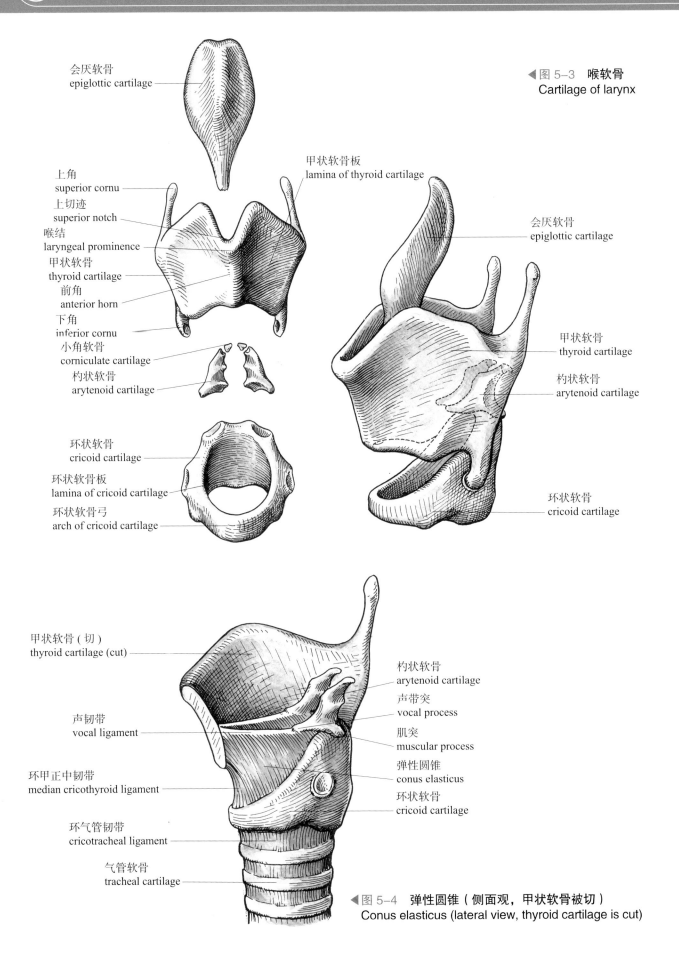

会厌软骨
epiglottic cartilage

甲状软骨板
lamina of thyroid cartilage

▲图 5-3　喉软骨
Cartilage of larynx

上角
superior cornu

上切迹
superior notch

喉结
laryngeal prominence

甲状软骨
thyroid cartilage

前角
anterior horn

下角
inferior cornu

小角软骨
corniculate cartilage

杓状软骨
arytenoid cartilage

环状软骨
cricoid cartilage

环状软骨板
lamina of cricoid cartilage

环状软骨弓
arch of cricoid cartilage

会厌软骨
epiglottic cartilage

甲状软骨
thyroid cartilage

杓状软骨
arytenoid cartilage

环状软骨
cricoid cartilage

甲状软骨（切）
thyroid cartilage (cut)

声韧带
vocal ligament

环甲正中韧带
median cricothyroid ligament

环气管韧带
cricotracheal ligament

气管软骨
tracheal cartilage

杓状软骨
arytenoid cartilage

声带突
vocal process

肌突
muscular process

弹性圆锥
conus elasticus

环状软骨
cricoid cartilage

▲图 5-4　弹性圆锥（侧面观，甲状软骨被切）
Conus elasticus (lateral view, thyroid cartilage is cut)

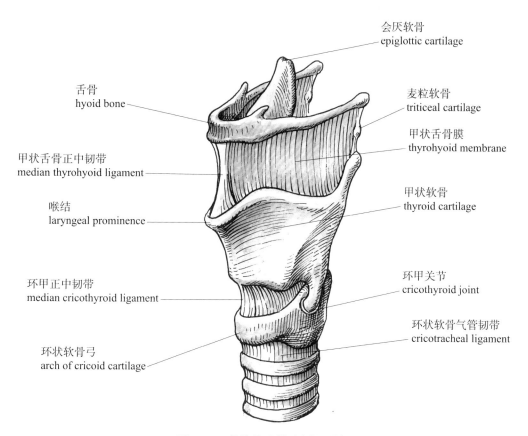

会厌软骨
epiglottic cartilage

舌骨
hyoid bone

麦粒软骨
triticeal cartilage

甲状舌骨膜
thyrohyoid membrane

甲状舌骨正中韧带
median thyrohyoid ligament

甲状软骨
thyroid cartilage

喉结
laryngeal prominence

环甲正中韧带
median cricothyroid ligament

环甲关节
cricothyroid joint

环状软骨气管韧带
cricotracheal ligament

环状软骨弓
arch of cricoid cartilage

图 5-5　喉软骨连结（侧面观）
Joints of the laryngeal cartilages (lateral view)

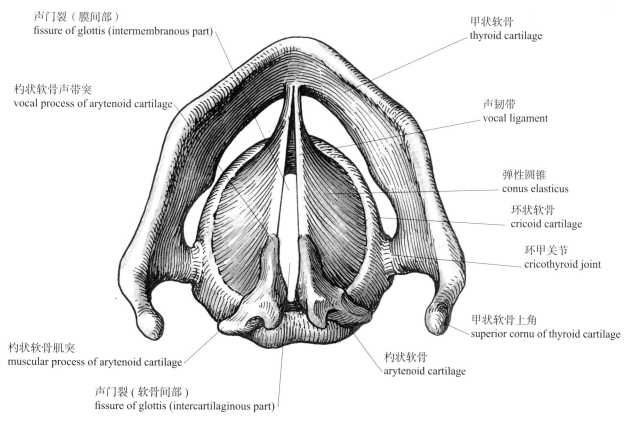

声门裂（膜间部）
fissure of glottis (intermembranous part)

甲状软骨
thyroid cartilage

杓状软骨声带突
vocal process of arytenoid cartilage

声韧带
vocal ligament

弹性圆锥
conus elasticus

环状软骨
cricoid cartilage

环甲关节
cricothyroid joint

甲状软骨上角
superior cornu of thyroid cartilage

杓状软骨肌突
muscular process of arytenoid cartilage

杓状软骨
arytenoid cartilage

声门裂（软骨间部）
fissure of glottis (intercartilaginous part)

图 5-6　喉软骨和弹性圆锥（上面观）
Laryngeal cartilages and conus elasticus (superior view)

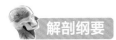

解剖纲要

弹性圆锥起自甲状软骨前角后面，呈扇形向后、向下止于杓状软骨声带突和环状软骨上缘。其上缘游离增厚为声韧带，位于甲状软骨至声带突之间。声韧带连同声带肌及覆盖于其表面的喉黏膜一起构成声带。

弹性圆锥中部弹性纤维增厚称环甲正中韧带。急性喉阻塞时，可在环甲正中韧带处进行穿刺，以建立暂时的通气道。

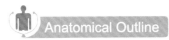

Anatomical Outline

The conus elasticus originates from the back of the anterior horn of the thyroid cartilage and extends backward and downward in a fan-shaped to the vocal processes of arytenoid cartilage and the superior edge of cricoid cartilage. The upper margin is free and thickened to form the vocal ligament, located between the thyroid cartilage and the vocal processes. The vocal ligament together with the vocal muscles and the laryngeal mucosa covering the surface form the vocal cords.

The thickened elastic fibers in the middle part of the elastic cone, is called as the median cricothyroid ligament. Acute laryngeal obstruction can be punctured in order to establish a temporary airway.

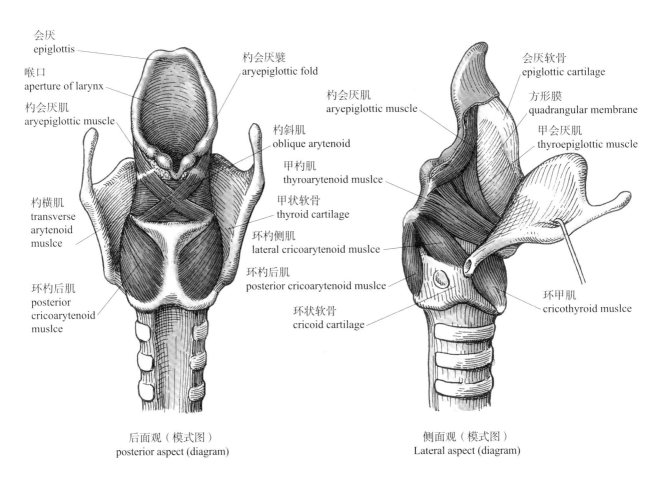

后面观（模式图）
posterior aspect (diagram)

侧面观（模式图）
Lateral aspect (diagram)

图 5-7　喉肌
Laryngeal muscles

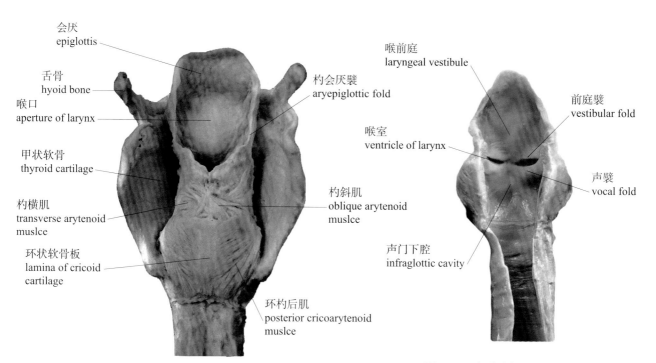

图 5-8 喉肌（后面观）
Laryngeal muscles (posterior view)

图 5-9 喉腔（打开后面观）
Laryngeal cavity (opened posterior view)

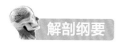 解剖纲要

喉腔上起喉口，与咽腔相通；下连气管。侧壁的前庭襞和声襞将喉腔分为喉前庭、喉中间腔和声门下腔。

喉中间腔向两侧经前庭襞和声襞间的裂隙至喉室。声门裂是喉腔最狭窄之处，位于两侧声襞及杓状软骨底和声带突之间。

Anatomical Outline

Laryngeal cavity ranges from the aperture of larynx above, connected to pharyngeal cavity, downward to the trachea. The laryngeal cavity is divided into laryngeal vestibule, intermediate cavity of larynx and infraglottic cavity by vestibular fold and vocal fold on the lateral wall of the larynx.

The intermediate cavity of larynx extends to the ventricle of larynx on both sides through the fissures between the vestibular folds and the vocal folds. The fissure of glottis is the narrowest part of the larynx, and it lies between the vocal folds and the base of the arytenoid cartilages and the vocal processes.

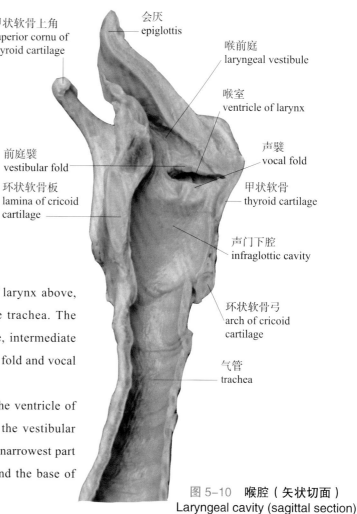

图 5-10 喉腔（矢状切面）
Laryngeal cavity (sagittal section)

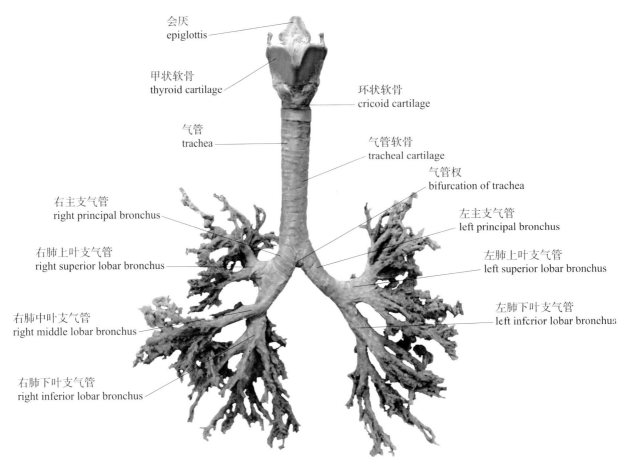

会厌
epiglottis

甲状软骨
thyroid cartilage

环状软骨
cricoid cartilage

气管
trachea

气管软骨
tracheal cartilage

气管杈
bifurcation of trachea

右主支气管
right principal bronchus

左主支气管
left principal bronchus

右肺上叶支气管
right superior lobar bronchus

左肺上叶支气管
left superior lobar bronchus

右肺中叶支气管
right middle lobar bronchus

左肺下叶支气管
left inferior lobar bronchus

右肺下叶支气管
right inferior lobar bronchus

图 5-11 气管和支气管
Trachea and bronchi

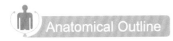 解剖纲要

气管起于环状软骨下缘，约平第 6 颈椎体下缘；向下至胸骨角平面，约平第 4 胸椎体下缘，分叉形成左、右主支气管。气管隆嵴位于气管杈的内面，略偏向左侧，是支气管镜检查时判断气管分叉的重要标志。

左、右主支气管的区别：左支气管细而长，斜行；右支气管短而粗，走行相对较直。

在肺门处，左、右主支气管分为次级支气管，进入肺叶，称为肺叶支气管。肺叶支气管进入肺叶后，继续分出肺段支气管。各级支气管在肺叶内分支形成树状，称为支气管树。

Anatomical Outline

The trachea originates from the inferior margin of the cricoid cartilage at the level of the lower margin of the 6th cervical vertebral body; it descends to the sternal angle plane at the level of lower margin of 4th thoracic vertebral body, and then bifurcates to form the left and right main bronchi. The carina of trachea is located inside the bifurcation of trachea, slightly to the left, which is an important sign of tracheal bifurcation during bronchoscopy.

The difference between right and left principal bronchi: left one is thin and long, oblique; right one is short and thick, with relatively horizontal course.

At the hilum, the left and right main bronchi are divided into secondary bronchi and enter the lobes of the lung, called lobar bronchi which continue to branch, forming smaller bronchi called segmental bronchi. These branches resemble a tree and so are called the bronchial tree.

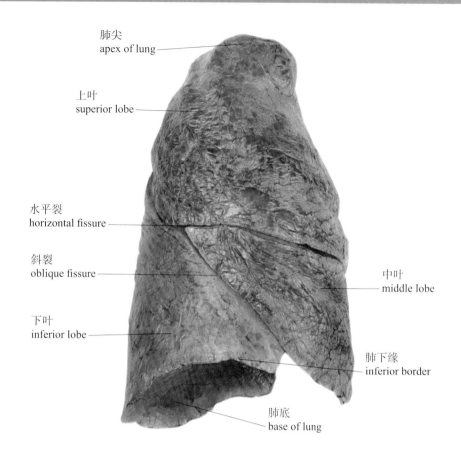

肺尖
apex of lung

上叶
superior lobe

水平裂
horizontal fissure

斜裂
oblique fissure

下叶
inferior lobe

中叶
middle lobe

肺下缘
inferior border

肺底
base of lung

图 5-12 右肺肋面
Costal surface of right lung

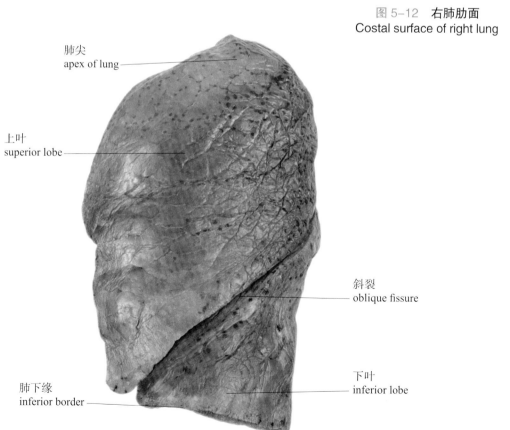

肺尖
apex of lung

上叶
superior lobe

斜裂
oblique fissure

肺下缘
inferior border

下叶
inferior lobe

图 5-13 左肺肋面
Costal surface of left lung

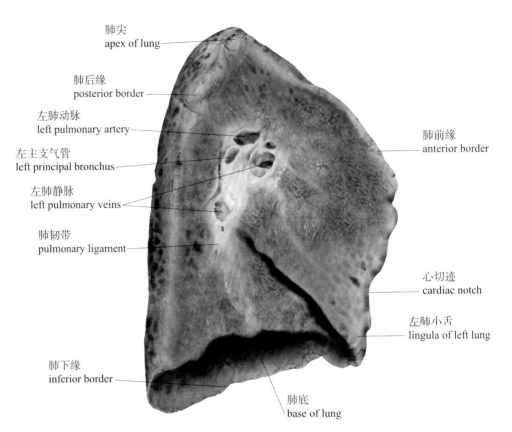

肺尖
apex of lung

肺后缘
posterior border

左肺动脉
left pulmonary artery

左主支气管
left principal bronchus

左肺静脉
left pulmonary veins

肺韧带
pulmonary ligament

肺下缘
inferior border

肺前缘
anterior border

心切迹
cardiac notch

左肺小舌
lingula of left lung

肺底
base of lung

图 5-14　左肺纵隔面
Mediastinal surface of left lung

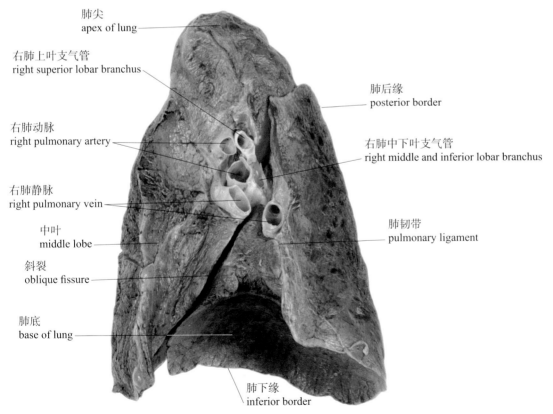

肺尖
apex of lung

右肺上叶支气管
right superior lobar branchus

右肺动脉
right pulmonary artery

右肺静脉
right pulmonary vein

中叶
middle lobe

斜裂
oblique fissure

肺底
base of lung

肺后缘
posterior border

右肺中下叶支气管
right middle and inferior lobar branchus

肺韧带
pulmonary ligament

肺下缘
inferior border

图 5-15　右肺纵隔面
Mediastinal surface of right lung

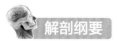

解剖纲要

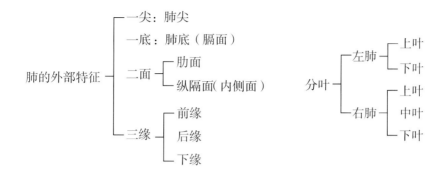

```
                    ┌─ 一尖：肺尖
                    │
                    ├─ 一底：肺底（膈面）
                    │                              ┌─ 左肺 ─┬─ 上叶
                    │        ┌─ 肋面                │         └─ 下叶
肺的外部特征 ─┤  二面 ─┤                    分叶 ─┤
                    │        └─ 纵隔面(内侧面)       │         ┌─ 上叶
                    │                              └─ 右肺 ─┼─ 中叶
                    │        ┌─ 前缘                          └─ 下叶
                    └─ 三缘 ─┼─ 后缘
                             └─ 下缘
```

Anatomical Outline

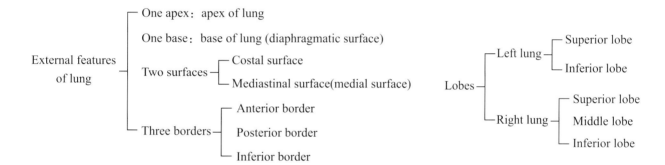

```
                         ┌─ One apex：apex of lung
                         │
                         ├─ One base：base of lung (diaphragmatic surface)
                         │                                        ┌─ Left lung ─┬─ Superior lobe
External features ─┤                 ┌─ Costal surface            │              └─ Inferior lobe
    of lung          │  Two surfaces ─┤                   Lobes ─┤
                         │                 └─ Mediastinal surface(medial surface)  ┌─ Superior lobe
                         │                                        └─ Right lung ─┼─ Middle lobe
                         │                 ┌─ Anterior border                      └─ Inferior lobe
                         └─ Three borders ─┼─ Posterior border
                                           └─ Inferior border
```

解剖纲要

　　肺门位于肺纵隔面，内有支气管、血管、神经、淋巴管等出入。出入肺门的结构被结缔组织包裹，统称为肺根。肺根内的结构排列：

　　自前向后：肺静脉、肺动脉、主支气管。

　　自上而下：左肺：肺动脉、主支气管、肺静脉；右肺：上叶支气管、肺动脉、中下叶支气管、肺静脉。

Anatomical Outline

　　The hilum of lung is located on the mediastinal surface with access to the bronchi, blood vessels, nerves, lymphatic vessels, etc. The structure of the entrance and exit of the hilum are encapsulated by connective tissue, collectively known as the lung root. The structural arrangement in the roots of lung:

　　From anterior to posterior: pulmonary veins, pulmonary arteries, and principle bronchi.

　　From superior to inferior: left lung: pulmonary artery, principle bronchus, pulmonary vein; right lung: superior lobe bronchus, pulmonary artery, middle-inferior lobe bronchus and pulmonary vein.

Part 2 Splanchnology 第二篇 内脏学

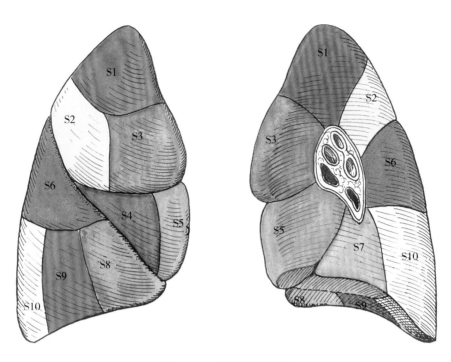

图 5-16　右肺叶和肺段
Lobes and segments of right lung

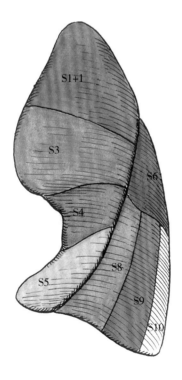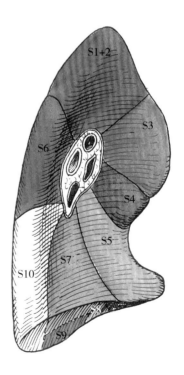

图 5-17　左肺叶和肺段
Lobes and segments of left lung

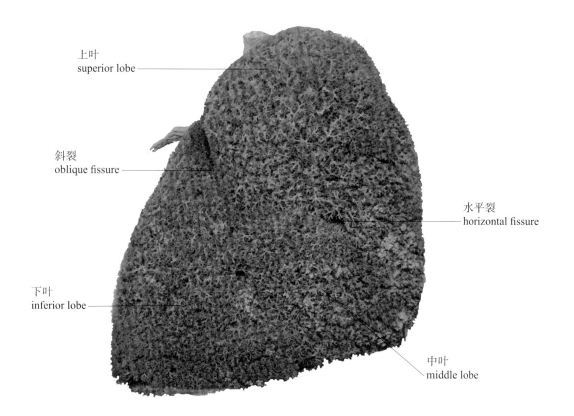

上叶
superior lobe

斜裂
oblique fissure

水平裂
horizontal fissure

下叶
inferior lobe

中叶
middle lobe

图 5-18 右肺铸型（肋面）
Cast of right lung (costal surface)

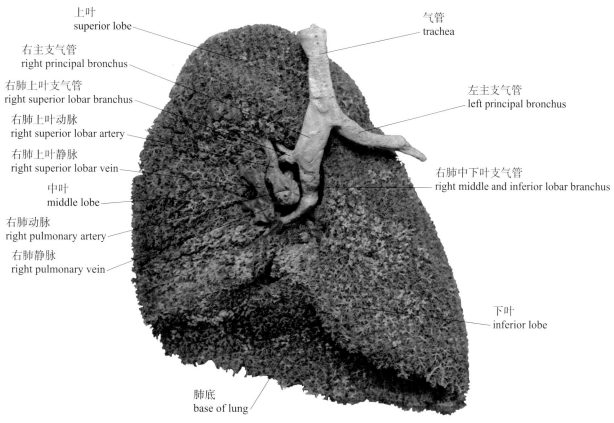

上叶
superior lobe

气管
trachea

右主支气管
right principal bronchus

左主支气管
left principal bronchus

右肺上叶支气管
right superior lobar branchus

右肺上叶动脉
right superior lobar artery

右肺上叶静脉
right superior lobar vein

右肺中下叶支气管
right middle and inferior lobar branchus

中叶
middle lobe

右肺动脉
right pulmonary artery

右肺静脉
right pulmonary vein

下叶
inferior lobe

肺底
base of lung

图 5-19 右肺铸型（纵隔面）
Cast of right lung (mediastinal surface)

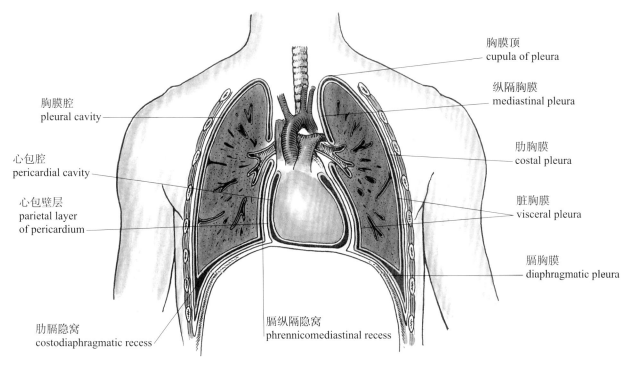

胸膜顶
cupula of pleura

纵隔胸膜
mediastinal pleura

胸膜腔
pleural cavity

肋胸膜
costal pleura

心包腔
pericardial cavity

脏胸膜
visceral pleura

心包壁层
parietal layer
of pericardium

膈胸膜
diaphragmatic pleura

肋膈隐窝
costodiaphragmatic recess

膈纵隔隐窝
phrennicomediastinal recess

图 5-20　胸膜和胸膜腔（冠状切面）
Pleura and pleural cavity (coronal section)

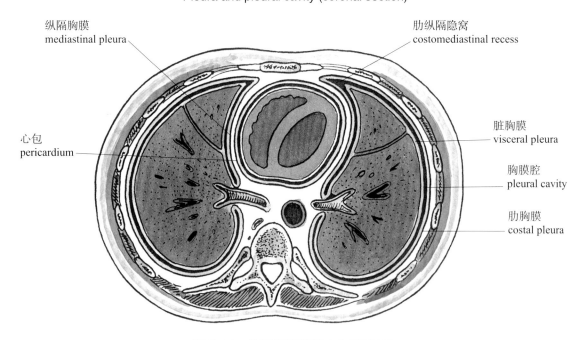

纵隔胸膜
mediastinal pleura

肋纵隔隐窝
costomediastinal recess

心包
pericardium

脏胸膜
visceral pleura

胸膜腔
pleural cavity

肋胸膜
costal pleura

图 5-21　胸膜和胸膜腔（水平切面）
Pleura and pleural cavity (horizontal section)

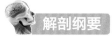 解剖纲要

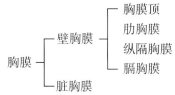

壁胸膜与脏胸膜之间密闭的腔隙为胸膜腔。左、右各一，呈负压。其内有少许浆液，可减少摩擦。

第二篇 内脏学
Part 2 Splanchnology

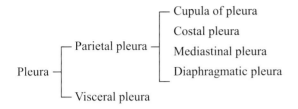
Anatomical Outline

Pleura ─┬─ Parietal pleura ─┬─ Cupula of pleura
        │   ├─ Costal pleura
        │   ├─ Mediastinal pleura
        │   └─ Diaphragmatic pleura
        └─ Visceral pleura

The airtight space between the parietal pleura and the visceral pleura is pleural cavity. There is one on each side. It is negative pressure in pleural cavity. There is little amount of serous fluid to reduce friction.

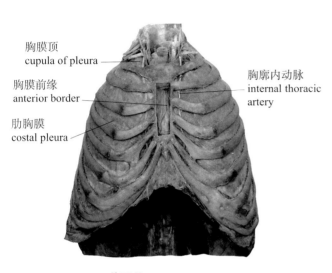

胸膜顶 cupula of pleura
胸膜前缘 anterior border
肋胸膜 costal pleura
胸廓内动脉 internal thoracic artery

前面观 Anterior view

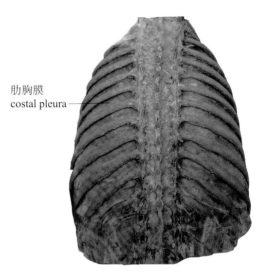

肋胸膜 costal pleura

后面观 Posterior view

图 5-22 壁胸膜
Parietal pleura

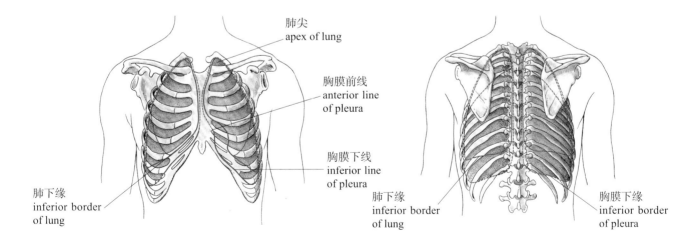

肺尖 apex of lung
胸膜前线 anterior line of pleura
胸膜下线 inferior line of pleura
肺下缘 inferior border of lung
肺下缘 inferior border of lung
胸膜下缘 inferior border of pleura

图 5-23 胸膜和肺的体表投影（前面观）
Surface projection of the pleura and the lung (anterior view)

图 5-24 胸膜和肺的体表投影（后面观）
Surface projection of the pleura and the lung (posterior view)

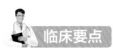
临床要点

任何原因引起的胸膜破损，致使空气进入胸膜腔，称为气胸。此时胸膜腔压力升高，甚至负压变成正压，使肺压缩，静脉回心血流受阻，产生不同程度的肺、心功能障碍。

Key Points of the Clinic

The pleura is broken down from any reason, air entering the pleural cavity, it is called the pneumothorax. At this time, pleural pressure increases, or even negative pressure changes into positive, which result in compression of the lung, blocking of venous blood reflux and producing varying degrees of dysfunction of lung and heart.

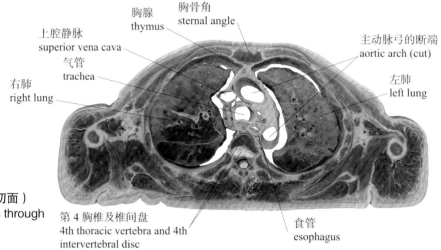

▶ 图 5–25　纵隔（平胸骨角的横切面）
Mediastinum (transverse section through the level of sternal angle)

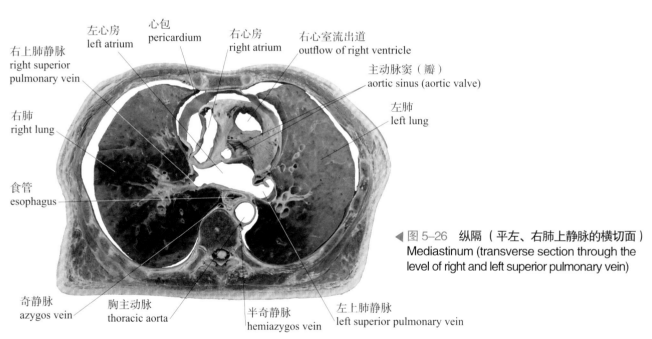

◀ 图 5–26　纵隔（平左、右肺上静脉的横切面）
Mediastinum (transverse section through the level of right and left superior pulmonary vein)

解剖纲要

　　纵隔区分（四分法）：以胸骨角水平面分为上纵隔和下纵隔，下纵隔再以心包为界分为前纵隔、中纵隔和后纵隔。

 Anatomical Outline

　　Division of the mediastinum（inquartation）：The mediastinum is divided into the superior mediastinum and the inferior mediastinum by the sternal angle horizontal plane. The inferior mediastinum is subdivided into the anterior mediastinum, the middle mediastinum and the posterior mediastinum by the pericardium.

第六章　泌尿系统

Chapter 6 Urinary system

第二篇　内脏学
Part 2 Splanchnology

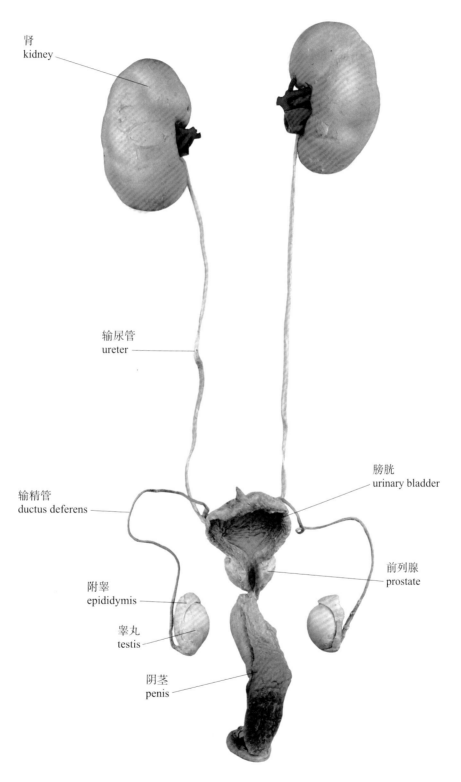

肾
kidney

输尿管
ureter

膀胱
urinary bladder

输精管
ductus deferens

前列腺
prostate

附睾
epididymis

睾丸
testis

阴茎
penis

图 6-1　男性泌尿生殖系统
Male urogenital system

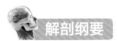 解剖纲要

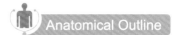 Anatomical Outline

泌尿系统组成及主要功能

组成	主要功能
肾	生成尿液、分泌激素
输尿管	输送尿液至膀胱
膀胱	储存尿液
尿道	将尿液排出体外

Composition and main functions of the urinary system

Composition	Main functions
Kidney	Produce urine and secrete hormones
Ureter	Convey the urine to the urinary bladder
Urinary bladder	Store the urine
Urethra	Excrete the urine

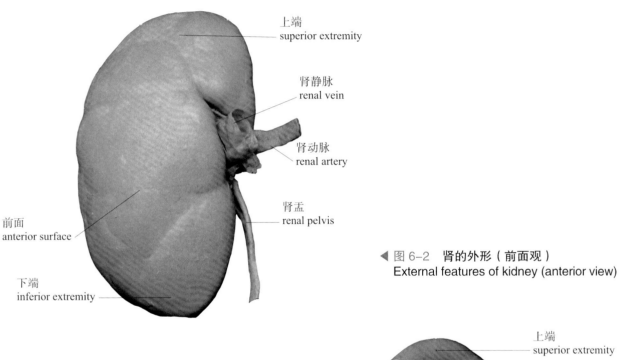

上端
superior extremity

肾静脉
renal vein

肾动脉
renal artery

肾盂
renal pelvis

前面
anterior surface

下端
inferior extremity

◀ 图 6-2　肾的外形（前面观）
External features of kidney (anterior view)

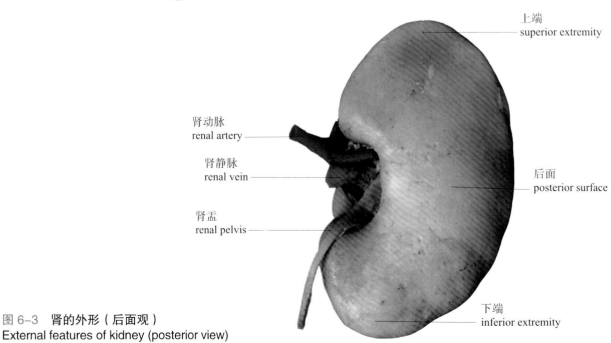

上端
superior extremity

肾动脉
renal artery

肾静脉
renal vein

肾盂
renal pelvis

后面
posterior surface

下端
inferior extremity

▶ 图 6-3　肾的外形（后面观）
External features of kidney (posterior view)

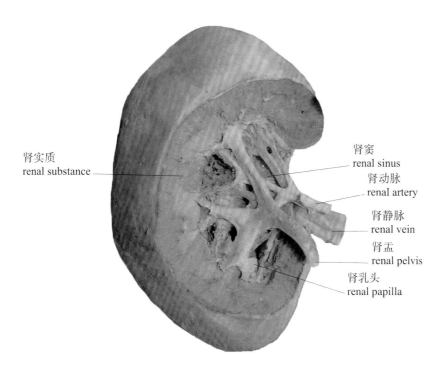

图 6-4 肾窦及其内容
Renal sinus and its contents

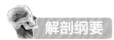 解剖纲要

肾蒂内各结构的排列关系：

自前向后：肾静脉、肾动脉、肾盂末端；自上而下：肾动脉、肾静脉、肾盂。肾窦为由肾门伸入肾实质的凹陷，容纳肾血管、肾小盏、肾大盏、肾盂和脂肪等。

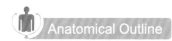 Anatomical Outline

Arrangement of structures in renal pedicle:

From anterior to posterior: renal vein, renal artery, terminal part of the renal pelvis; from superior to inferior: renal artery, renal vein, renal pelvis. The renal sinus is a depression of renal parenchyma, which contains renal vessels, minor renal calyces, major renal calyces, renal pelvis and adipose tissue.

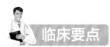 临床要点

肾区：位于腰背部，竖脊肌外侧缘与第 12 肋的夹角处，为肾门的体表投影点。肾病变时，触压或叩击此处会引起疼痛。

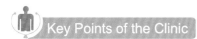 Key Points of the Clinic

Renal region: It is located in the area between the lateral margin of the erector spine and the 12th rib. It is the superficial projection of the renal hilum. If there is a disease in the kidney, press or knock here may cause pain.

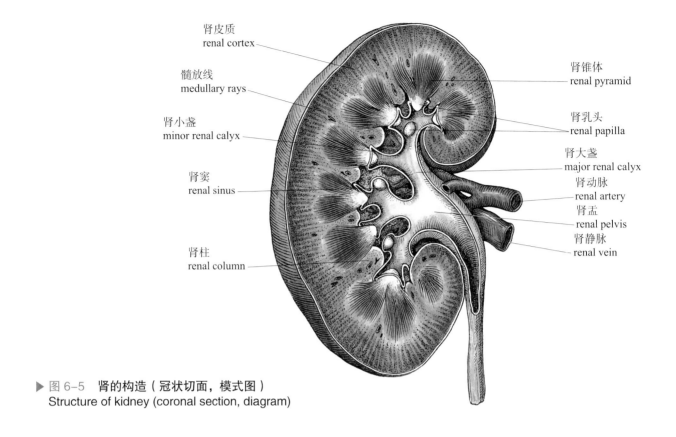

肾皮质
renal cortex

髓放线
medullary rays

肾小盏
minor renal calyx

肾窦
renal sinus

肾柱
renal column

肾锥体
renal pyramid

肾乳头
renal papilla

肾大盏
major renal calyx

肾动脉
renal artery

肾盂
renal pelvis

肾静脉
renal vein

▶ 图 6-5　肾的构造（冠状切面，模式图）
Structure of kidney (coronal section, diagram)

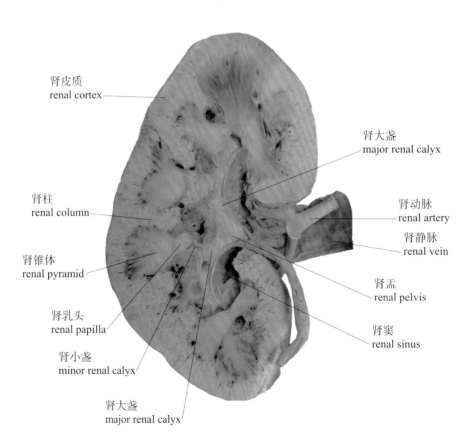

肾皮质
renal cortex

肾柱
renal column

肾锥体
renal pyramid

肾乳头
renal papilla

肾小盏
minor renal calyx

肾大盏
major renal calyx

肾大盏
major renal calyx

肾动脉
renal artery

肾静脉
renal vein

肾盂
renal pelvis

肾窦
renal sinus

图 6-6　肾的构造（冠状切面）
Structure of kidney (coronal section)

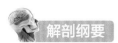

肾的结构

肾实质	肾皮质	位于表层，可见许多细小颗粒，伸入肾锥体之间的皮质称肾柱
	肾髓质	位于深层，由15~20个肾锥体构成，肾锥体的尖端称肾乳头，朝向肾窦，顶端有乳头孔
肾窦	肾小盏	7~8个，漏斗形，包绕肾乳头
	肾大盏	2~3个肾小盏汇合而成
	肾盂	扁漏斗状，由2~3个肾大盏组成

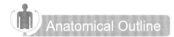

The structure of the kidney

Renal parenchyma	Renal cortex	It is located on the surface of the kidney. There are many fine granules. The parts from renal cortex dipping in between the pyramids are named renal columns
	Renal medulla	It is beneath the cortex. It consists of 15-20 renal pyramids. The apex of the pyramid is called renal papilla, which is toward renal sinus. The foramina on the apex are called the papillary foramina
Renal sinus	Minor renal calyx	There are 7-8, funnel-shaped, encircling the renal papilla
	Major renal calyx	Two or three minor renal calyces converge into one major renal calyx
	Renal pelvis	The renal pelvis is formed by integration of 2-3 major calyces. It is a flat funnel-shaped sac

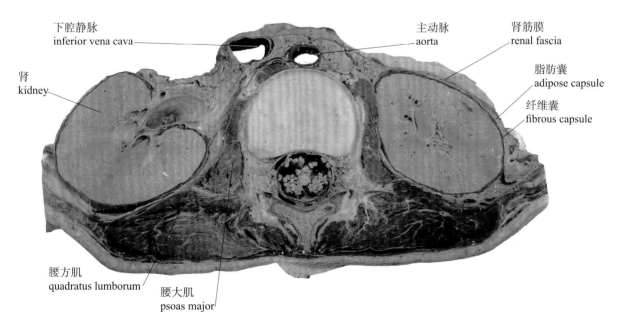

图 6-7　肾的被膜
Coverings of kidney

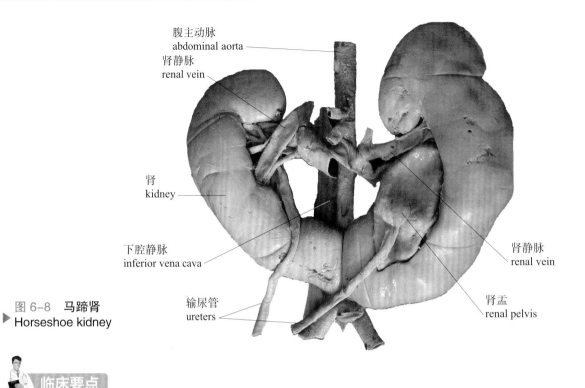

腹主动脉 abdominal aorta
肾静脉 renal vein
肾 kidney
下腔静脉 inferior vena cava
输尿管 ureters
肾静脉 renal vein
肾盂 renal pelvis

图 6-8　马蹄肾
▶ Horseshoe kidney

临床要点

马蹄肾：肾畸形的一种。两侧肾的下端互相连接呈马蹄形，出现率为 1%~3%，易引起肾盂积水、感染或肾结石。

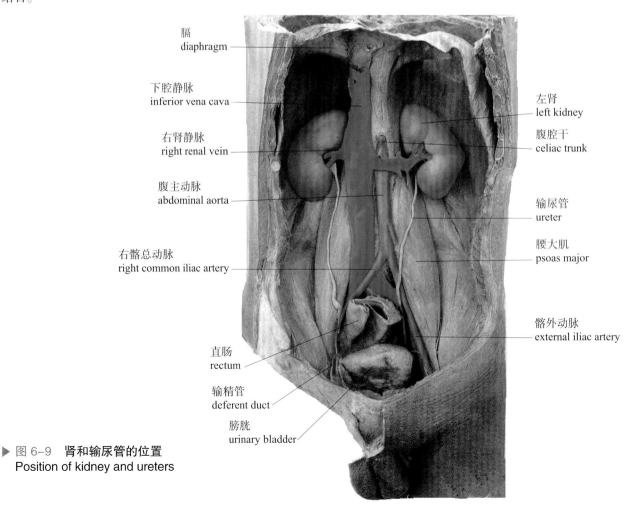

膈 diaphragm
下腔静脉 inferior vena cava
右肾静脉 right renal vein
腹主动脉 abdominal aorta
右髂总动脉 right common iliac artery
直肠 rectum
输精管 deferent duct
膀胱 urinary bladder
左肾 left kidney
腹腔干 celiac trunk
输尿管 ureter
腰大肌 psoas major
髂外动脉 external iliac artery

▶ 图 6-9　肾和输尿管的位置
Position of kidney and ureters

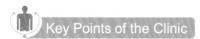 Key Points of the Clinic

Horseshoe kidney: a kind of renal malformation. The lower ends of the two kidneys are connected in the shape of horseshoe and the occurrence rate is 1-3%. Horseshoe kidney is easy to cause hydronephrosis, infection or kidney stones.

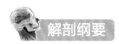 解剖纲要

输尿管狭窄及其位置和意义

狭窄	部位	意义
上狭窄	肾盂输尿管移行处	结石易嵌顿部位。主要的临床表现为绞痛和血尿
中狭窄	骨盆上口，输尿管跨过髂血管处	
下狭窄	壁内部，穿膀胱壁处	

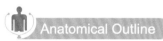 Anatomical Outline

The constriction of the ureter and its location and significance

Constriction	Position	Significance
Superior constriction	The junction of the ureter and the renal pelvis	The constricted areas are potential sites of obstruction by stones.The main clinical manifestations are colic and hematuria
Middle constriction	In the upper part of the pelvis, at the point where ureter crosses the iliac vessels	
Inferior constriction	The intramural part, through the bladder wall	

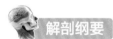 解剖纲要

膀胱是储存尿液的肌性囊状器官，其形状、大小、位置和壁的厚度随尿液充盈程度而异。空虚的膀胱呈三棱锥体形，分尖、体、底和颈四部。

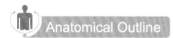 Anatomical Outline

Urinary bladder is a muscular cystic organ that stores urine. Its shape, size, location and wall thickness vary with the degree of urine filling. The empty bladder is triangular-shaped, with apex, body, fundus, and neck.

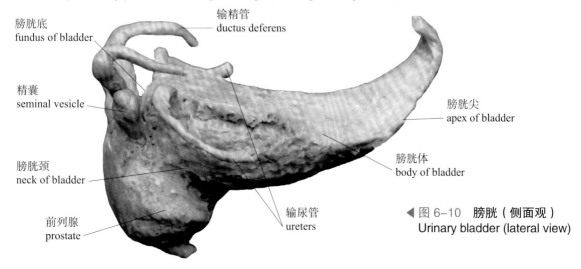

膀胱底 fundus of bladder
输精管 ductus deferens
精囊 seminal vesicle
膀胱颈 neck of bladder
前列腺 prostate
输尿管 ureters
膀胱尖 apex of bladder
膀胱体 body of bladder

◀ 图 6-10　膀胱（侧面观）
Urinary bladder (lateral view)

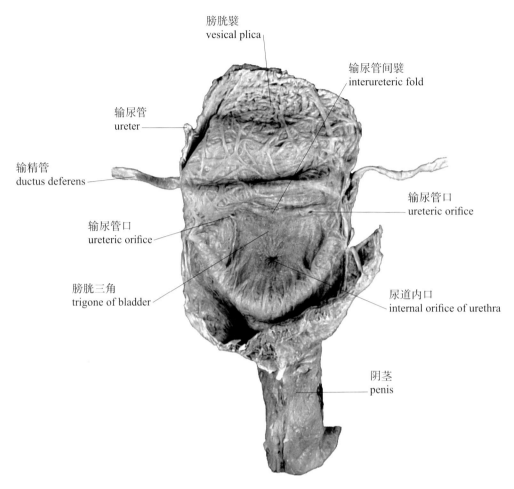

图 6-11　膀胱三角（前面观）
Trigone of bladder (anterior view)

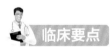 临床要点

　　1. 膀胱三角：在膀胱底内面，位于左、右输尿管口和尿道内口之间的三角区。膀胱三角是肿瘤、结核和炎症的好发部位，膀胱镜检查时应特别注意。

　　2. 两个输尿管口之间的皱襞称输尿管间襞，膀胱镜下所见为一苍白带，是临床寻找输尿管口的标志。

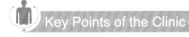 Key Points of the Clinic

　　1. Trigone of bladder: the triangular area among the left and right ureteral orifices and the internal orifice of the urethral on the inner surface of the fundus of bladder. Trigone of the bladder is susceptible to tumor, tuberculosis, and inflammation.

　　2. The folds between the two ureteral orifices are called interureteric fold, and the pallid bands seen under cystoscopy are clinical marker of looking for ureteral orifices.

第七章　生殖系统
Chapter 7 Reproductive system

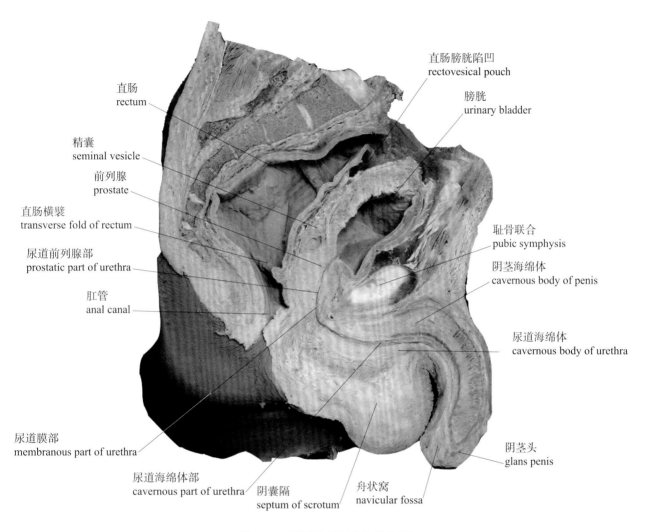

直肠
rectum

精囊
seminal vesicle

前列腺
prostate

直肠横襞
transverse fold of rectum

尿道前列腺部
prostatic part of urethra

肛管
anal canal

尿道膜部
membranous part of urethra

尿道海绵体部
cavernous part of urethra

阴囊隔
septum of scrotum

直肠膀胱陷凹
rectovesical pouch

膀胱
urinary bladder

耻骨联合
pubic symphysis

阴茎海绵体
cavernous body of penis

尿道海绵体
cavernous body of urethra

阴茎头
glans penis

舟状窝
navicular fossa

图 7-1　**男性盆部正中矢状切面**
Median sagittal section of male pelvis

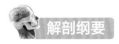 解剖纲要

男性、女性生殖系统的组成和功能

分部		男性生殖系统		女性生殖系统	
		组成	功能	组成	功能
内生殖器	生殖腺	睾丸	产生精子及雄性激素	卵巢	产生卵子及雌性激素
	生殖管道	附睾、输精管、射精管、男性尿道	输送精子	输卵管、子宫、阴道	输送卵子、孕育胎儿、排出月经
	附属腺	精囊腺、前列腺、尿道球腺	产生精液	前庭大腺	分泌液体、润滑阴道口
外生殖器		阴囊、阴茎	以性交功能为主	女外阴	以性交功能为主

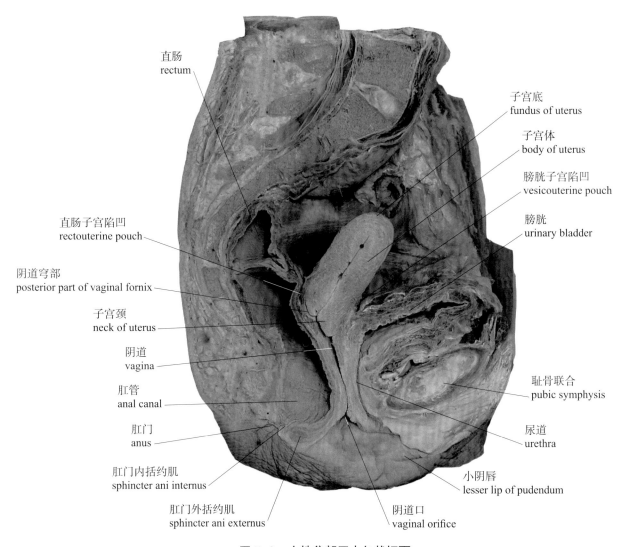

直肠
rectum

子宫底
fundus of uterus

子宫体
body of uterus

膀胱子宫陷凹
vesicouterine pouch

膀胱
urinary bladder

直肠子宫陷凹
rectouterine pouch

阴道穹部
posterior part of vaginal fornix

子宫颈
neck of uterus

阴道
vagina

肛管
anal canal

肛门
anus

肛门内括约肌
sphincter ani internus

肛门外括约肌
sphincter ani externus

耻骨联合
pubic symphysis

尿道
urethra

小阴唇
lesser lip of pudendum

阴道口
vaginal orifice

图 7-2 女性盆部正中矢状切面
Median sagittal section of female pelvis

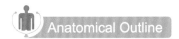 Anatomical Outline

Composition and function of the male and female reproductive system

Division		Male reproductive system		Female reproductive system	
		Composition	Function	Composition	Function
Internal genital organs	Gonad	Testes	Produce sperm and androgen	Ovary	Produce ovum and estrogen
	Ducts	Epididymis, ductus, ejaculatory duct, male urethra	Transfer the sperm	Uterine tube, uterus, vagina	Ovum delivery, fertilization, fetal development, menstrual discharge
	Accessory gland	Seminal vesicle, prostate, bulbourethral gland	Produce seminal fluid	Greater vestibular glands	Secrete liquid to lubricate the vagina
External genital organs		Scrotum and penis	Sexual intercourse	Vulva (female pudendum)	Sexual intercourse

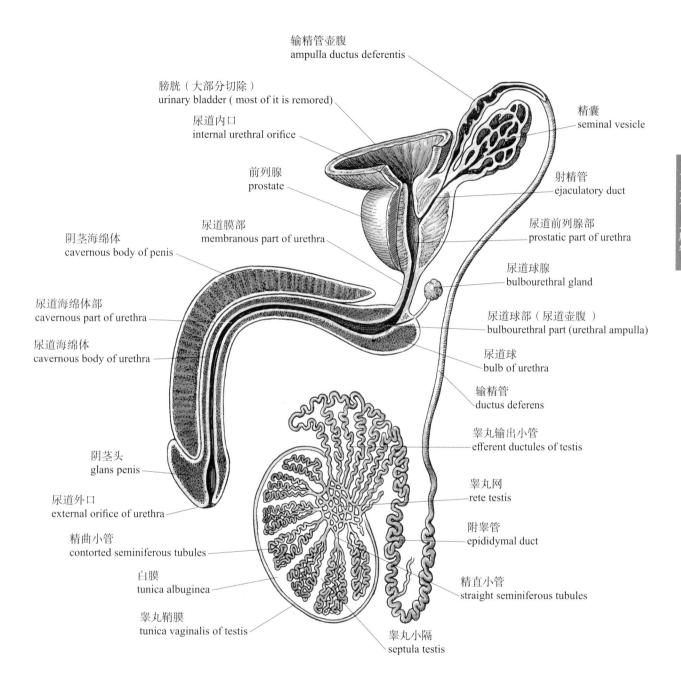

输精管壶腹
ampulla ductus deferentis

膀胱（大部分切除）
urinary bladder（most of it is remored）

尿道内口
internal urethral orifice

前列腺
prostate

尿道膜部
membranous part of urethra

阴茎海绵体
cavernous body of penis

尿道海绵体部
cavernous part of urethra

尿道海绵体
cavernous body of urethra

阴茎头
glans penis

尿道外口
external orifice of urethra

精曲小管
contorted seminiferous tubules

白膜
tunica albuginea

睾丸鞘膜
tunica vaginalis of testis

精囊
seminal vesicle

射精管
ejaculatory duct

尿道前列腺部
prostatic part of urethra

尿道球腺
bulbourethral gland

尿道球部（尿道壶腹）
bulbourethral part (urethral ampulla)

尿道球
bulb of urethra

输精管
ductus deferens

睾丸输出小管
efferent ductules of testis

睾丸网
rete testis

附睾管
epididymal duct

精直小管
straight seminiferous tubules

睾丸小隔
septula testis

图 7-3 男性生殖器（示意图）
Male reproductive organs (schematic diagram)

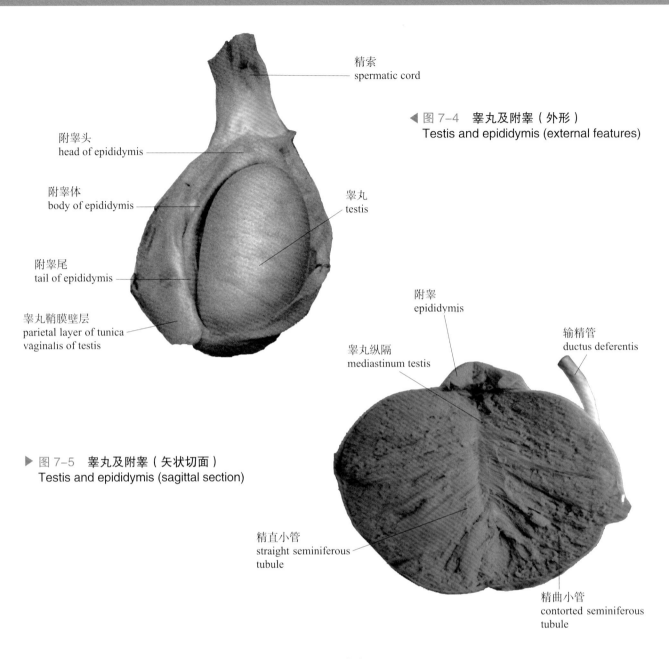

精索
spermatic cord

◀ 图 7-4　睾丸及附睾（外形）
Testis and epididymis (external features)

附睾头
head of epididymis

附睾体
body of epididymis

睾丸
testis

附睾尾
tail of epididymis

睾丸鞘膜壁层
parietal layer of tunica
vaginalis of testis

附睾
epididymis

输精管
ductus deferentis

睾丸纵隔
mediastinum testis

▶ 图 7-5　睾丸及附睾（矢状切面）
Testis and epididymis (sagittal section)

精直小管
straight seminiferous
tubule

精曲小管
contorted seminiferous
tubule

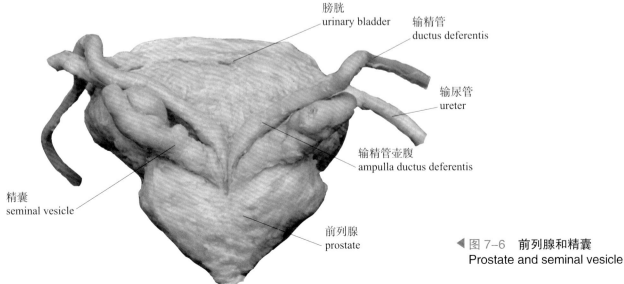

膀胱
urinary bladder

输精管
ductus deferentis

输尿管
ureter

输精管壶腹
ampulla ductus deferentis

精囊
seminal vesicle

前列腺
prostate

◀ 图 7-6　前列腺和精囊
Prostate and seminal vesicle

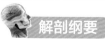 解剖纲要

输精管的分部及各部特点

分部	位置及特点
睾丸部	位于睾丸后缘、附睾内侧，最短
精索部	位置表浅，易于触及，为结扎输精管的理想部位
腹股沟管部	穿行于腹股沟管内，是精索的主要内容物
盆部	位于盆腔，最长，走行弯曲，近末端有输精管壶腹

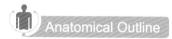 Anatomical Outline

The division and features of the ductus deferens

Parts	Position and features
Testicular part	It is located at the posterior border of the testis and the medial side of the epididymis, shortest part
Funicular part	Superficial, it is easy to be palpated. It is the place where the vasectomy is performed
Inguinal part	It passes through the inguinal canal. It is the main content of the spermatic cord
Pelvic part	It is located in the pelvis. The longest part. The terminal portion is dilated and called the ampulla ductus deferens

 解剖纲要

前列腺的分部：前列腺底、前列腺体、前列腺尖。

前列腺的分叶：前叶（1）、中叶（1）、后叶（1）、侧叶（2）。

 Anatomical Outline

Parts of the prostate: base prostatae, body prostatae, apex prostatae.

Lobes of the prostate: anterior lobe (1), middle lobe (1), posterior lobe (1), lateral lobe (2).

 临床要点

前列腺结缔组织增生而引起的前列腺肥大，常发生在中叶和侧叶，从而压迫尿道，造成排尿困难甚至尿潴留。后叶位于中叶和两侧叶的后方，是前列腺肿瘤的易发部位。前列腺体后面平坦，中间有一纵行浅沟，称前列腺沟，活体直肠指诊可扪及此沟。前列腺肥大时，此沟消失。

 Key Points of the Clinic

Hyperplasia of connective tissue in the prostate often occurs in the middle lobe and lateral lobes, which can compress the urethra and cause dysuria or even urinary retention. The posterior lobe, located behind the middle and lateral lobes, is a predisposing site of prostate tumors. The posterior surface of the prostate is flat. There is a sulcus along the midline on the posterior surface of the prostate gland. The sulcus can be palpated by rectal examination. This sulcus disappears in a condition of prostatauxe.

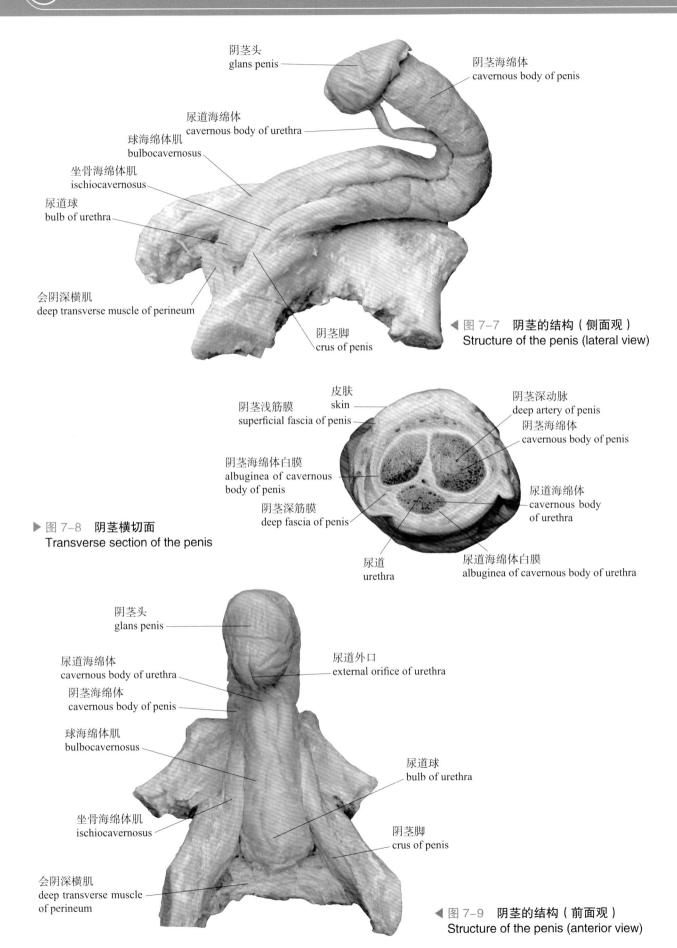

阴茎头
glans penis

阴茎海绵体
cavernous body of penis

尿道海绵体
cavernous body of urethra

球海绵体肌
bulbocavernosus

坐骨海绵体肌
ischiocavernosus

尿道球
bulb of urethra

会阴深横肌
deep transverse muscle of perineum

阴茎脚
crus of penis

◀ 图 7-7　阴茎的结构（侧面观）
Structure of the penis (lateral view)

皮肤
skin

阴茎浅筋膜
superficial fascia of penis

阴茎深动脉
deep artery of penis

阴茎海绵体
cavernous body of penis

阴茎海绵体白膜
albuginea of cavernous
body of penis

阴茎深筋膜
deep fascia of penis

尿道海绵体
cavernous body
of urethra

尿道
urethra

尿道海绵体白膜
albuginea of cavernous body of urethra

▶ 图 7-8　阴茎横切面
Transverse section of the penis

阴茎头
glans penis

尿道海绵体
cavernous body of urethra

尿道外口
external orifice of urethra

阴茎海绵体
cavernous body of penis

球海绵体肌
bulbocavernosus

尿道球
bulb of urethra

坐骨海绵体肌
ischiocavernosus

阴茎脚
crus of penis

会阴深横肌
deep transverse muscle
of perineum

◀ 图 7-9　阴茎的结构（前面观）
Structure of the penis (anterior view)

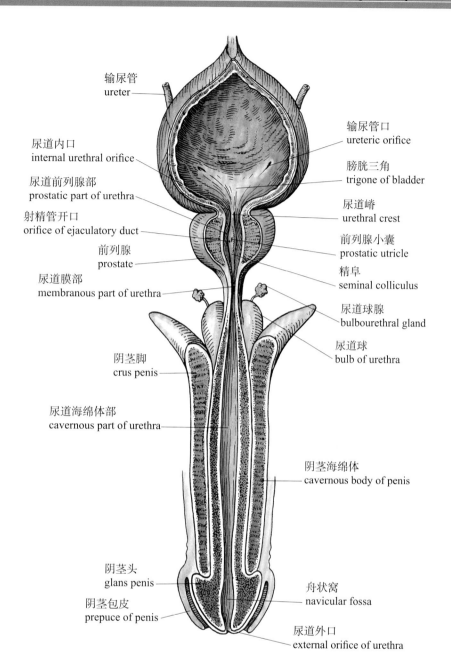

图 7-10 膀胱和男性尿道（前面观）
Urinary bladder and male urethra (anterior view)

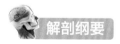 解剖纲要

男性尿道的形态结构

二口	二弯曲	三部	三狭窄	三膨大
尿道内口：起自膀胱	耻骨下弯：恒定	前列腺部：穿前列腺实质	尿道内口	前列腺部
尿道外口：开口于阴茎头	耻骨前弯：可变直或消失	膜部：穿尿生殖膈	尿道膜部	尿道球部
—	—	海绵体部：穿尿道海绵体	尿道外口（最窄）	舟状窝

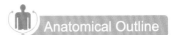

Morphological structure of the male urethra

Two orifices	Two curvatures	Three portions	Three strictures	Three enlargements
Internal orifice of the urethra: from the urinary bladder	Subpubic curvature: fixed curve	Prostatic portion: pierces the prostate	Internal orifice	Prostatic portion
External orifice of the urethra: opens at the glans of penis	Prepubic curvature: may straighten or disappear	Membranous portion: pierces the urogenital diaphragm	Membranous portion	Bulbous portion
—	—	Cavernous portion: runs through the cavernous body of the urethra	External orifice (the narrowest part)	Navicular fossa

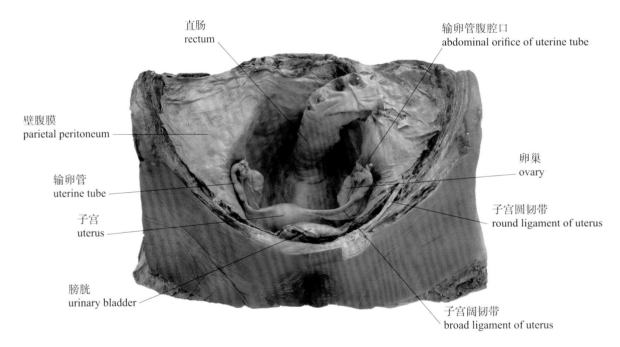

图 7-11　原位女性内生殖器
Original location of female internal genital organs

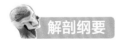

输卵管分部与特点

分部	特点
输卵管子宫部	位于子宫壁内，内径最细，与子宫腔通
输卵管峡部	短直而狭窄，为输卵管结扎常选部位
输卵管壶腹部	占输卵管全长的 2/3，粗而弯曲，卵子通常在此部与精子结合成受精卵
输卵管漏斗部	末端边缘有输卵管伞，与腹膜腔通

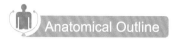 Anatomical Outline

Divisions and characteristic of the uterine tube

Division	Characteristic
Uterine part of fallopian tube	It lies in the wall of the uterus, the narrowest part of the uterine tube, opening to the uterine cavity
Isthmus of uterine the tube	It is short and straight. It is the place where the ligation of the uterine tube is performed usually
Ampulla of uterine tube	It is the longest and widest part of the uterine tube. Fertilization usually occurs in this region
Infundibulum of uterine tube	Tubal umbrella with terminal margin, it communicates with the pertoneal cavity

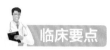 临床要点

通常情况，卵子与精子在输卵管壶腹部结合成受精卵，经输卵管子宫口进入子宫，植入子宫内膜中发育成胎儿。若受精卵未能迁移入子宫而在输卵管或腹膜腔内发育，即为宫外孕。

Key Points of the Clinic

Usually, the fertilized ovum is formed at the ampulla of the uterine tube and then moves to the uterus where the fetus develops. If the fertilized ovum fails to migrate into the uterus and develops in the fallopian tube or peritoneal cavity, that is an ectopic pregnancy.

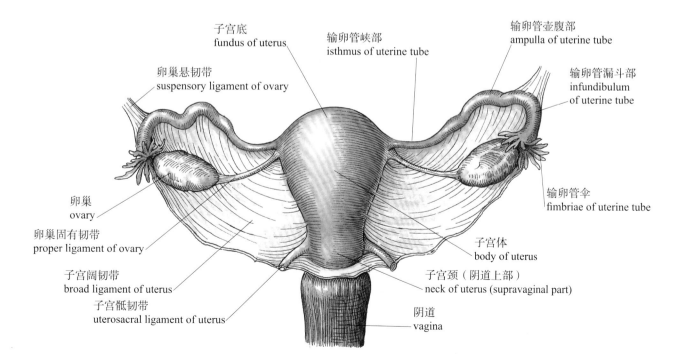

图 7-12　子宫外形（后面观）
Features of uterus (posterior view)

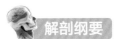解剖纲要

成人未孕子宫呈前后稍扁、倒置的梨形。子宫位于小骨盆中央，膀胱与直肠之间，下端接阴道。当膀胱空虚时，成人子宫呈轻度的前倾前屈位。前倾：子宫的长轴与阴道的长轴形成一个向前开放的角，略大于 90°。前屈：子宫体与子宫颈之间形成的一个向前开放的钝角，约 170°。

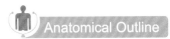Anatomical Outline

In the nulliparous adult, the uterus is slightly flat and an inverted pear-shaped organ. It is located in the center of the pelvic cavity, between the bladder and rectum. The lower part inserts into the vagina. When the bladder is empty, the adult uterus shows a mild anteversion and anteflexion. Anteversion: the long axis of the uterus and the long axis of the vagina form an angle that opens forward, slightly more than 90°. Anteflexion: the body of the uterus is bent downward at its junction with the cervix of the uterus forming an obtuse angle of about 170°.

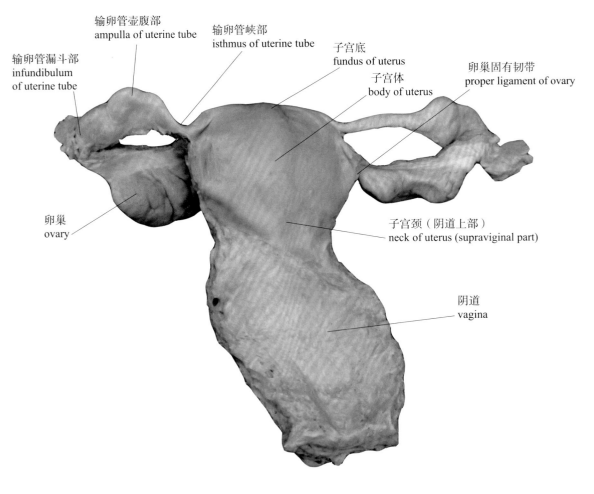

图 7-13 女性内生殖器（前面观）
Female internal genital organs(anterior view)

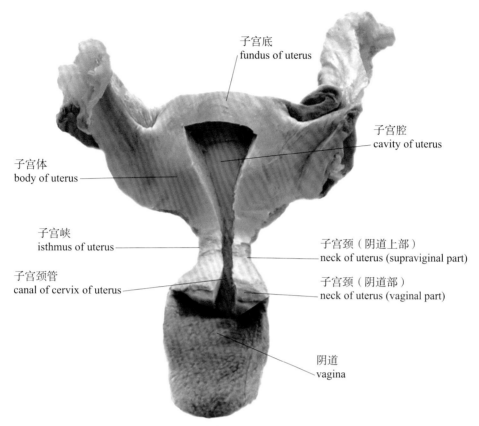

图 7-14　女性内生殖器（示子宫腔）
Female internal genital organs (showing cavity of uterus)

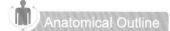 解剖纲要

子宫的固定装置：韧带、阴道和盆底肌。

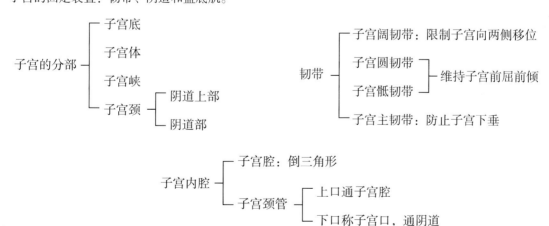

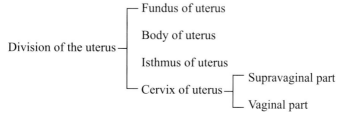 Anatomical Outline

Supports of the uterus：the normal position of the uterus is maintained by ligaments, vagina and the major muscles of the pelvic floor.

Division of the uterus ┬ Fundus of uterus
　　　　　　　　　　 ├ Body of uterus
　　　　　　　　　　 ├ Isthmus of uterus
　　　　　　　　　　 └ Cervix of uterus ┬ Supravaginal part
　　　　　　　　　　　　　　　　　　　 └ Vaginal part

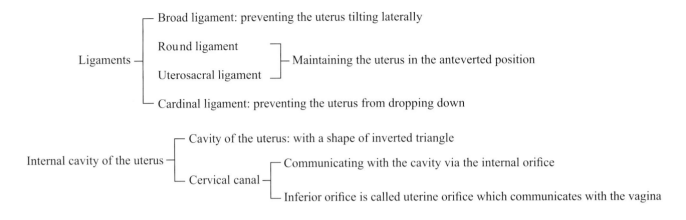

Ligaments
- Broad ligament: preventing the uterus tilting laterally
- Round ligament ┐
- Uterosacral ligament ┘ — Maintaining the uterus in the anteverted position
- Cardinal ligament: preventing the uterus from dropping down

Internal cavity of the uterus
- Cavity of the uterus: with a shape of inverted triangle
- Cervical canal
  - Communicating with the cavity via the internal orifice
  - Inferior orifice is called uterine orifice which communicates with the vagina

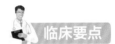 临床要点

　　子宫峡为子宫体的下部与子宫颈阴道上部相接处较狭细的部分。非妊娠时，子宫峡不明显，长约1 cm；妊娠期，子宫峡逐渐伸展变长，形成"子宫下段"，至妊娠末期，可延长至7~11 cm，壁薄，为剖宫术常用的切口部位。

Key Points of the Clinic

　　Isthmus of the uterus is the constricted part of the uterus between the body and cervix. Normally, it is about 1 cm in length. During pregnancy, it gradually extends and becomes longer, forming as "lower uterine segment". At the end of pregnancy, it can be extended to 7-11 cm, where the thin wall is the common incision site of cesarean section.

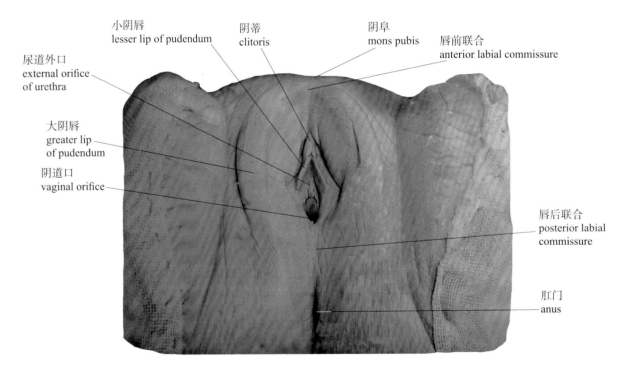

图 7-15　女性外生殖器
Female external genital organs

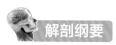 解剖纲要

阴道前庭是位于两侧小阴唇之间的裂隙，前部有尿道外口，后部有阴道口，阴道口两侧各有一个前庭大腺导管的开口。

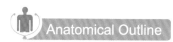 Anatomical Outline

A vaginal vestibule is a cleft between the lesser lips of the pudendum. The external orifice of the urethra is located anterior and the vaginal orifice is behind it. The orifices of the greater vestibular glands are on both sides of the vaginal orifice.

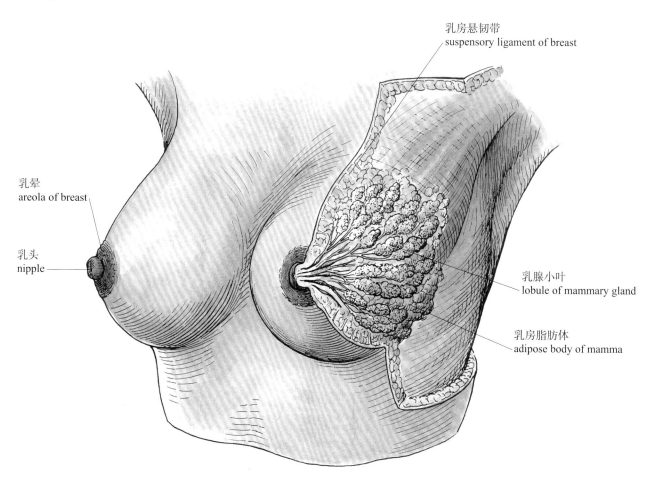

乳房悬韧带
suspensory ligament of breast

乳晕
areola of breast

乳头
nipple

乳腺小叶
lobule of mammary gland

乳房脂肪体
adipose body of mamma

图 7-16 女性乳房
Female mamma

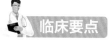 临床要点

乳腺叶和输乳管均以乳头为中心呈放射状排列，乳腺手术时宜做放射状切口，以减少对乳腺叶和输乳管的损伤。

乳房悬韧带（又称 Cooper 韧带）向深面连于胸筋膜，向浅面连于皮肤和乳头，对乳房起支持和固定作用。当乳腺癌侵及此韧带时，纤维组织增生，韧带缩短，牵引皮肤向内凹陷，致使皮肤表面出现许多点状小凹陷。另外，淋巴回流受阻引起皮肤淋巴水肿，使局部皮肤呈橘皮样改变，是乳腺癌早期常有的一个体征。

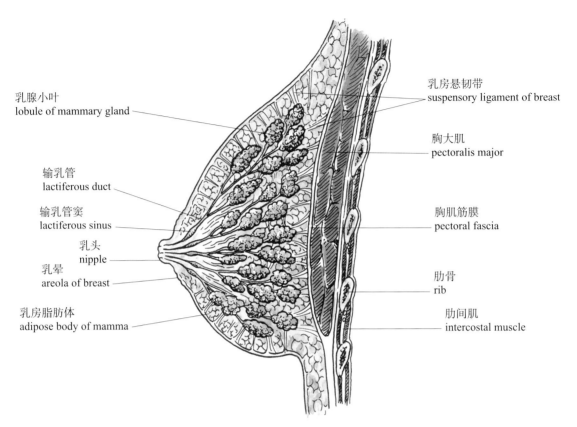

乳腺小叶
lobule of mammary gland

输乳管
lactiferous duct

输乳管窦
lactiferous sinus

乳头
nipple

乳晕
areola of breast

乳房脂肪体
adipose body of mamma

乳房悬韧带
suspensory ligament of breast

胸大肌
pectoralis major

胸肌筋膜
pectoral fascia

肋骨
rib

肋间肌
intercostal muscle

图 7-17　女性乳房（矢状切面）
Female mamma (sagittal section)

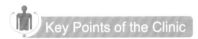 Key Points of the Clinic

Both the lobes of the mammary gland and the lactiferous ducts are arranged radially around the nipple. The radial incision should be made to reduce the damage to the lobes and ducts in breast surgery.

The suspensory ligament of the breast (also known as Cooper's ligament) connects to the pectoral fascia (deep) and the skin and nipple (superficial), supports and fixes the breast. When the breast cancer invades this ligament, the ligament becomes short and pulls the skin inward. In this condition, there are some dot-shaped small concaves on the skin. Also, the obstruction of lymphatic reflux causing the skin lymphedema, making the local skin orange-like changes, is a common sign in the early stage of breast cancer.

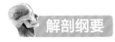 解剖纲要

广义的会阴指封闭小骨盆下口的所有软组织，呈菱形。

两侧坐骨结节的连线将会阴分为前、后两个三角区。前方为尿生殖区，男性有尿道通过，女性有尿道和阴道通过；后方为肛区，有肛管通过。

会阴的结构，除男、女生殖器外，主要是肌和筋膜。

尿生殖膈：由尿生殖膈上、下筋膜与会阴深横肌和尿道括约肌共同组成。

盆膈：由盆膈上、下筋膜及其间的肛提肌和尾骨肌共同组成。

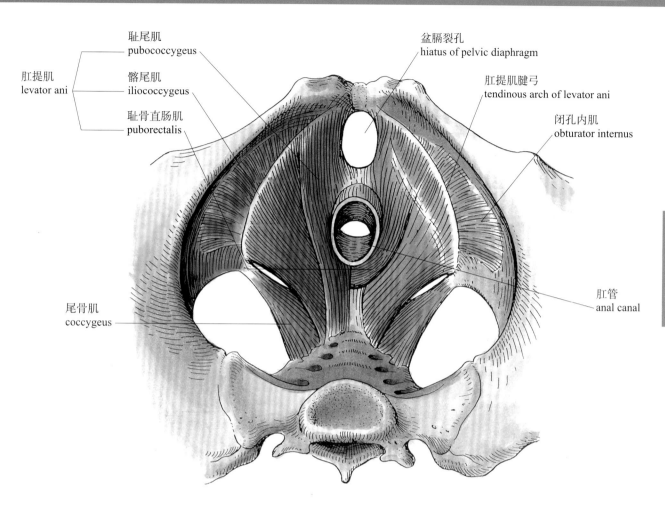

图 7-18 盆膈肌
Muscles of pelvic diaphram

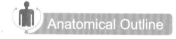 Anatomical Outline

The generalized perineum refers to the closure of all soft tissue of the lower pelvic orifice in a rhombus shape.

The transverse line drawing between the both ischial tuberosities divides the perineum into the anterior and posterior triangular regions. The anterior one, urogenital region, there are urethra in male, vagina and urethra in the female. The posteror one, anal region, there is anal canal.

The structures of the perineum, besides the male and female genitalia, are mainly muscle and fascia.

The superior and inferior fascia of the urogenital diaphragm and the deep transverse muscle of perineum and the urethral sphincter together form the urogenital diaphragm.

The inferior and superior fascia of the pelvic diaphragm and levator ani and coccygeus form the pelvic diaphragm.

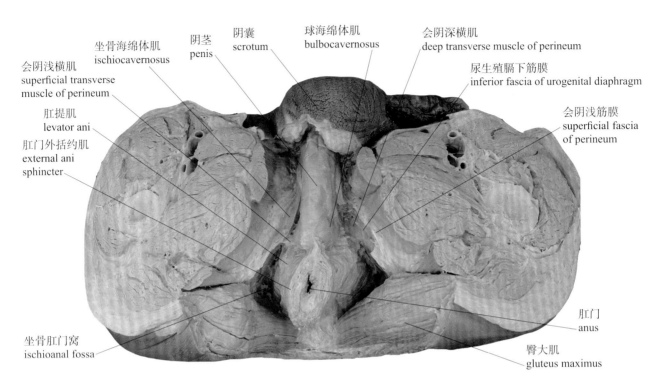

会阴浅横肌
superficial transverse
muscle of perineum

坐骨海绵体肌
ischiocavernosus

阴茎
penis

阴囊
scrotum

球海绵体肌
bulbocavernosus

会阴深横肌
deep transverse muscle of perineum

尿生殖膈下筋膜
inferior fascia of urogenital diaphragm

会阴浅筋膜
superficial fascia
of perineum

肛提肌
levator ani

肛门外括约肌
external ani
sphincter

坐骨肛门窝
ischioanal fossa

肛门
anus

臀大肌
gluteus maximus

图 7-19 男性会阴肌
Muscles of the male perineum

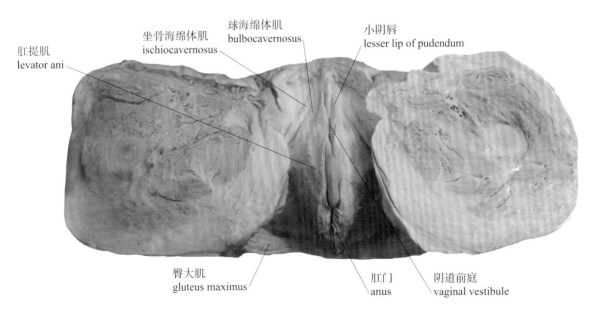

肛提肌
levator ani

坐骨海绵体肌
ischiocavernosus

球海绵体肌
bulbocavernosus

小阴唇
lesser lip of pudendum

臀大肌
gluteus maximus

肛门
anus

阴道前庭
vaginal vestibule

图 7-20 女会阴
Female perineum

第八章 腹膜

Chapter 8 Peritoneum

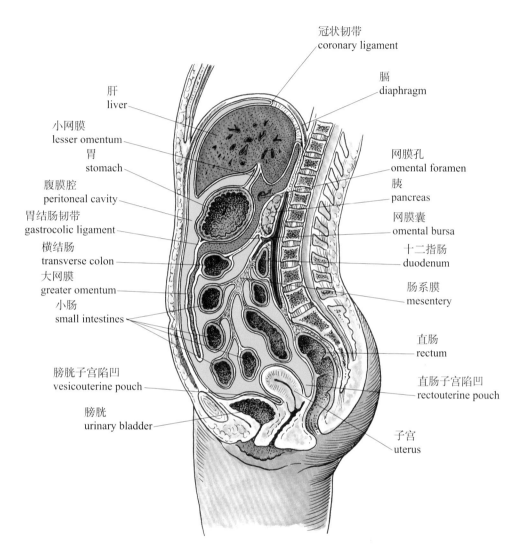

图 8-1 腹膜和腹膜腔（女性经腹部和盆部的正中矢状切面）
Peritoneum and peritoneal cavity (median sagittal section through the abdomen and pelvis in female)

解剖纲要

1. 小网膜：为由肝门移行于胃小弯和十二指肠上部的双层腹膜结构。分为肝胃韧带和肝十二指肠韧带两部分。肝十二指肠韧带内有胆总管（右前）、肝固有动脉（左前）和肝门静脉（后方）通过。

2. 大网膜：为连于胃大弯与横结肠之间的四层腹膜结构，形似围裙，覆盖在空肠、回肠和横结肠的前方。

3. 网膜囊：小网膜和胃后壁与腹后壁的腹膜之间的扁窄间隙，为腹膜腔的一部分。

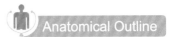

Anatomical Outline

1. Lesser omentum: It is a double-layer peritoneal structure that is moved from the hepatic hilums to the small curvature of the stomach and the upper portion of duodenum. It is divided into two parts: hepatogastric ligament and hepatoduodenal ligament. The common bile duct (right anterior), the hepatic proper artery (left anterior) and the hepatic portal vein (posterior) pass through within the hepatoduodenal ligament.

2. Greater omentum： It is a four-layer peritoneal structure connected to the great curvature of the stomach and the transverse colon, resembling an apron covering the front of the jejunum, ileum and transverse colon.

3. Omental bursa： It is a flat narrow space between the peritoneum of the lesser omentum and the posterior gastric wall and the posterior abdominal wall, which is part of the peritoneal cavity.

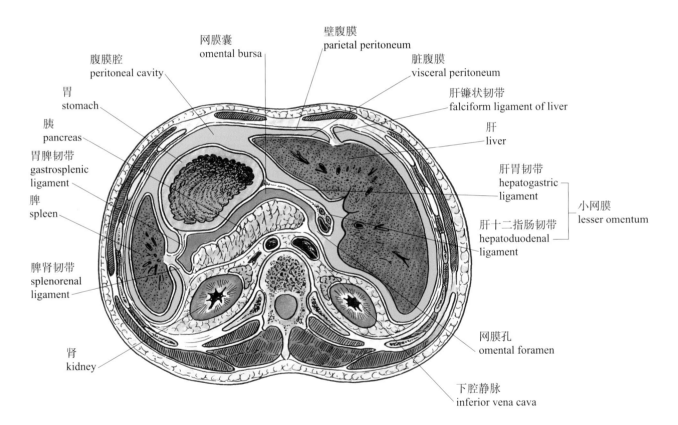

图 8-2　经网膜孔的腹部横切面
Transverse section of abdomen through the level of omental foramen

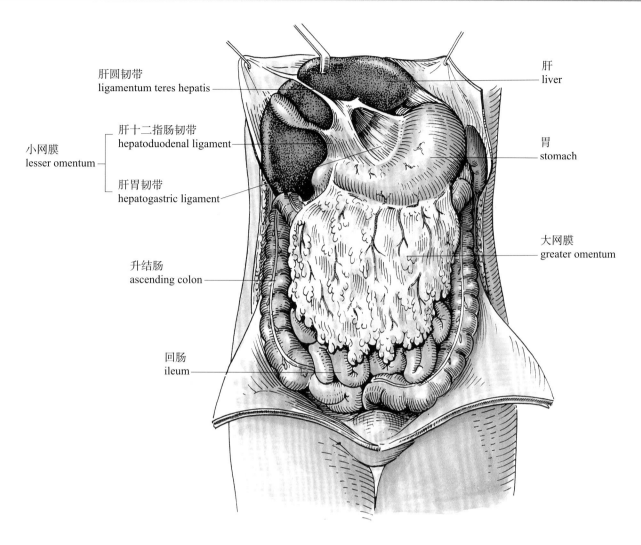

图 8-3 网膜
Omentum

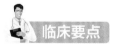 临床要点

大网膜含巨噬细胞，有重要的防御功能。当腹膜腔内有炎症时，大网膜可包围病灶以防止炎症扩散蔓延，故有腹腔卫士之称。小儿的大网膜较短，一般在脐平面以上，因此当有阑尾炎或其他下腹部炎症时，病灶区不易被大网膜包裹而局限化，常导致弥漫性腹膜炎。

大网膜的血管常用作心冠状动脉搭桥术中的供体血管。整形外科常使用带血管蒂的大网膜片铺盖胸、腹壁或颅骨创面，作为植皮的基础。

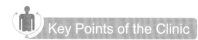 Key Points of the Clinic

The greater omentum contains macrophages and has important defensive function. When there is inflammation in the peritoneal cavity, the greater omentum can surround the lesion to prevent the spread of inflammation, so it is known as the guard of the abdominal cavity. In children, the greater omentum is short and generally above the level of the umbilicus. Therefore, when appendicitis or other inflammation of the lower abdomen, it is not easily confined by the greater omentum, which often leads to diffuse peritonitis.

The vessels of the greater omentum are commonly used as donor's vessels in the surgery of coronary artery bypass. In plastic surgery, greater omentum with vascular pedicle is often used to cover the wound surface of thoracic, abdominal wall or skull as the basis of skin graft.

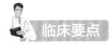

腹膜陷凹主要位于盆腔内。男性有直肠膀胱陷凹，女性有膀胱子宫陷凹和直肠子宫陷凹。直肠子宫陷凹又称 Douglas 腔。凹底与阴道后穹隆之间仅隔以阴道后壁和腹膜。站立或坐位时，男性的直肠膀胱陷凹和女性的直肠子宫陷凹是腹膜腔的最低部位，故腹膜腔内的积液多聚积于此。临床上可进行直肠穿刺和阴道后穹隆穿刺以进行诊断和治疗。

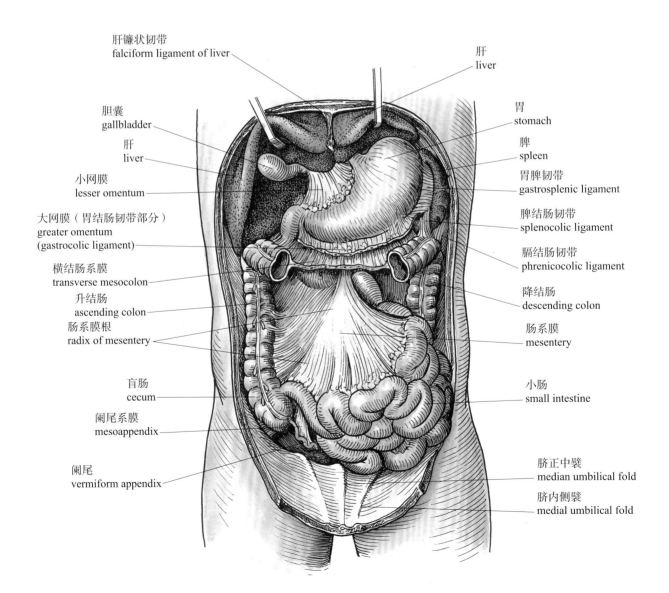

图 8-4　肠系膜和韧带
Mesenteries and ligaments

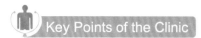 Key Points of the Clinic

Peritoneal pouches are mainly in the pelvic cavity. In the male, the rectovesical pouch lies between the rectum and urinary bladder. In the female, there are two pouches, vesicouterine pouch, and rectouterine pouch. The rectouterine pouch is also named the Douglas cavity. The posterior wall of the vagina and peritoneum are only separated between the concave bottom and the posterior fornix of vagina. Standing or sitting, the rectovesical pouch in male and rectouterine pouch in female are the lowest part of the peritoneal cavity respectively, where the peritoneal effusion mostly accumulates. Rectal puncture and posterior vaginal fornix puncture can be performed clinically for diagnosis and treatment.

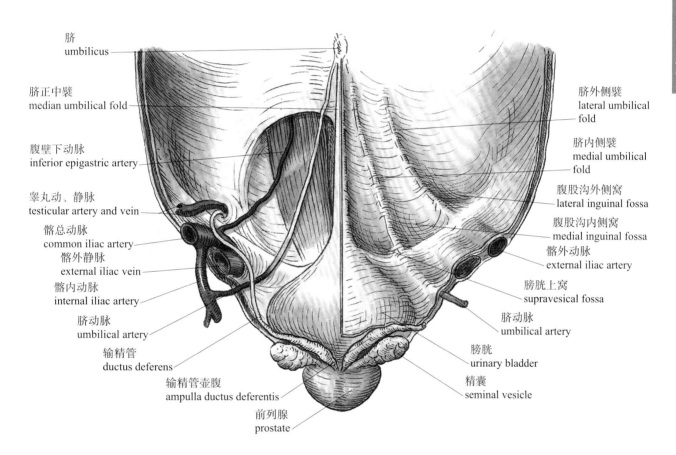

图 8-5　腹前壁内面的腹膜皱襞和凹窝
Peritoneal folds and fossa on the inner surface of the anterior abdominal wall

第三篇
脉管系统
Part 3 Angiology System

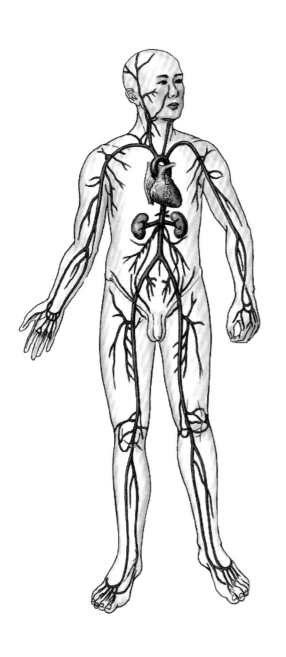

第九章　心血管系统
Chapter 9 Cardiovascular system

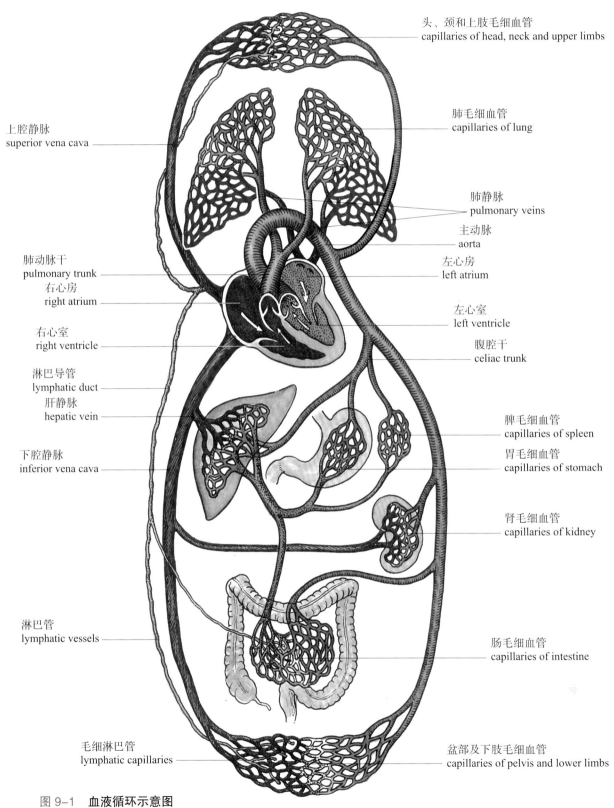

头、颈和上肢毛细血管
capillaries of head, neck and upper limbs

肺毛细血管
capillaries of lung

肺静脉
pulmonary veins

主动脉
aorta

左心房
left atrium

左心室
left ventricle

腹腔干
celiac trunk

脾毛细血管
capillaries of spleen

胃毛细血管
capillaries of stomach

肾毛细血管
capillaries of kidney

肠毛细血管
capillaries of intestine

盆部及下肢毛细血管
capillaries of pelvis and lower limbs

上腔静脉
superior vena cava

肺动脉干
pulmonary trunk

右心房
right atrium

右心室
right ventricle

淋巴导管
lymphatic duct

肝静脉
hepatic vein

下腔静脉
inferior vena cava

淋巴管
lymphatic vessels

毛细淋巴管
lymphatic capillaries

图 9-1　血液循环示意图
Schematic diagram of blood circulation

第一节 心 Section 1 Heart

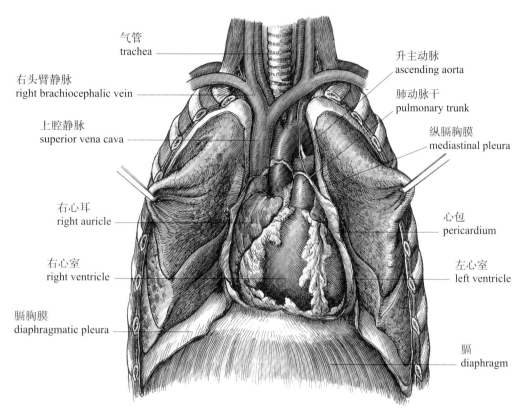

气管
trachea

升主动脉
ascending aorta

右头臂静脉
right brachiocephalic vein

肺动脉干
pulmonary trunk

上腔静脉
superior vena cava

纵膈胸膜
mediastinal pleura

右心耳
right auricle

心包
pericardium

右心室
right ventricle

左心室
left ventricle

膈胸膜
diaphragmatic pleura

膈
diaphragm

图 9-2 心的位置
Position of heart

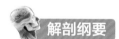 解剖纲要

心脏的"三左"位置

左偏：心脏位置偏向中线左侧。正中矢状切将心脏分为两部分，2/3 位于正中线左侧，1/3 位于正中线右侧。

左斜：心尖朝向左前下方，心底朝向右后上方，心脏长轴左斜约 45°。

左旋：右半心位于右前方，左半心位于左后方，室间隔向左侧旋转约 45°。

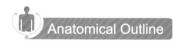 Anatomical Outline

"Three left" position of the heart

Left declination: The heart lies slightly to the left of the midline. A midsagittal section would divide the heart into two parts: two thirds are to the left of midline; one thirds is to the right of the midline.

Left oblique: The apex points at anteroinferior and left. The base is oriented to posterosuperior and right. The long axis of the heart sits at a left oblique angle about 45°.

Left rotation: The right half of the heart lies in the right front, the left half of the heart lies in the left rear, and the interventricular septum rotates about 45° to the left.

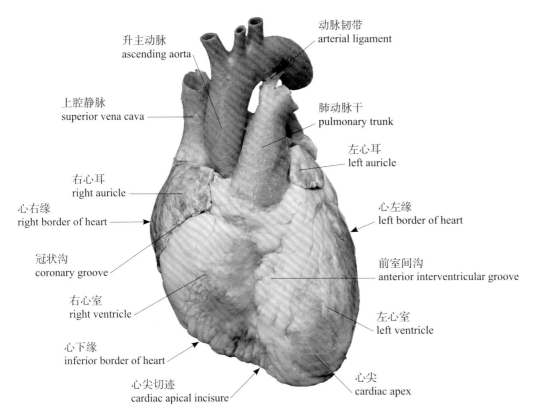

升主动脉
ascending aorta

动脉韧带
arterial ligament

上腔静脉
superior vena cava

肺动脉干
pulmonary trunk

左心耳
left auricle

右心耳
right auricle

心左缘
left border of heart

心右缘
right border of heart

冠状沟
coronary groove

右心室
right ventricle

前室间沟
anterior interventricular groove

左心室
left ventricle

心下缘
inferior border of heart

心尖切迹
cardiac apical incisure

心尖
cardiac apex

图 9-3　心的外形（胸肋面）
External features of heart (sternocostal surface)

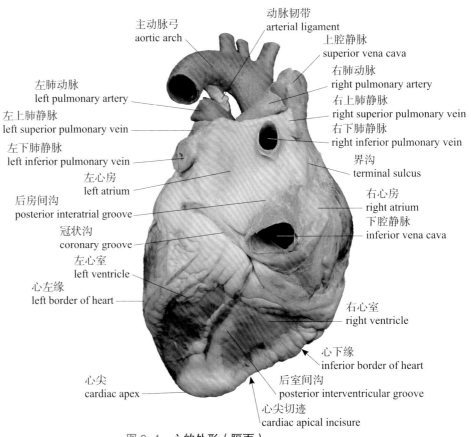

主动脉弓
aortic arch

动脉韧带
arterial ligament

上腔静脉
superior vena cava

右肺动脉
right pulmonary artery

左肺动脉
left pulmonary artery

右上肺静脉
right superior pulmonary vein

左上肺静脉
left superior pulmonary vein

右下肺静脉
right inferior pulmonary vein

左下肺静脉
left inferior pulmonary vein

界沟
terminal sulcus

左心房
left atrium

右心房
right atrium

后房间沟
posterior interatrial groove

下腔静脉
inferior vena cava

冠状沟
coronary groove

左心室
left ventricle

心左缘
left border of heart

右心室
right ventricle

心下缘
inferior border of heart

心尖
cardiac apex

后室间沟
posterior interventricular groove

心尖切迹
cardiac apical incisure

图 9-4　心的外形（膈面）
External features of heart (diaphragmatic surface)

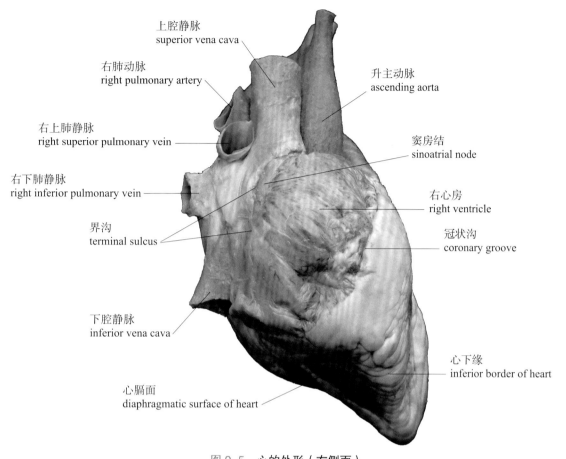

图 9-5　心的外形（右侧面）
External features of heart (right side)

上腔静脉
superior vena cava

右肺动脉
right pulmonary artery

升主动脉
ascending aorta

右上肺静脉
right superior pulmonary vein

窦房结
sinoatrial node

右下肺静脉
right inferior pulmonary vein

右心房
right ventricle

界沟
terminal sulcus

冠状沟
coronary groove

下腔静脉
inferior vena cava

心下缘
inferior border of heart

心膈面
diaphragmatic surface of heart

第三篇　脉管系统
Part 3 Angiology System

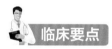 临床要点

1. 心尖位于左胸前壁第 5 肋间隙与左锁骨中线内侧 1 ~ 2cm 深处，此处可触及心尖搏动；当左心室增大时（如患高血压病），心尖位置可外移至锁骨中线外侧。

2. 左心房后方与食管相邻、上方与左主支气管相邻，左心房增大时（如二尖瓣狭窄）可压迫上述结构。

3. 后房间沟、后室间沟与冠状沟的相交处称房室交点（或称房室交界区），其深面有诸多重要结构，如房室结、右纤维三角、右冠状动脉 "U" 形弯曲、冠状窦开口等。

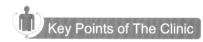 Key Points of The Clinic

1. The apex of the heart is located 1-2 cm medial to the intersection of the fifth intercostal space and the left midclavicular line, where the apex impulse can be palpable. However, the apex may move laterally out of the left midclavicular line, when the left ventricle has pathophysiological enlargement due to some diseases, such as hypertension.

2. The posterior left atrium is adjacent to the esophagus and the left main bronchus. The left atrium is enlarged because of illnesses (such as mitral stenosis), which can compress the esophagus and the left main bronchus.

3. Atrioventricular junction (atrioventricular junctional area), is an area where the coronal groove meets the posterior interatrial and interventricular grooves, containing many important components of the heart, such as the atrioventricular node, the right fibrous trigone, the U-shaped curve of the right coronary artery, the open of the coronal sinus, et al.

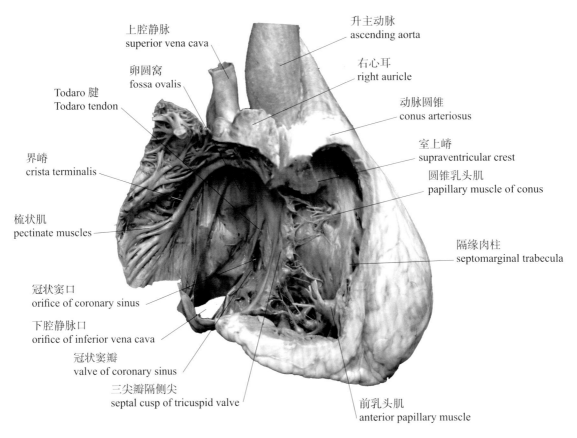

上腔静脉
superior vena cava

升主动脉
ascending aorta

卵圆窝
fossa ovalis

右心耳
right auricle

Todaro 腱
Todaro tendon

动脉圆锥
conus arteriosus

界嵴
crista terminalis

室上嵴
supraventricular crest

圆锥乳头肌
papillary muscle of conus

梳状肌
pectinate muscles

隔缘肉柱
septomarginal trabecula

冠状窦口
orifice of coronary sinus

下腔静脉口
orifice of inferior vena cava

冠状窦瓣
valve of coronary sinus

三尖瓣隔侧尖
septal cusp of tricuspid valve

前乳头肌
anterior papillary muscle

图 9-6　右心房和右心室（内面观）
Right atrium and ventricle (internal view)

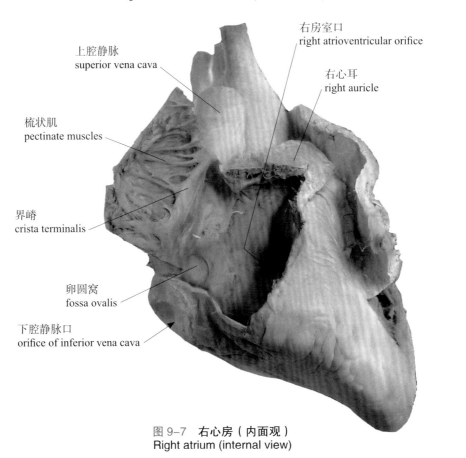

上腔静脉
superior vena cava

右房室口
right atrioventricular orifice

右心耳
right auricle

梳状肌
pectinate muscles

界嵴
crista terminalis

卵圆窝
fossa ovalis

下腔静脉口
orifice of inferior vena cava

图 9-7　右心房（内面观）
Right atrium (internal view)

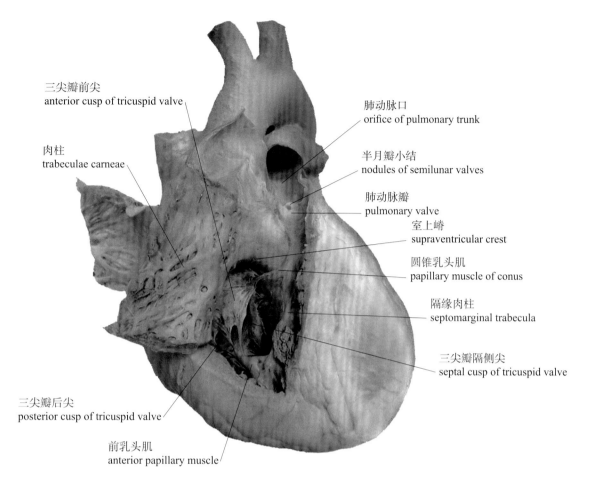

三尖瓣前尖
anterior cusp of tricuspid valve

肉柱
trabeculae carneae

肺动脉口
orifice of pulmonary trunk

半月瓣小结
nodules of semilunar valves

肺动脉瓣
pulmonary valve

室上嵴
supraventricular crest

圆锥乳头肌
papillary muscle of conus

隔缘肉柱
septomarginal trabecula

三尖瓣隔侧尖
septal cusp of tricuspid valve

三尖瓣后尖
posterior cusp of tricuspid valve

前乳头肌
anterior papillary muscle

图 9–8　右心室（内面观）
Right ventricle (internal view)

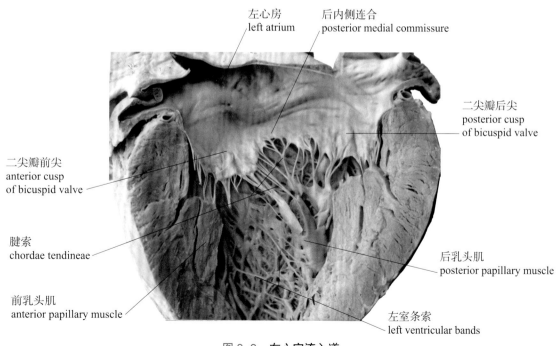

左心房
left atrium

后内侧连合
posterior medial commissure

二尖瓣后尖
posterior cusp
of bicuspid valve

二尖瓣前尖
anterior cusp
of bicuspid valve

腱索
chordae tendineae

前乳头肌
anterior papillary muscle

后乳头肌
posterior papillary muscle

左室条索
left ventricular bands

图 9–9　左心室流入道
Inflow tract of left ventricle

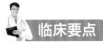 临床要点

1. 左、右心耳腔面凹凸不平，当心功能障碍（如心房纤颤）时，心内血流缓慢，易导致血栓形成。

2. 右心房内，冠状窦口前内缘、三尖瓣隔侧尖附着缘和 Todaro 腱之间的三角区，称 Koch 三角。其前部心内膜深面为房室结。

3. 左心室前壁介于前室间沟、左房室沟和左冠状动脉旋支的左缘支三者之间，此区域内血管较少，是手术进入左室腔的唯一壁面，被称为外科手术壁。

4. 瓣膜病是风湿病的常见合并症，可引起瓣膜口狭窄或关闭不全，多发生在二尖瓣和主动脉瓣。在彩色多普勒超声检查中易被看到。

Key Points of the Clinic

1.The internal surface of the left/right auricle is uneven. Beware of dysfunction (such as atrial fibrillation), slow blood flow in the heart, easy to lead to thrombosis.

2. In the right atrium a triangular area is enclosed by the anterior boundary of the coronary sinus, the attaching the boundary of the septal cusp of the tricuspid valve and the Todaro tendon, called the Koch triangle. The anterior edocardium of the koch triangle is the atrioventricular node.

3. On the anterior wall of the left ventricle, there is an area called the surgical wall, through which we may open the left ventricle during surgery, where enclosed by anterior interventricular sulcus, left atrioventricular sulcus and left marginal branch of the left coronal artery. The region has few blood vessels and is the only wall that enters the left ventricle.

4. Valvular disease, a common complication of rheumatism, can cause valve stenosis or incomplete closure, mostly in the mitral and aortic valves. It can be observed by color Doppler ultrasonography.

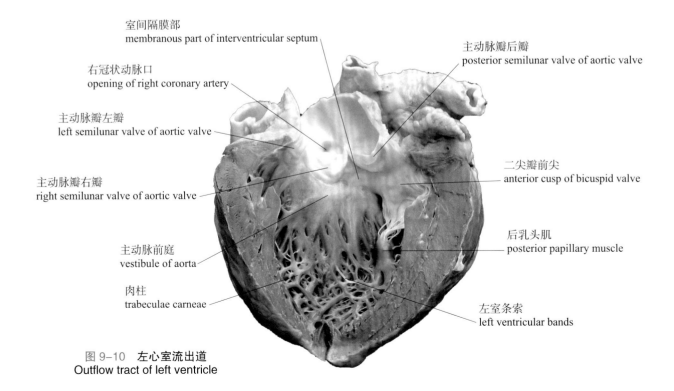

室间隔膜部
membranous part of interventricular septum

右冠状动脉口
opening of right coronary artery

主动脉瓣左瓣
left semilunar valve of aortic valve

主动脉瓣右瓣
right semilunar valve of aortic valve

主动脉前庭
vestibule of aorta

肉柱
trabeculae carneae

主动脉瓣后瓣
posterior semilunar valve of aortic valve

二尖瓣前尖
anterior cusp of bicuspid valve

后乳头肌
posterior papillary muscle

左室条索
left ventricular bands

图 9-10　左心室流出道
Outflow tract of left ventricle

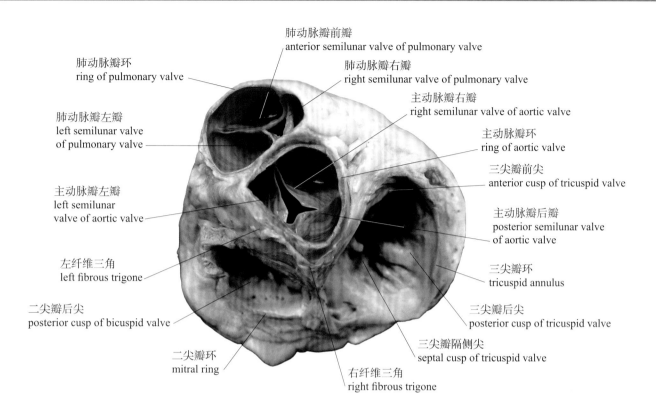

肺动脉瓣前瓣
anterior semilunar valve of pulmonary valve

肺动脉瓣右瓣
right semilunar valve of pulmonary valve

肺动脉瓣环
ring of pulmonary valve

主动脉瓣右瓣
right semilunar valve of aortic valve

肺动脉瓣左瓣
left semilunar valve
of pulmonary valve

主动脉瓣环
ring of aortic valve

三尖瓣前尖
anterior cusp of tricuspid valve

主动脉瓣左瓣
left semilunar
valve of aortic valve

主动脉瓣后瓣
posterior semilunar valve
of aortic valve

左纤维三角
left fibrous trigone

三尖瓣环
tricuspid annulus

二尖瓣后尖
posterior cusp of bicuspid valve

三尖瓣后尖
posterior cusp of tricuspid valve

二尖瓣环
mitral ring

右纤维三角
right fibrous trigone

三尖瓣隔侧尖
septal cusp of tricuspid valve

图 9-11　心纤维支架（上面观）
Fibrous skeleton of heart (superior view)

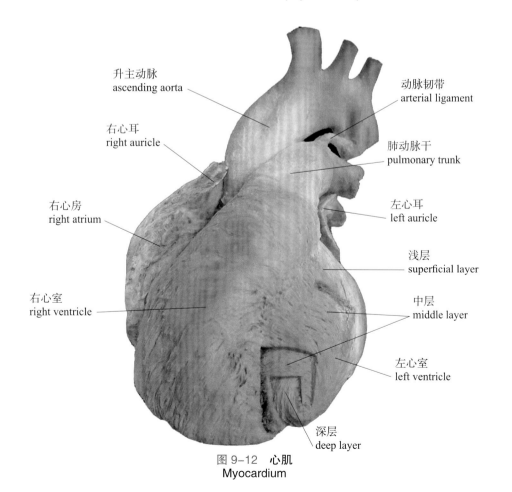

升主动脉
ascending aorta

动脉韧带
arterial ligament

右心耳
right auricle

肺动脉干
pulmonary trunk

右心房
right atrium

左心耳
left auricle

浅层
superficial layer

右心室
right ventricle

中层
middle layer

左心室
left ventricle

深层
deep layer

图 9-12　心肌
Myocardium

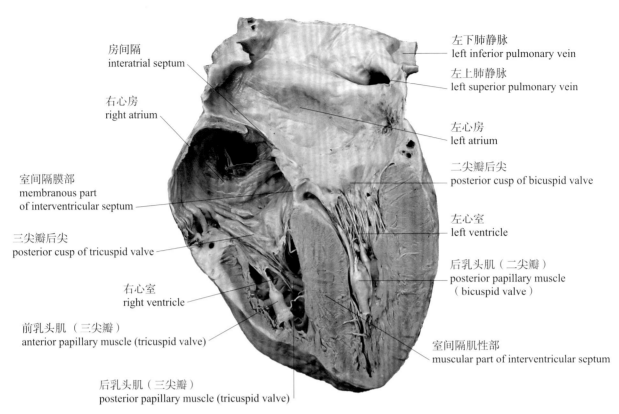

房间隔
interatrial septum

左下肺静脉
left inferior pulmonary vein

左上肺静脉
left superior pulmonary vein

右心房
right atrium

左心房
left atrium

二尖瓣后尖
posterior cusp of bicuspid valve

室间隔膜部
membranous part
of interventricular septum

左心室
left ventricle

三尖瓣后尖
posterior cusp of tricuspid valve

后乳头肌（二尖瓣）
posterior papillary muscle
（bicuspid valve）

右心室
right ventricle

前乳头肌（三尖瓣）
anterior papillary muscle (tricuspid valve)

室间隔肌性部
muscular part of interventricular septum

后乳头肌（三尖瓣）
posterior papillary muscle (tricuspid valve)

图 9-13 通过心间隔的心脏纵切面
Longitudinal section through the cardiac septum

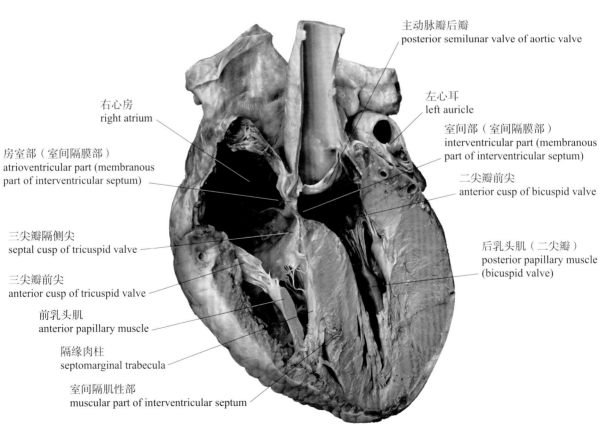

主动脉瓣后瓣
posterior semilunar valve of aortic valve

右心房
right atrium

左心耳
left auricle

房室部（室间隔膜部）
atrioventricular part (membranous
part of interventricular septum)

室间部（室间隔膜部）
interventricular part (membranous
part of interventricular septum)

二尖瓣前尖
anterior cusp of bicuspid valve

三尖瓣隔侧尖
septal cusp of tricuspid valve

三尖瓣前尖
anterior cusp of tricuspid valve

后乳头肌（二尖瓣）
posterior papillary muscle
(bicuspid valve)

前乳头肌
anterior papillary muscle

隔缘肉柱
septomarginal trabecula

室间隔肌性部
muscular part of interventricular septum

图 9-14 室间隔与房室隔
Interventricular septum and atrioventricular septum

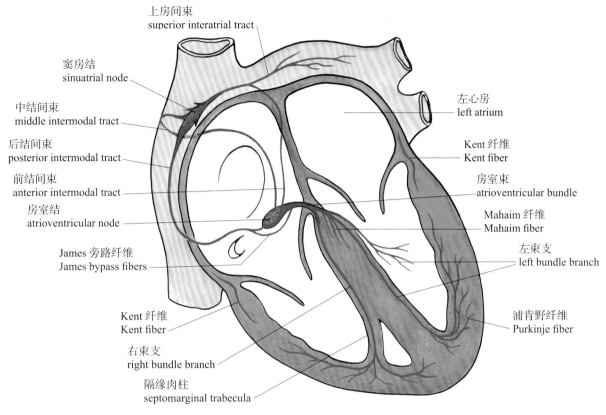

上房间束
superior interatrial tract

窦房结
sinuatrial node

中结间束
middle intermodal tract

后结间束
posterior intermodal tract

前结间束
anterior intermodal tract

房室结
atrioventricular node

James 旁路纤维
James bypass fibers

Kent 纤维
Kent fiber

右束支
right bundle branch

隔缘肉柱
septomarginal trabecula

左心房
left atrium

Kent 纤维
Kent fiber

房室束
atrioventricular bundle

Mahaim 纤维
Mahaim fiber

左束支
left bundle branch

浦肯野纤维
Purkinje fiber

图 9-15 心传导系
Conduction of heart

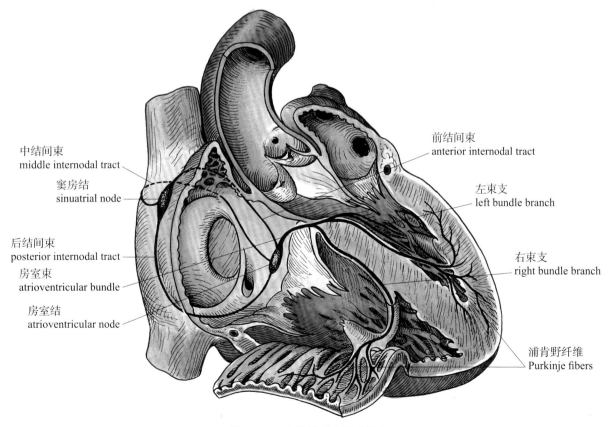

中结间束
middle internodal tract

窦房结
sinuatrial node

后结间束
posterior internodal tract

房室束
atrioventricular bundle

房室结
atrioventricular node

前结间束
anterior internodal tract

左束支
left bundle branch

右束支
right bundle branch

浦肯野纤维
Purkinje fibers

图 9-16 心传导系（模式图）
Conduction system of heart (diagram)

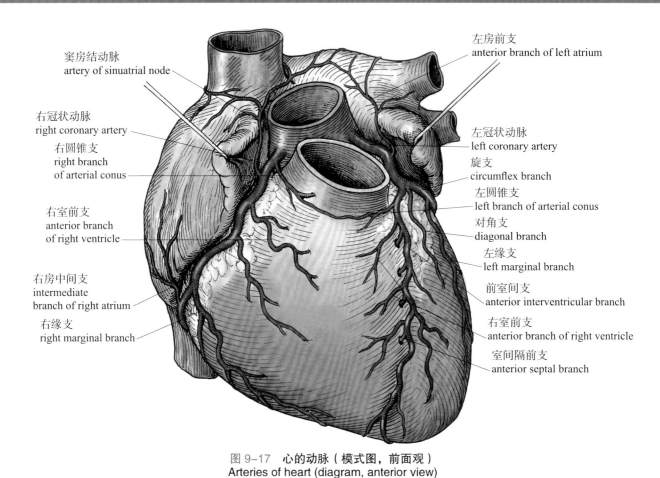

窦房结动脉
artery of sinuatrial node

右冠状动脉
right coronary artery

右圆锥支
right branch
of arterial conus

右室前支
anterior branch
of right ventricle

右房中间支
intermediate
branch of right atrium

右缘支
right marginal branch

左房前支
anterior branch of left atrium

左冠状动脉
left coronary artery

旋支
circumflex branch

左圆锥支
left branch of arterial conus

对角支
diagonal branch

左缘支
left marginal branch

前室间支
anterior interventricular branch

右室前支
anterior branch of right ventricle

室间隔前支
anterior septal branch

图 9-17　心的动脉（模式图，前面观）
Arteries of heart (diagram, anterior view)

右冠状动脉
right coronary artery

右室前支
anterior branch
of right ventricle

右缘支
right marginal branch

左冠状动脉
left coronary artery

对角支
diagonal branch

前室间支
anterior interventricular branch

图 9-18　心的动脉（前面观）
Arteries of heart (anterior view)

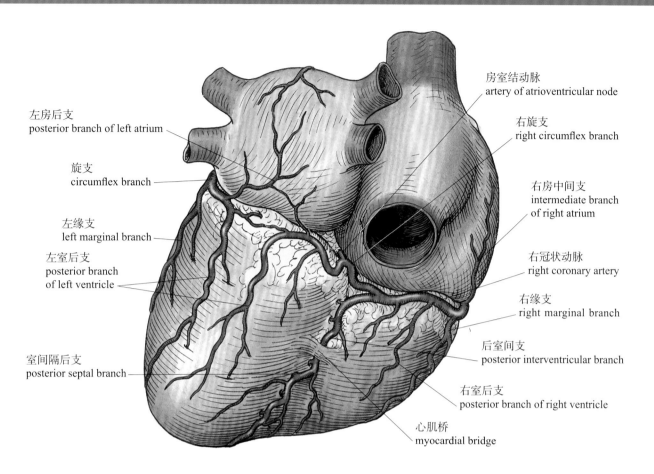

左房后支
posterior branch of left atrium

旋支
circumflex branch

左缘支
left marginal branch

左室后支
posterior branch
of left ventricle

室间隔后支
posterior septal branch

房室结动脉
artery of atrioventricular node

右旋支
right circumflex branch

右房中间支
intermediate branch
of right atrium

右冠状动脉
right coronary artery

右缘支
right marginal branch

后室间支
posterior interventricular branch

右室后支
posterior branch of right ventricle

心肌桥
myocardial bridge

图 9-19　心的动脉（模式图，后面观）
Arteries of heart (diagram, posterior view)

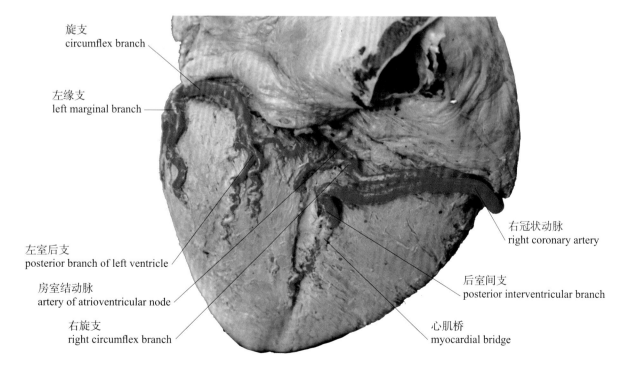

旋支
circumflex branch

左缘支
left marginal branch

左室后支
posterior branch of left ventricle

房室结动脉
artery of atrioventricular node

右旋支
right circumflex branch

右冠状动脉
right coronary artery

后室间支
posterior interventricular branch

心肌桥
myocardial bridge

图 9-20　心的动脉（后面观）
Arteries of heart (posterior view)

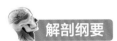 解剖纲要

冠状动脉分支

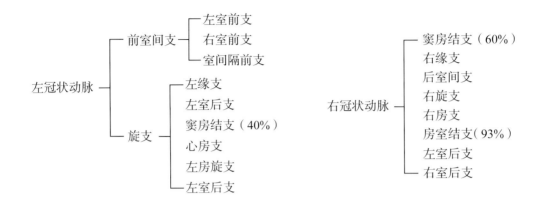

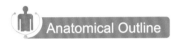 Anatomical Outline

The branches of coronary artery

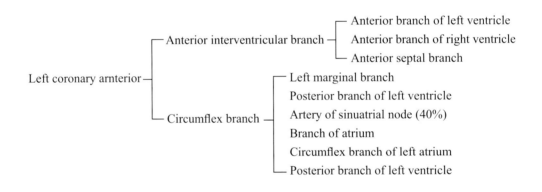

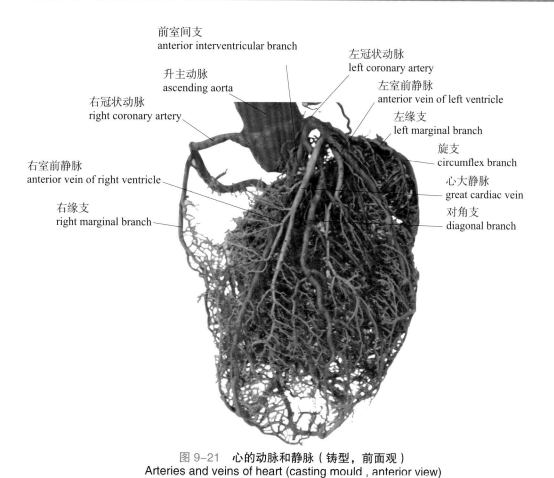

前室间支
anterior interventricular branch

升主动脉
ascending aorta

右冠状动脉
right coronary artery

左冠状动脉
left coronary artery

左室前静脉
anterior vein of left ventricle

左缘支
left marginal branch

旋支
circumflex branch

心大静脉
great cardiac vein

对角支
diagonal branch

右室前静脉
anterior vein of right ventricle

右缘支
right marginal branch

图 9-21　心的动脉和静脉（铸型，前面观）
Arteries and veins of heart (casting mould , anterior view)

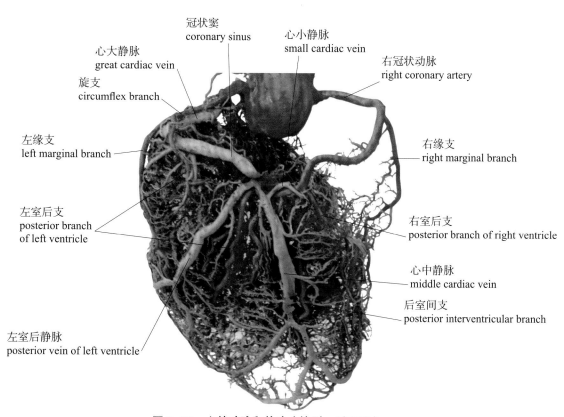

冠状窦
coronary sinus

心小静脉
small cardiac vein

心大静脉
great cardiac vein

右冠状动脉
right coronary artery

旋支
circumflex branch

左缘支
left marginal branch

右缘支
right marginal branch

左室后支
posterior branch
of left ventricle

右室后支
posterior branch of right ventricle

心中静脉
middle cardiac vein

后室间支
posterior interventricular branch

左室后静脉
posterior vein of left ventricle

图 9-22　心的动脉和静脉（铸型，后面观）
Arteries and veins of heart (casting mould , posterior view)

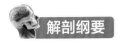解剖纲要

冠状动脉的分布类型

1. 右优势型 (65.7%)：右冠状动脉在膈面除发出后室间支外，还有分支分布于左室膈面的部分或全部。

2. 均衡型 (28.7%)：两侧心室的膈面分别由本侧的冠状动脉供血，它们的分布区域不越过房室交点和后室间沟，后室间支为左或右冠状动脉末梢，或同时来自两侧冠状动脉。

3. 左优势型 (5.6%)：左冠状动脉除发出分支分布于左室膈面外，还越过房室交点和后室间沟分布于右室膈面的一部分，后室间支和房室结支均发自左冠状动脉。

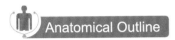Anatomical Outline

Distribution types of the coronary artery

1. Right dominance (65.7%): In addition to the posterior interventricular branches of the right coronary artery on the diaphragmatic surface, it also supplies the part or most of the diaphragmatic surface of the left ventricle.

2. Co-dominance (28.7%): The diaphragmatic surfaces of both ventricles are supplied by ipsilateral coronary arteries. Their distribution areas do not cross atrioventricular crux and posterior interventricular sulcus. Posterior interventricular branches are left or right coronary artery endings, or come from both coronary arteries.

3. Left dominance (5.6%): The left coronary artery not only distributes on the diaphragmatic surface of the left ventricle, but also distributes on the diaphragmatic surface of the right ventricle across the atv-ventricular crux and posterior interventricular sulcus. The posterior interventricular branch and artery of atrioventricular node originate from the left coronary artery.

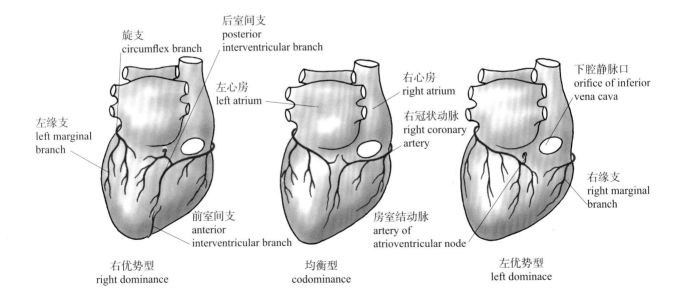

图 9-23　冠状动脉的分布类型（后面观）
Distribution types of coronary artery (posterior view)

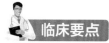 **临床要点**

1. 冠状动脉性心脏病，是由冠状动脉部分或全部阻塞造成的心肌缺血所引发的，常引起心绞痛，严重者造成大片心肌坏死，导致心肌梗死。

2. 冠状动脉造影术是一种诊断冠状动脉功能的 X 线记录技术。采用一根长导管经股动脉或肱动脉进入升主动脉。导管尖端正好进入冠状动脉口，注入少量不透 X 线的造影剂以显示活动的冠状动脉血管造影图像。此技术用于发现临床上心绞痛或心肌梗死时的冠状动脉狭窄或闭塞位置；同时，可利用球囊血管成形术或支架以扩张此部位的冠状动脉。

3. 冠状动脉分流术是用来为狭窄或阻塞冠状动脉远端的心肌重新建立可靠血液供应的手段，最常用的方法是游离胸廓内动脉，并与阻塞远侧段的冠状动脉相吻合。

Key Points of the Clinic

1. Coronary heart disease (CAD) is the myocardial ischemia caused by partial or total occlusion of coronary artery, which often causes angina pectoris. In severe cases, it causes massive myocardial necrosis and leads to myocardial infarction.

2. The coronary angiography is an important method to check the function of the coronary artery in clinic. A long catheter is used to enter the ascending aorta via the femoral or brachial artery. The tip of the catheter is inserted right into the opening of the coronary artery and a small amount of opaque contrast is injected to show the angiographic image of a moving coronary artery. This technique is used to find the location of coronary artery stenosis or occlusion in clinical angina pectoris or myocardial infarction. At the same time, balloon angioplasty or stents can be used to dilate the coronary arteries in this area.

3. Coronary bypass surgery is a method to re-establish a reliable blood supply to the heart muscle which are supplied by the distal end of a narrowed or blocked coronary artery. The most common method is to dissociate the internal thoracic artery and anastomose it with the blocked distal coronary artery.

第三篇 脉管系统 Part 3 Angiology System

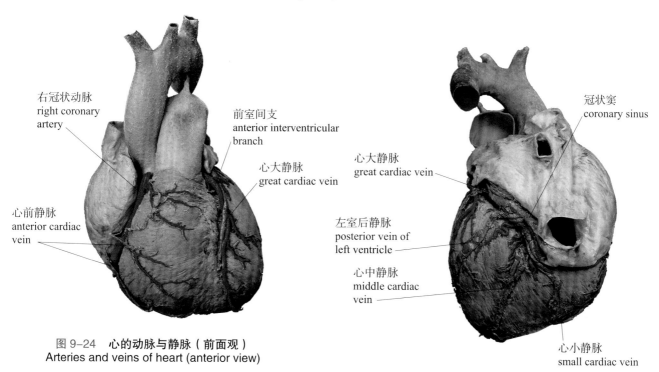

图 9-24 心的动脉与静脉（前面观）
Arteries and veins of heart (anterior view)

图 9-25 心的静脉（后面观）
Veins of heart (posterior view)

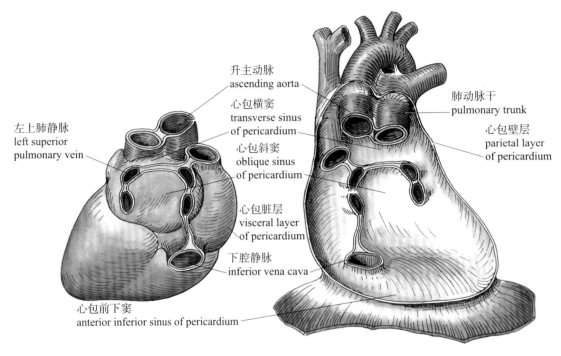

升主动脉
ascending aorta

心包横窦
transverse sinus
of pericardium

心包斜窦
oblique sinus
of pericardium

左上肺静脉
left superior
pulmonary vein

心包脏层
visceral layer
of pericardium

肺动脉干
pulmonary trunk

心包壁层
parietal layer
of pericardium

下腔静脉
inferior vena cava

心包前下窦
anterior inferior sinus of pericardium

图 9-26　心包
Pericardium

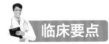　临床要点

1. 心包横窦为心包腔在主动脉、肺动脉后方与上腔静脉、左心房前壁前方间的细长的囊状间隙。心脏直视手术需阻断主动脉和肺动脉血流时，可通过横窦钳夹两个大动脉。

2. 心包斜窦是左心房后壁、左右肺静脉、下腔静脉与心包后壁之间的间隙，其后方与食管相邻。手术需阻断下腔静脉血流时，可经斜窦下部进行。

3. 心包积液指浆膜性心包和心包壁层之间的积液。如果大量液体积聚可造成心脏压塞，此时大量积聚的液体限制了心脏舒张期的充盈，导致血压降低、心动过速，若不进行心包穿刺解除心脏压塞，最后可出现心脏停搏。

Key Points of the Clinic

1. The transverse pericardial sinus is a slender cystic space between the pericardium behind the aorta and pulmonary artery and the superior vena cava and the anterior wall of the left atrium.When aorta and pulmonary artery blood flow are blocked in open heart surgery, the two major arteries can be clamped via transverse pericardial sinus.

2. The oblique sinus of the pericardium is the space between the posterior wall of the left atrium, left and right pulmonary veins, inferior vena cava and the posterior wall of the pericardium, and its rear is adjacent to the esophagus. During clinical cardiac operation, the blood flow of the inferior vena cava can be temporarily blocked through lower oblique sinus.

3. Pericardial effusion means fluid accumulation between layers of serous and parietal pericardium. If large amounts of fluid accumulation can cause cardiac tamponade, at this time a large number of accumulation of liquid limit the cardiac diastolic filling, lead to lower blood pressure, tachycardia. If pericardiocentesis is not performed to relieve cardiac tamponade, finally can appear cardiac arrest.

Part 3 Angiology System

第三篇 脉管系统

第二节 动脉 Section 2 Artery

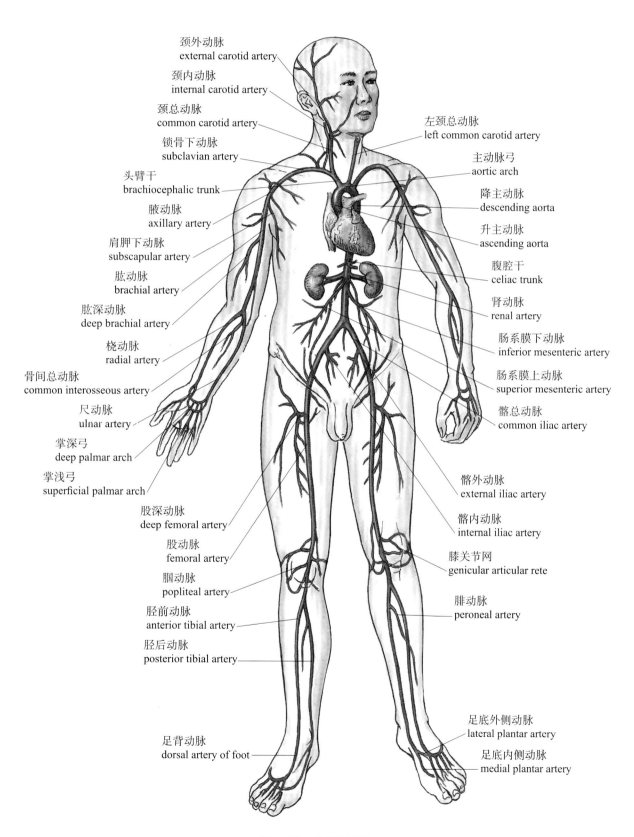

颈外动脉
external carotid artery

颈内动脉
internal carotid artery

颈总动脉
common carotid artery

锁骨下动脉
subclavian artery

头臂干
brachiocephalic trunk

腋动脉
axillary artery

肩胛下动脉
subscapular artery

肱动脉
brachial artery

肱深动脉
deep brachial artery

桡动脉
radial artery

骨间总动脉
common interosseous artery

尺动脉
ulnar artery

掌深弓
deep palmar arch

掌浅弓
superficial palmar arch

股深动脉
deep femoral artery

股动脉
femoral artery

腘动脉
popliteal artery

胫前动脉
anterior tibial artery

胫后动脉
posterior tibial artery

足背动脉
dorsal artery of foot

左颈总动脉
left common carotid artery

主动脉弓
aortic arch

降主动脉
descending aorta

升主动脉
ascending aorta

腹腔干
celiac trunk

肾动脉
renal artery

肠系膜下动脉
inferior mesenteric artery

肠系膜上动脉
superior mesenteric artery

髂总动脉
common iliac artery

髂外动脉
external iliac artery

髂内动脉
internal iliac artery

膝关节网
genicular articular rete

腓动脉
peroneal artery

足底外侧动脉
lateral plantar artery

足底内侧动脉
medial plantar artery

图 9-27 体循环动脉
Arteries of systemic circulation

体循环的动脉

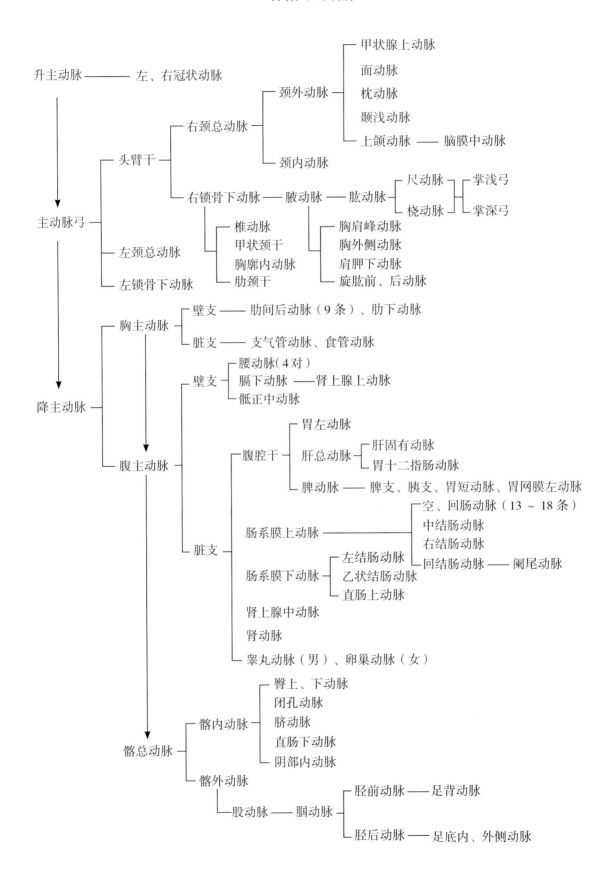

Arteries of the systemic circulation

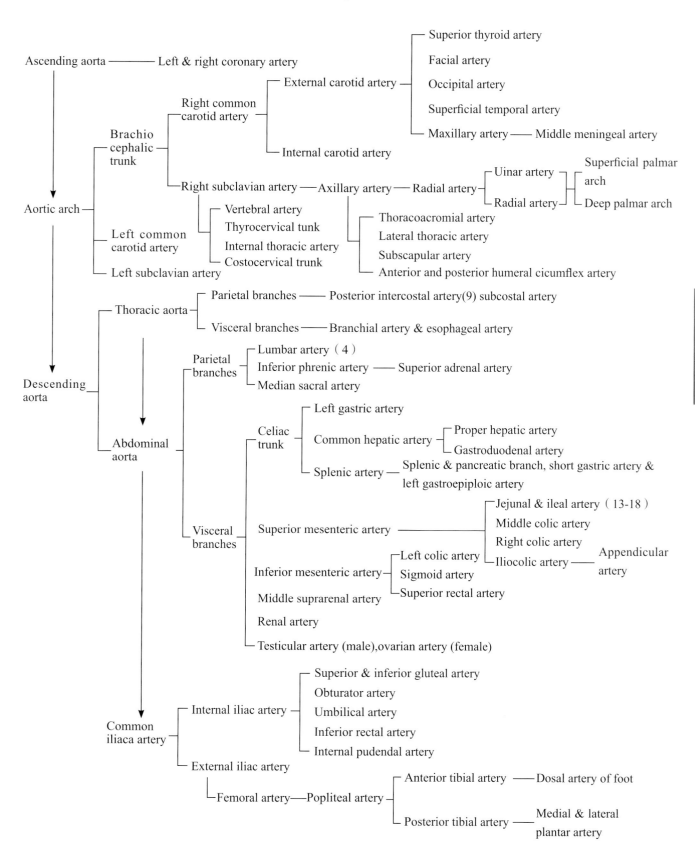

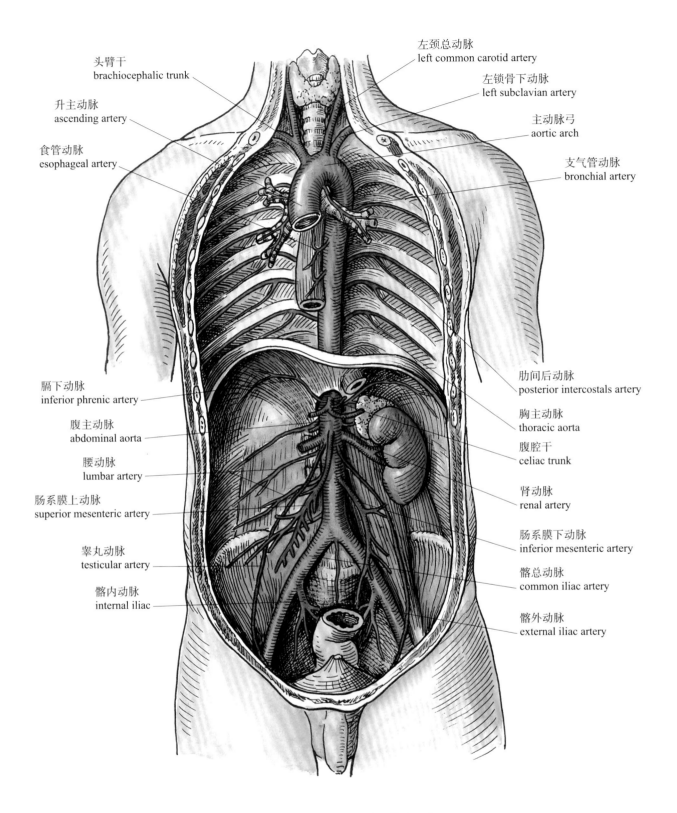

头臂干
brachiocephalic trunk

升主动脉
ascending artery

食管动脉
esophageal artery

左颈总动脉
left common carotid artery

左锁骨下动脉
left subclavian artery

主动脉弓
aortic arch

支气管动脉
bronchial artery

肋间后动脉
posterior intercostals artery

胸主动脉
thoracic aorta

腹腔干
celiac trunk

肾动脉
renal artery

肠系膜下动脉
inferior mesenteric artery

髂总动脉
common iliac artery

髂外动脉
external iliac artery

膈下动脉
inferior phrenic artery

腹主动脉
abdominal aorta

腰动脉
lumbar artery

肠系膜上动脉
superior mesenteric artery

睾丸动脉
testicular artery

髂内动脉
internal iliac

图 9-28　主动脉及其分支（模式图）
Aorta and its branches (diagram)

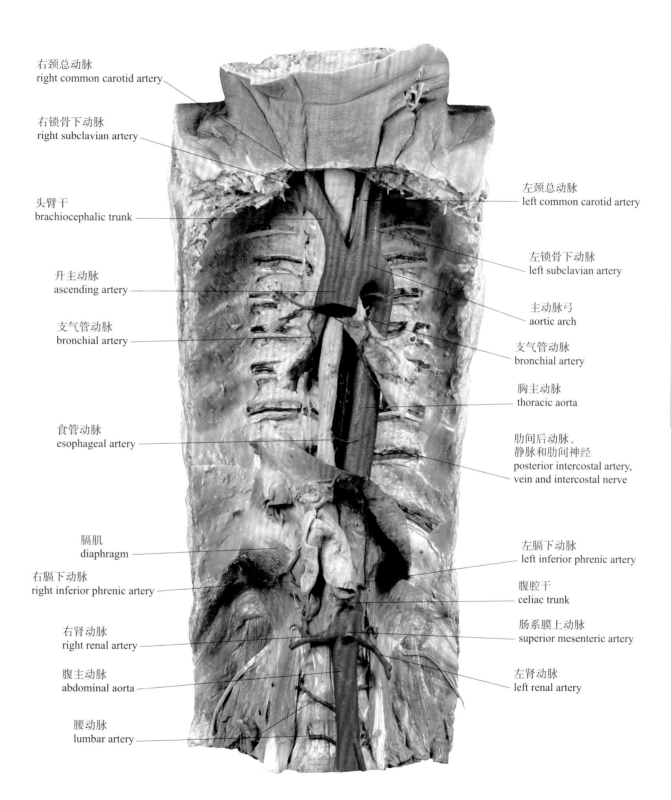

右颈总动脉
right common carotid artery

右锁骨下动脉
right subclavian artery

头臂干
brachiocephalic trunk

升主动脉
ascending artery

支气管动脉
bronchial artery

食管动脉
esophageal artery

膈肌
diaphragm

右膈下动脉
right inferior phrenic artery

右肾动脉
right renal artery

腹主动脉
abdominal aorta

腰动脉
lumbar artery

左颈总动脉
left common carotid artery

左锁骨下动脉
left subclavian artery

主动脉弓
aortic arch

支气管动脉
bronchial artery

胸主动脉
thoracic aorta

肋间后动脉、
静脉和肋间神经
posterior intercostal artery,
vein and intercostal nerve

左膈下动脉
left inferior phrenic artery

腹腔干
celiac trunk

肠系膜上动脉
superior mesenteric artery

左肾动脉
left renal artery

图 9-29 主动脉及其分支
Aorta and its branches

Part 3 Angiology System 第三篇 脉管系统

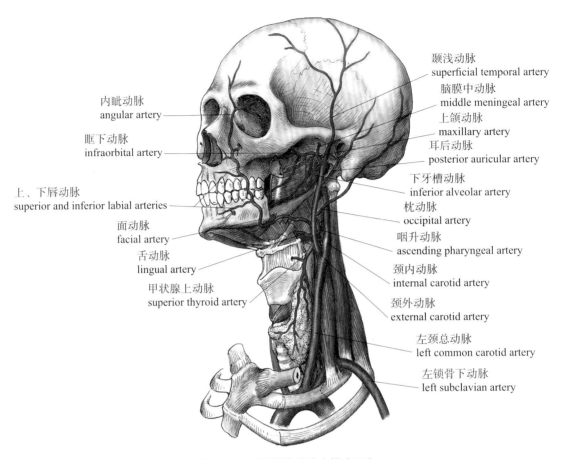

内眦动脉
angular artery

眶下动脉
infraorbital artery

上、下唇动脉
superior and inferior labial arteries

面动脉
facial artery

舌动脉
lingual artery

甲状腺上动脉
superior thyroid artery

颞浅动脉
superficial temporal artery

脑膜中动脉
middle meningeal artery

上颌动脉
maxillary artery

耳后动脉
posterior auricular artery

下牙槽动脉
inferior alveolar artery

枕动脉
occipital artery

咽升动脉
ascending pharyngeal artery

颈内动脉
internal carotid artery

颈外动脉
external carotid artery

左颈总动脉
left common carotid artery

左锁骨下动脉
left subclavian artery

图 9-30 头颈部的动脉（模式图）
Arteries of head and neck (diagram)

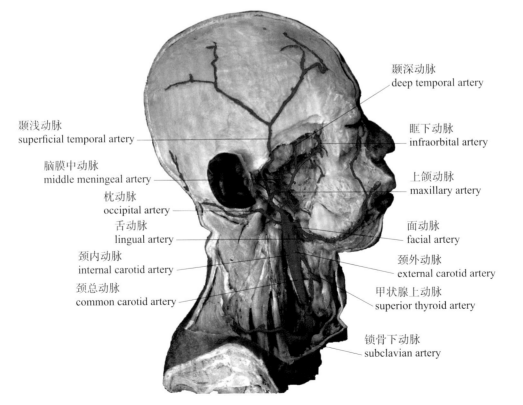

颞浅动脉
superficial temporal artery

脑膜中动脉
middle meningeal artery

枕动脉
occipital artery

舌动脉
lingual artery

颈内动脉
internal carotid artery

颈总动脉
common carotid artery

颞深动脉
deep temporal artery

眶下动脉
infraorbital artery

上颌动脉
maxillary artery

面动脉
facial artery

颈外动脉
external carotid artery

甲状腺上动脉
superior thyroid artery

锁骨下动脉
subclavian artery

图 9-31 头颈部的动脉
Arteries of head and neck

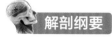

解剖纲要

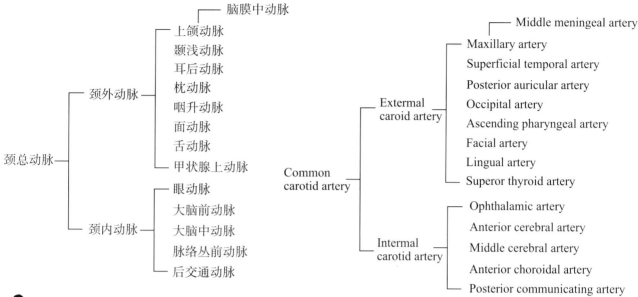

颈总动脉
├─ 颈外动脉
│ ├─ 上颌动脉 ── 脑膜中动脉
│ ├─ 颞浅动脉
│ ├─ 耳后动脉
│ ├─ 枕动脉
│ ├─ 咽升动脉
│ ├─ 面动脉
│ ├─ 舌动脉
│ └─ 甲状腺上动脉
└─ 颈内动脉
   ├─ 眼动脉
   ├─ 大脑前动脉
   ├─ 大脑中动脉
   ├─ 脉络丛前动脉
   └─ 后交通动脉

Anatomical Outline

Common carotid artery
├─ External carotid artery
│ ├─ Maxillary artery ── Middle meningeal artery
│ ├─ Superficial temporal artery
│ ├─ Posterior auricular artery
│ ├─ Occipital artery
│ ├─ Ascending pharyngeal artery
│ ├─ Facial artery
│ ├─ Lingual artery
│ └─ Superor thyroid artery
└─ Internal carotid artery
   ├─ Ophthalamic artery
   ├─ Anterior cerebral artery
   ├─ Middle cerebral artery
   ├─ Anterior choroidal artery
   └─ Posterior communicating artery

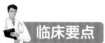

临床要点

动脉搏动点和特殊结构

1. 颈总动脉：在胸锁乳突肌前缘，平环状软骨弓的侧方，向后内将动脉压向第6颈椎横突。

2. 面动脉：在咬肌前缘，下颌骨下缘，将动脉压向下颌骨。

3. 颞浅动脉：在外耳门前上方，颧弓根部，将动脉压向颧弓。

4. 颈动脉窦：为颈总动脉末端和颈内动脉起始部的膨大，窦壁外膜下含压力感受器，为动脉血压调节的重要感受装置。

5. 颈动脉小球：位于颈动脉分叉的后方，可感受血液中 CO_2 分压、O_2 分压和 pH 变化，反射性调节呼吸。

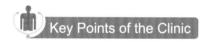

Key Points of the Clinic

Arterial pulsation points and special sturcture

1. The common carotid artery: It is present at the crossing point of the anterior border of sternocleidomastoid muscle and the arch of cricoid cartilage, presses the artery posteriorly to the transverse process of the 6th cervical vertebrate.

2. The facial artery: It is present at the crossing point of the anterior border of masseter and the lower border of the mandible, presses the artery to the mandible.

3. The superficial temporal artery: It is present at the root of zygomatic arch (anterior to the external acoustic meatus), presses the artery toward zygomatic arch.

4. Carotid sinus: It's a dilated segment located at the end of the common carotid artery and the beginning of the internal carotid artery. The wall of carotid sinus contains baroreceptors sensitive to changes in blood pressure, which plays an important role in regulating the arterial blood pressure.

5. Carotid glomus (carotid body): It is a group of chemoreceptors adjacent to bifurcation of carotid artery. The carotid glomus is sensitive to changes of concentrations of CO_2, O_2 and pH of the blood, and is responsible for the reflex regulation of respiration.

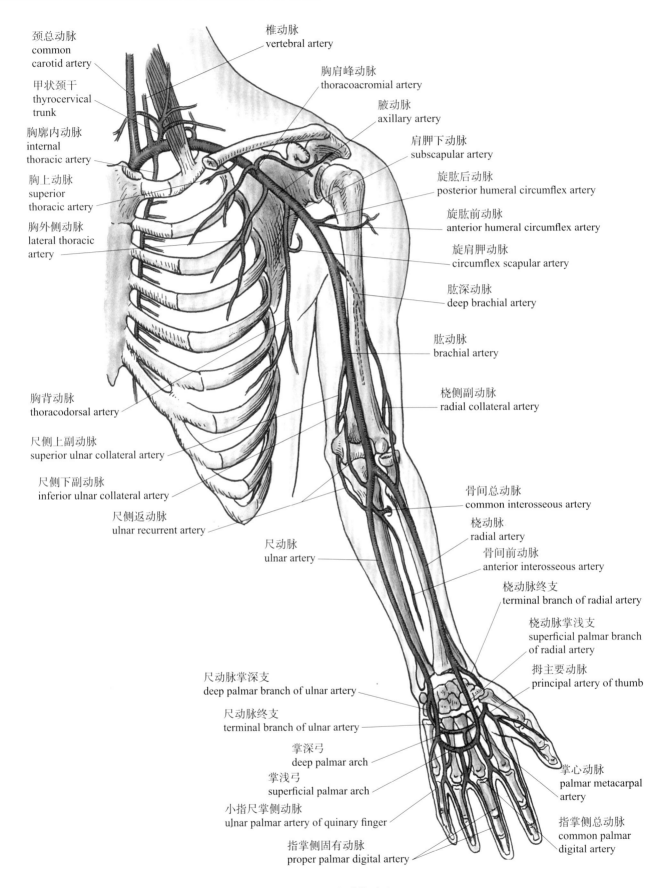

颈总动脉
common carotid artery

甲状颈干
thyrocervical trunk

胸廓内动脉
internal thoracic artery

胸上动脉
superior thoracic artery

胸外侧动脉
lateral thoracic artery

胸背动脉
thoracodorsal artery

尺侧上副动脉
superior ulnar collateral artery

尺侧下副动脉
inferior ulnar collateral artery

尺侧返动脉
ulnar recurrent artery

尺动脉掌深支
deep palmar branch of ulnar artery

尺动脉终支
terminal branch of ulnar artery

掌深弓
deep palmar arch

掌浅弓
superficial palmar arch

小指尺掌侧动脉
ulnar palmar artery of quinary finger

指掌侧固有动脉
proper palmar digital artery

椎动脉
vertebral artery

胸肩峰动脉
thoracoacromial artery

腋动脉
axillary artery

肩胛下动脉
subscapular artery

旋肱后动脉
posterior humeral circumflex artery

旋肱前动脉
anterior humeral circumflex artery

旋肩胛动脉
circumflex scapular artery

肱深动脉
deep brachial artery

肱动脉
brachial artery

桡侧副动脉
radial collateral artery

骨间总动脉
common interosseous artery

桡动脉
radial artery

骨间前动脉
anterior interosseous artery

桡动脉终支
terminal branch of radial artery

桡动脉掌浅支
superficial palmar branch of radial artery

拇主要动脉
principal artery of thumb

掌心动脉
palmar metacarpal artery

指掌侧总动脉
common palmar digital artery

尺动脉
ulnar artery

图 9-32　上肢的动脉
Arteries of upper limb

解剖纲要

上肢动脉

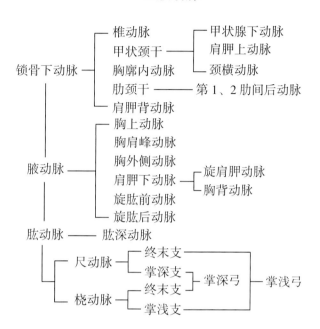

Anatomical Outline

Arteries of the systemic circulation

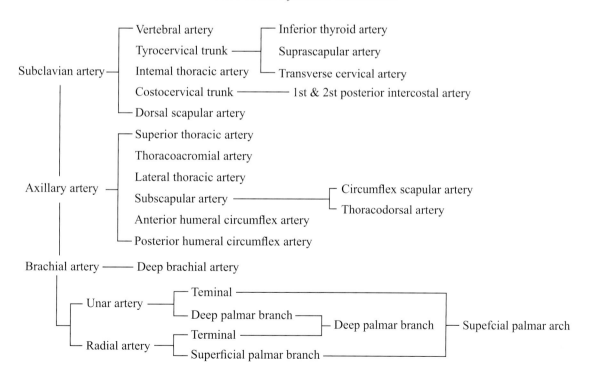

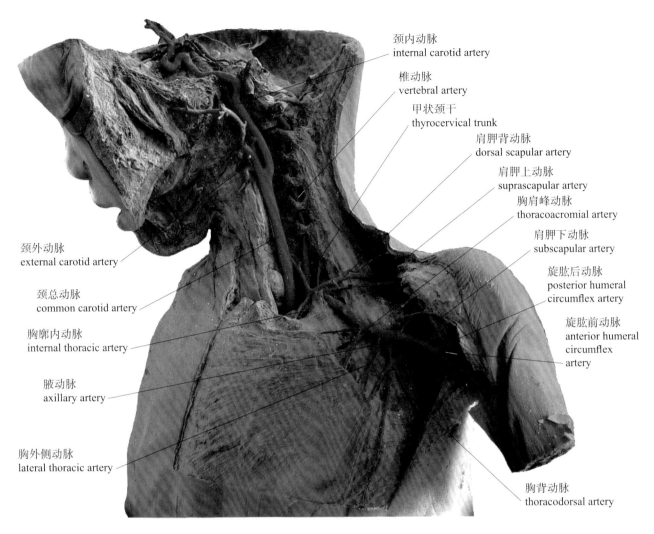

颈内动脉
internal carotid artery

椎动脉
vertebral artery

甲状颈干
thyrocervical trunk

肩胛背动脉
dorsal scapular artery

肩胛上动脉
suprascapular artery

胸肩峰动脉
thoracoacromial artery

肩胛下动脉
subscapular artery

旋肱后动脉
posterior humeral
circumflex artery

旋肱前动脉
anterior humeral
circumflex
artery

颈外动脉
external carotid artery

颈总动脉
common carotid artery

胸廓内动脉
internal thoracic artery

腋动脉
axillary artery

胸外侧动脉
lateral thoracic artery

胸背动脉
thoracodorsal artery

图 9-33　锁骨下动脉和腋动脉
Subclavian artery and axillary artery

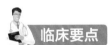 临床要点

1. 锁骨下动脉：上肢出血时，可于锁骨中点上方的锁骨上窝处向后下将该动脉压向第 1 肋止血。

2. 肱动脉：当前臂和手部出血时，可在臂中部将该动脉压向肱骨止血。

3. 桡动脉：下段位置表浅，仅被皮肤和筋膜遮盖，是临床触摸脉搏的部位。

Key Points of the Clinic

1. The subclavian artery: When the upper limbs bleed due to an injury, the subclavian artery can be blocked temporarily by pressing the artery towards the first rib in the supraclavicular fossa, located above the midpoint of the clavicle.

2. The brachial artery: When the forearms or the hands bleed, the brachial artery can be blocked temporarily by pressing the artery towards the humerus.

3. The radial artery: The lower segment of the artery is superficial, and only covered by skin and fascia, where we can palpate the arterial pulse in clinic.

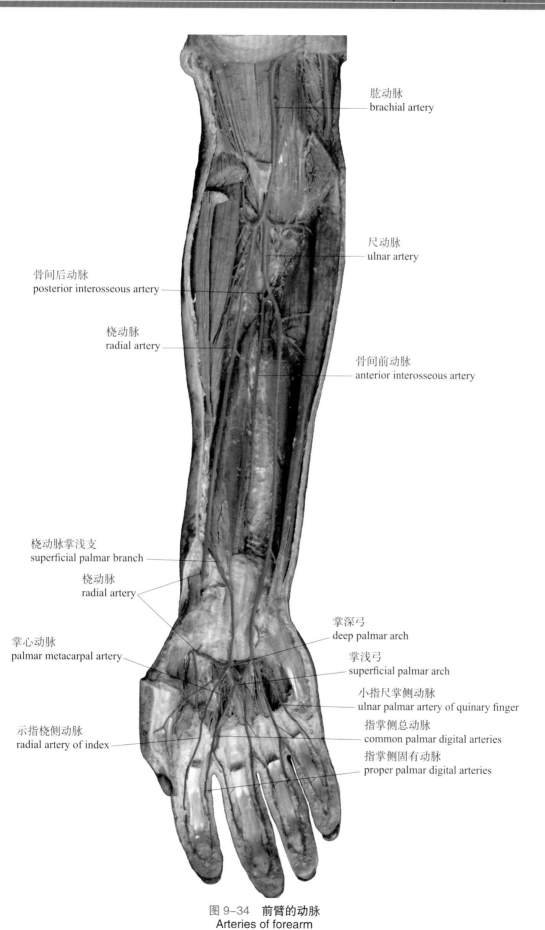

肱动脉
brachial artery

尺动脉
ulnar artery

骨间后动脉
posterior interosseous artery

桡动脉
radial artery

骨间前动脉
anterior interosseous artery

桡动脉掌浅支
superficial palmar branch

桡动脉
radial artery

掌深弓
deep palmar arch

掌浅弓
superficial palmar arch

掌心动脉
palmar metacarpal artery

小指尺掌侧动脉
ulnar palmar artery of quinary finger

指掌侧总动脉
common palmar digital arteries

示指桡侧动脉
radial artery of index

指掌侧固有动脉
proper palmar digital arteries

图 9-34　前臂的动脉
Arteries of forearm

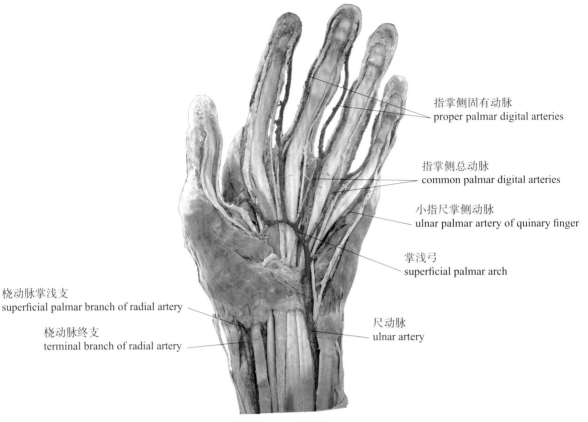

指掌侧固有动脉
proper palmar digital arteries

指掌侧总动脉
common palmar digital arteries

小指尺掌侧动脉
ulnar palmar artery of quinary finger

掌浅弓
superficial palmar arch

尺动脉
ulnar artery

桡动脉掌浅支
superficial palmar branch of radial artery

桡动脉终支
terminal branch of radial artery

图 9-35 掌浅弓
Superficial palmar arch

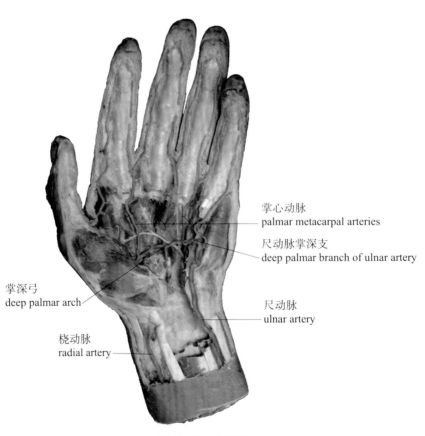

掌心动脉
palmar metacarpal arteries

尺动脉掌深支
deep palmar branch of ulnar artery

尺动脉
ulnar artery

掌深弓
deep palmar arch

桡动脉
radial artery

图 9-36 掌深弓
Deep palmar arch

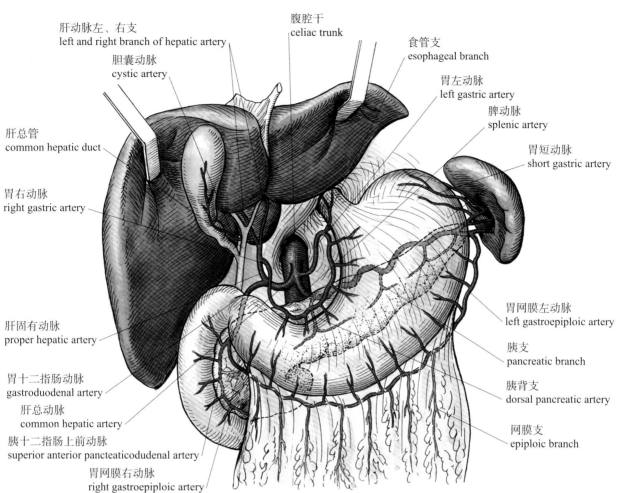

图 9-37　腹腔干及其分支（模式图）
Celiac trunk and its branches (diagram)

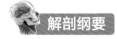　解剖纲要

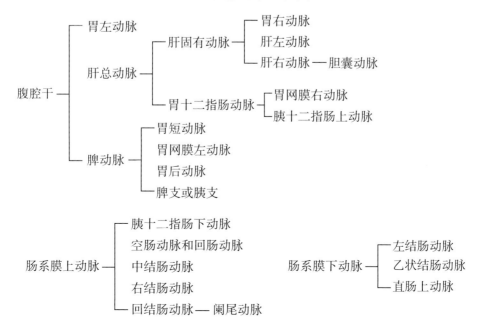

第三篇　脉管系统
Part 3 Angiology System

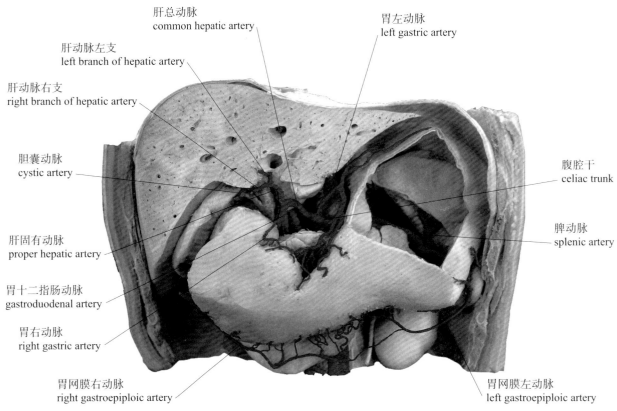

肝总动脉
common hepatic artery

胃左动脉
left gastric artery

肝动脉左支
left branch of hepatic artery

肝动脉右支
right branch of hepatic artery

胆囊动脉
cystic artery

腹腔干
celiac trunk

脾动脉
splenic artery

肝固有动脉
proper hepatic artery

胃十二指肠动脉
gastroduodenal artery

胃右动脉
right gastric artery

胃网膜右动脉
right gastroepiploic artery

胃网膜左动脉
left gastroepiploic artery

图 9-38　腹腔干及其分支
Celiac trunk and its branches

Anatomical Outline

The single visceral branches of the abdominal aorta

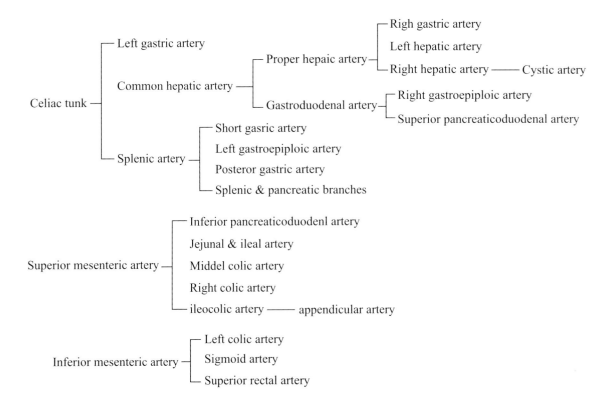

Celiac tunk ── Left gastric artery

Common hepatic artery ── Proper hepaic artery ── Righ gastric artery / Left hepatic artery / Right hepatic artery ── Cystic artery

Gastroduodenal artery ── Right gastroepiploic artery / Superior pancreaticoduodenal artery

Splenic artery ── Short gasric artery / Left gastroepiploic artery / Posteror gastric artery / Splenic & pancreatic branches

Superior mesenteric artery ── Inferior pancreaticoduodenl artery / Jejunal & ileal artery / Middel colic artery / Right colic artery / ileocolic artery ── appendicular artery

Inferior mesenteric artery ── Left colic artery / Sigmoid artery / Superior rectal artery

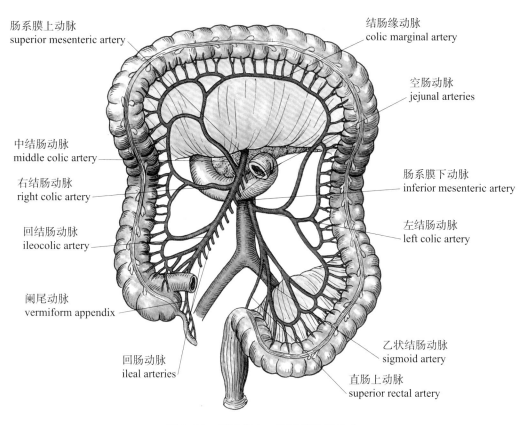

肠系膜上动脉
superior mesenteric artery

结肠缘动脉
colic marginal artery

空肠动脉
jejunal arteries

中结肠动脉
middle colic artery

右结肠动脉
right colic artery

肠系膜下动脉
inferior mesenteric artery

回结肠动脉
ileocolic artery

左结肠动脉
left colic artery

阑尾动脉
vermiform appendix

回肠动脉
ileal arteries

乙状结肠动脉
sigmoid artery

直肠上动脉
superior rectal artery

图 9-39 肠系膜上、下动脉及其分支
Superior mesenteric artery, inferior mesenteric artery and their branches

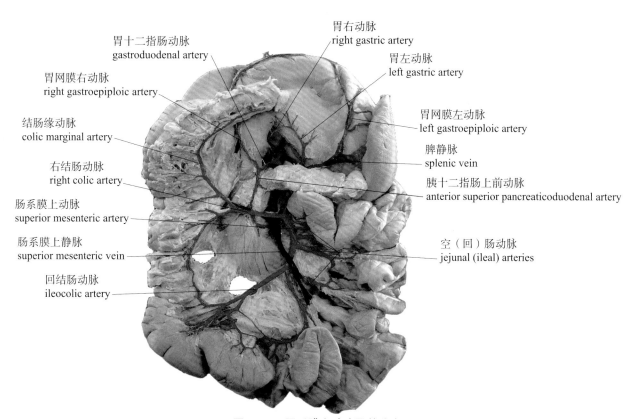

胃十二指肠动脉
gastroduodenal artery

胃右动脉
right gastric artery

胃左动脉
left gastric artery

胃网膜右动脉
right gastroepiploic artery

结肠缘动脉
colic marginal artery

胃网膜左动脉
left gastroepiploic artery

右结肠动脉
right colic artery

脾静脉
splenic vein

肠系膜上动脉
superior mesenteric artery

胰十二指肠上前动脉
anterior superior pancreaticoduodenal artery

肠系膜上静脉
superior mesenteric vein

空（回）肠动脉
jejunal (ileal) arteries

回结肠动脉
ileocolic artery

图 9-40 肠系膜上动脉及其分支
Superior mesenteric artery and its branches

第三篇 脉管系统
Part 3 Angiology System

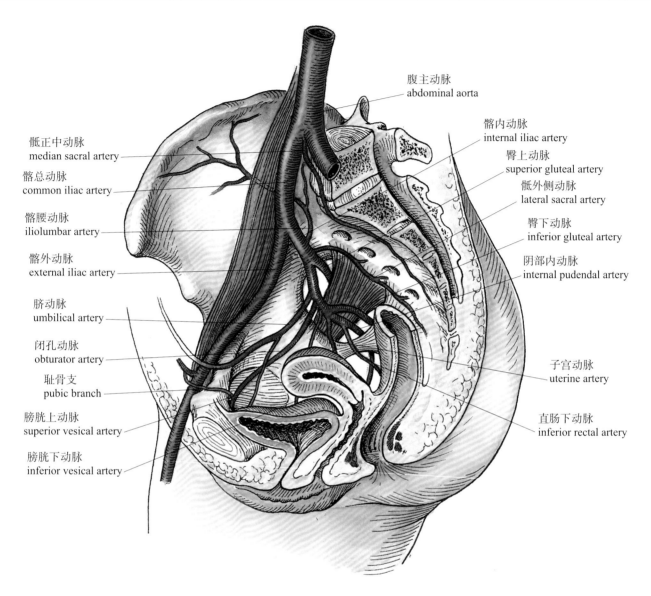

腹主动脉
abdominal aorta

骶正中动脉
median sacral artery

髂总动脉
common iliac artery

髂腰动脉
iliolumbar artery

髂外动脉
external iliac artery

脐动脉
umbilical artery

闭孔动脉
obturator artery

耻骨支
pubic branch

膀胱上动脉
superior vesical artery

膀胱下动脉
inferior vesical artery

髂内动脉
internal iliac artery

臀上动脉
superior gluteal artery

骶外侧动脉
lateral sacral artery

臀下动脉
inferior gluteal artery

阴部内动脉
internal pudendal artery

子宫动脉
uterine artery

直肠下动脉
inferior rectal artery

图 9-41 髂内动脉及其分支（女性，模式图）
Internal iliac artery and its branches (female, diagram)

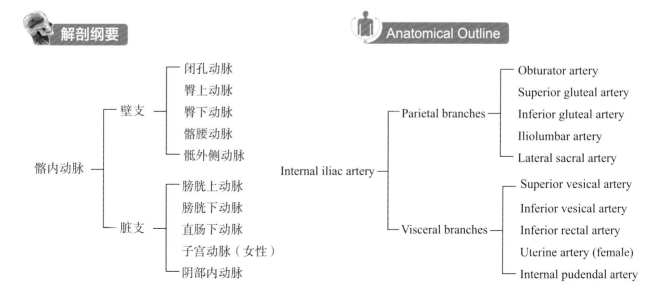

解剖纲要

髂内动脉 ┬ 壁支 ┬ 闭孔动脉
│   ├ 臀上动脉
│   ├ 臀下动脉
│   ├ 髂腰动脉
│   └ 骶外侧动脉
└ 脏支 ┬ 膀胱上动脉
       ├ 膀胱下动脉
       ├ 直肠下动脉
       ├ 子宫动脉（女性）
       └ 阴部内动脉

Anatomical Outline

Internal iliac artery ┬ Parietal branches ┬ Obturator artery
│   ├ Superior gluteal artery
│   ├ Inferior gluteal artery
│   ├ Iliolumbar artery
│   └ Lateral sacral artery
└ Visceral branches ┬ Superior vesical artery
                    ├ Inferior vesical artery
                    ├ Inferior rectal artery
                    ├ Uterine artery (female)
                    └ Internal pudendal artery

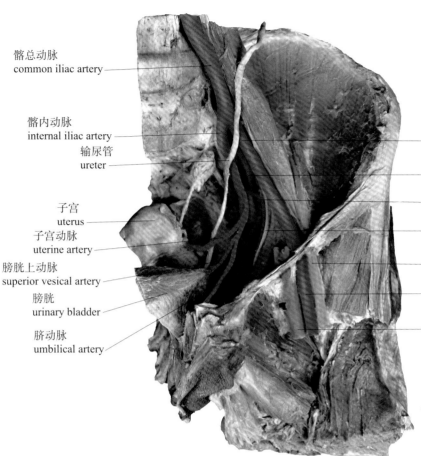

髂总动脉
common iliac artery

髂内动脉
internal iliac artery

输尿管
ureter

子宫
uterus

子宫动脉
uterine artery

膀胱上动脉
superior vesical artery

膀胱
urinary bladder

脐动脉
umbilical artery

髂外动脉
external iliac artery

臀上动脉
superior gluteal artery

闭孔动脉
obturator artery

闭孔神经
obturator nerve

股神经
femoral nerve

股动脉
femoral artery

股静脉
femoral vein

◀ 图 9-42 髂内动脉及其分支（女性）
Internal iliac artery and its branches
(female)

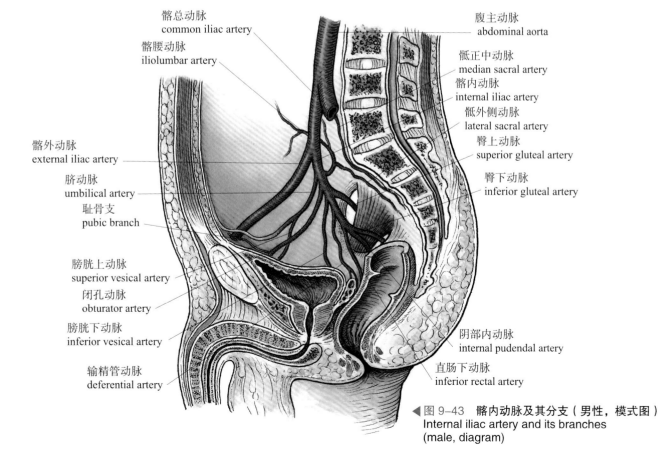

髂总动脉
common iliac artery

髂腰动脉
iliolumbar artery

髂外动脉
external iliac artery

脐动脉
umbilical artery

耻骨支
pubic branch

膀胱上动脉
superior vesical artery

闭孔动脉
obturator artery

膀胱下动脉
inferior vesical artery

输精管动脉
deferential artery

腹主动脉
abdominal aorta

骶正中动脉
median sacral artery

髂内动脉
internal iliac artery

骶外侧动脉
lateral sacral artery

臀上动脉
superior gluteal artery

臀下动脉
inferior gluteal artery

阴部内动脉
internal pudendal artery

直肠下动脉
inferior rectal artery

◀ 图 9-43 髂内动脉及其分支（男性，模式图）
Internal iliac artery and its branches
(male, diagram)

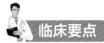

临床要点

1. 在子宫颈外侧 2cm 处，子宫动脉横向越过输尿管盆部的前上方，手术中结扎该动脉时，应特别小心避免误结扎输尿管。

2. 直肠上动脉是直肠供应动脉中最主要的一支，该动脉可自上而下穿肌层而达齿状线上方黏膜下层。直肠指检时可在该处触及动脉搏动。

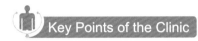

Key Points of the Clinic

1. At 2cm lateral to the cervix of the uterus, uterine artery crosses above and in front of the pelvic part of ureter. During surgical ligation of this artery, special care should be taken to avoid misligation of the ureter.

2. The superior rectal artery is the main artery supplying the rectum. The artery traverses the muscular layer from top to bottom and reaches the submucosa above the dentate line.During digital rectal examination, the artery can be palpated at this point.

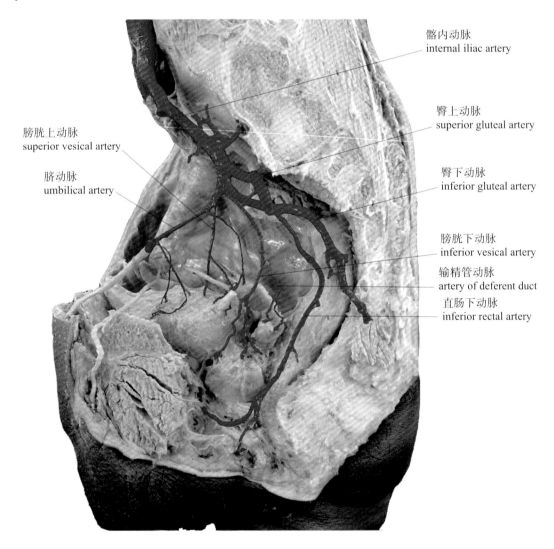

图 9-44 髂内动脉及其分支（男性）
Internal iliac artery and its branches (male)

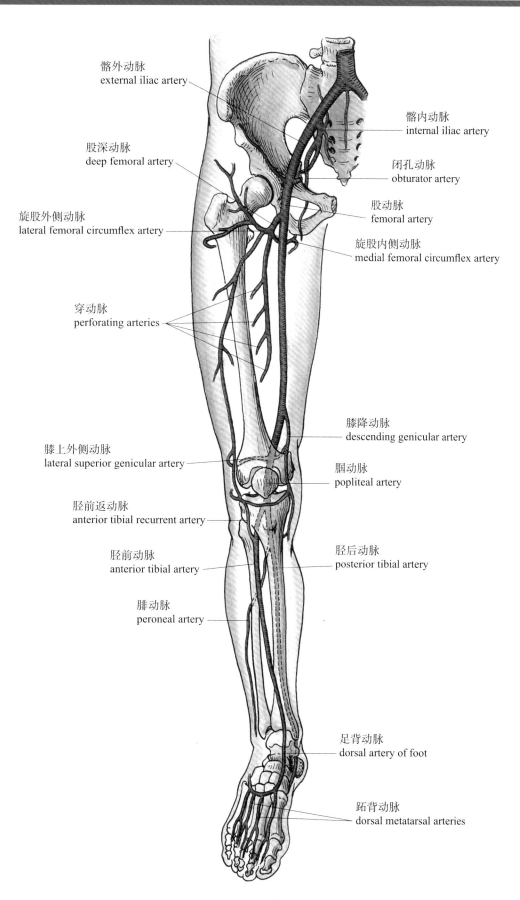

髂外动脉
external iliac artery

髂内动脉
internal iliac artery

股深动脉
deep femoral artery

闭孔动脉
obturator artery

旋股外侧动脉
lateral femoral circumflex artery

股动脉
femoral artery

旋股内侧动脉
medial femoral circumflex artery

穿动脉
perforating arteries

膝降动脉
descending genicular artery

膝上外侧动脉
lateral superior genicular artery

腘动脉
popliteal artery

胫前返动脉
anterior tibial recurrent artery

胫前动脉
anterior tibial artery

胫后动脉
posterior tibial artery

腓动脉
peroneal artery

足背动脉
dorsal artery of foot

跖背动脉
dorsal metatarsal arteries

图 9-45 下肢的动脉
Arteries of lower limb

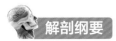 解剖纲要

下肢动脉

髂外动脉 —— 腹壁下动脉

胭动脉 —— 股动脉 —— 股深动脉 ┬ 旋股外侧动脉
　　　　　　　　　　　　　　　├ 旋股内侧动脉
　　　　　　　　　　　　　　　└ 穿动脉

胫前动脉　　　胫后动脉 —— 腓动脉
　　　　　　　　　　　├ 足底内侧动脉
足背动脉　　　　　　　└ 足底外侧动脉

足底动脉弓

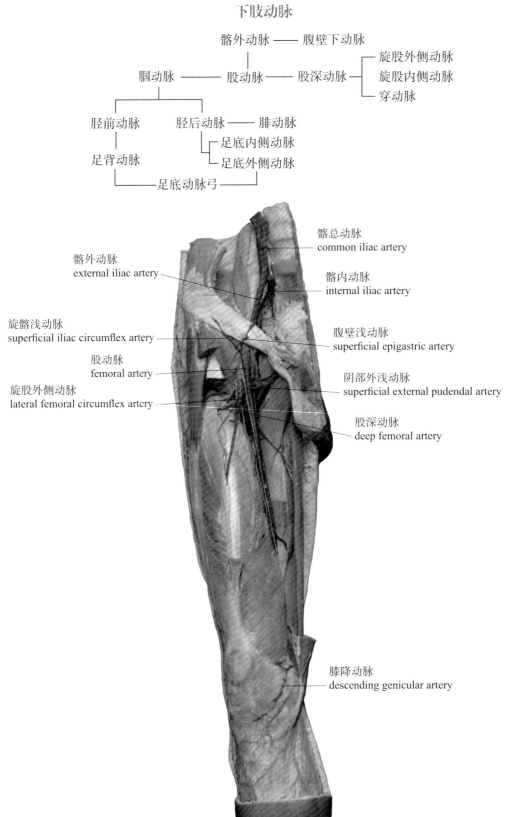

髂外动脉
external iliac artery

旋髂浅动脉
superficial iliac circumflex artery

股动脉
femoral artery

旋股外侧动脉
lateral femoral circumflex artery

髂总动脉
common iliac artery

髂内动脉
internal iliac artery

腹壁浅动脉
superficial epigastric artery

阴部外浅动脉
superficial external pudendal artery

股深动脉
deep femoral artery

膝降动脉
descending genicular artery

图 9-46　股动脉及其分支
Femoral artery and its branches

Anatomical Outline

Arteries of the low limb

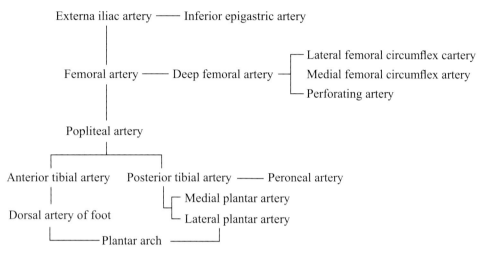

Externa iliac artery —— Inferior epigastric artery

Femoral artery —— Deep femoral artery ⎡ Lateral femoral circumflex cartery
⎢ Medial femoral circumflex artery
⎣ Perforating artery

Popliteal artery

Anterior tibial artery   Posterior tibial artery —— Peroneal artery

Dorsal artery of foot ⎡ Medial plantar artery
⎣ Lateral plantar artery

Plantar arch

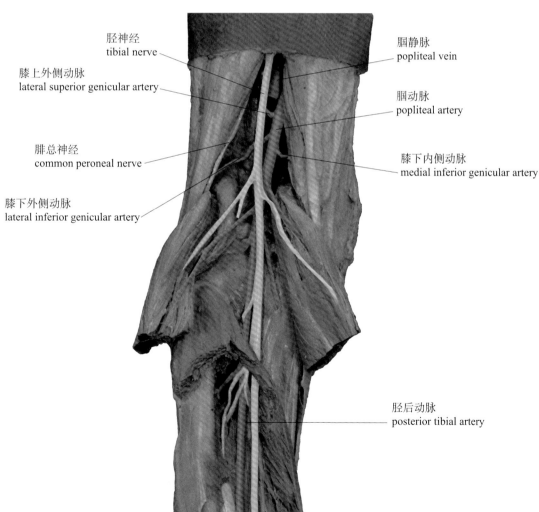

胫神经
tibial nerve

膝上外侧动脉
lateral superior genicular artery

腓总神经
common peroneal nerve

膝下外侧动脉
lateral inferior genicular artery

腘静脉
popliteal vein

腘动脉
popliteal artery

膝下内侧动脉
medial inferior genicular artery

胫后动脉
posterior tibial artery

图 9-47 **腘窝的动脉**
Arteries of popliteal fossa

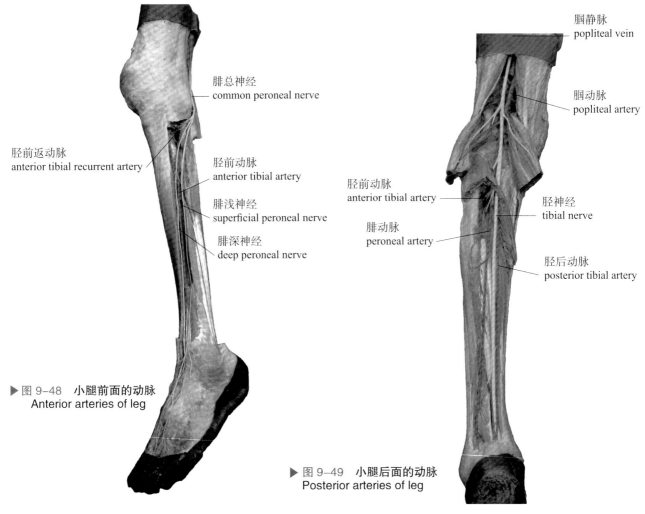

腓总神经
common peroneal nerve

胫前返动脉
anterior tibial recurrent artery

胫前动脉
anterior tibial artery

腓浅神经
superficial peroneal nerve

腓深神经
deep peroneal nerve

▶ 图 9–48　小腿前面的动脉
Anterior arteries of leg

腘静脉
popliteal vein

腘动脉
popliteal artery

胫前动脉
anterior tibial artery

胫神经
tibial nerve

腓动脉
peroneal artery

胫后动脉
posterior tibial artery

▶ 图 9–49　小腿后面的动脉
Posterior arteries of leg

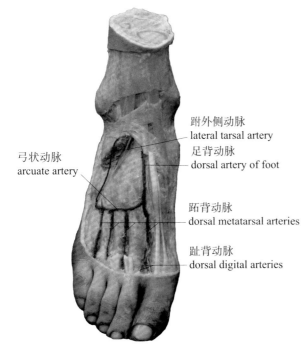

跗外侧动脉
lateral tarsal artery

足背动脉
dorsal artery of foot

弓状动脉
arcuate artery

跖背动脉
dorsal metatarsal arteries

趾背动脉
dorsal digital arteries

图 9–50　足背的动脉
Dorsal arteries of foot

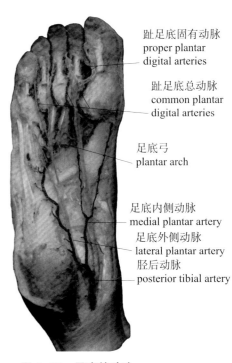

趾足底固有动脉
proper plantar
digital arteries

趾足底总动脉
common plantar
digital arteries

足底弓
plantar arch

足底内侧动脉
medial plantar artery

足底外侧动脉
lateral plantar artery

胫后动脉
posterior tibial artery

图 9–51　足底的动脉
Plantar arteries of foot

第三节 静脉 Section 3 Vein

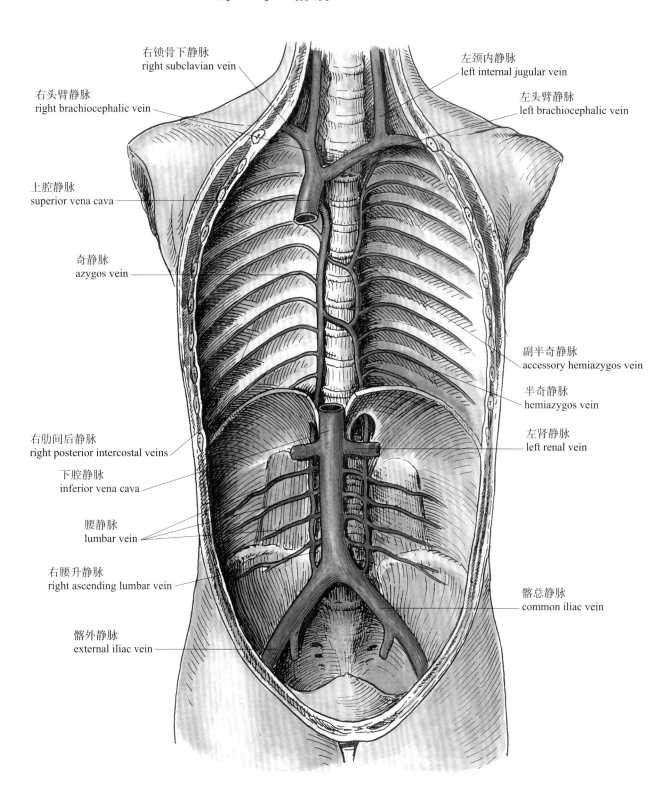

右锁骨下静脉
right subclavian vein

左颈内静脉
left internal jugular vein

右头臂静脉
right brachiocephalic vein

左头臂静脉
left brachiocephalic vein

上腔静脉
superior vena cava

奇静脉
azygos vein

副半奇静脉
accessory hemiazygos vein

半奇静脉
hemiazygos vein

右肋间后静脉
right posterior intercostal veins

左肾静脉
left renal vein

下腔静脉
inferior vena cava

腰静脉
lumbar vein

右腰升静脉
right ascending lumbar vein

髂总静脉
common iliac vein

髂外静脉
external iliac vein

图 9-52 腔静脉及其属支
Vena cava and their tributaries

上腔静脉系的血液流注

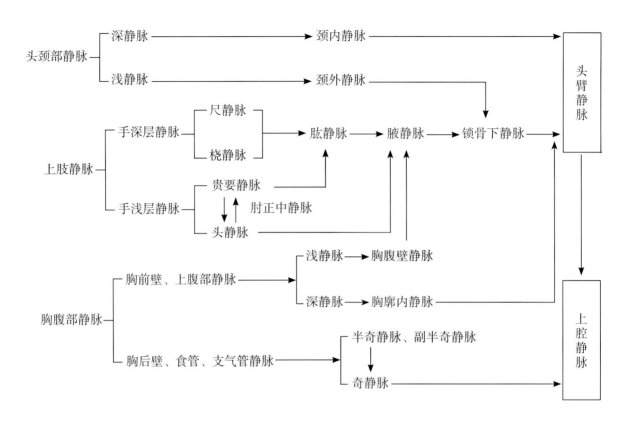

The venous drainage of the superior vena cava

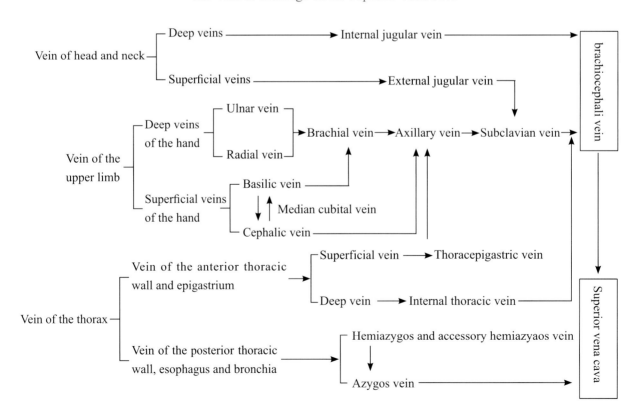

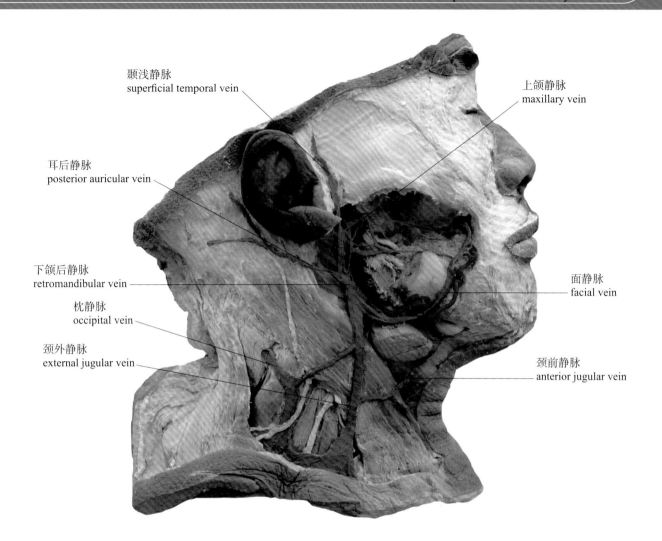

颞浅静脉
superficial temporal vein

上颌静脉
maxillary vein

耳后静脉
posterior auricular vein

下颌后静脉
retromandibular vein

枕静脉
occipital vein

颈外静脉
external jugular vein

面静脉
facial vein

颈前静脉
anterior jugular vein

图 9-53 头、颈部静脉
Veins of head and neck

第三篇 脉管系统
Part 3 Angiology System

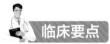 临床要点

1. 面部的"危险三角"：位于鼻根至两口角之间。此处的面静脉及其属支缺乏静脉瓣，且与颅内静脉窦交通，面部发生感染时，可扩散到颅内，导致颅内感染。

2. 颈静脉怒张：正常人站立位或坐位时，颈外静脉常不显露。当有心脏疾病或因上腔静脉阻塞引起中心静脉压升高时，在体表可见静脉充盈，称颈静脉怒张。

Key Points of the Clinic

1. "Danger triangle" of the face: It is located between the root of the nose and the corners of the mouth. The facial veins and their tributaries here lack venous valves, and communicate with the intracranial venous sinus. When an infection occurs on the face, it can spread to the stull, leading to intracranial infection.

2. Jugular vein distention (JVD): The external jugular vein is usually not exposed in standing or sitting position. When the central venous pressure is increased due to heart diseases or blockage of the superior vena cava, venous filling is seen on the body surface, called jugular vein distention.

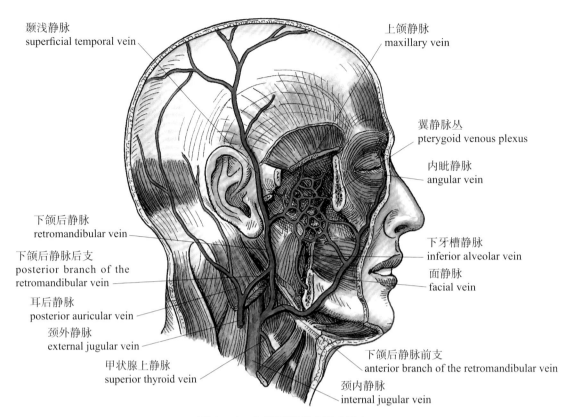

图 9-54　头部深静脉（模式图）
Deep veins of head (diagram)

颅内、外静脉的交通

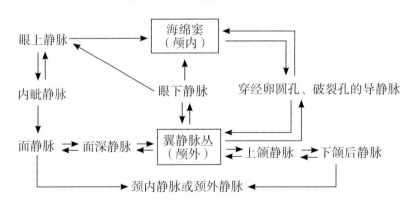

The communications between the intracranial and extracranial veins

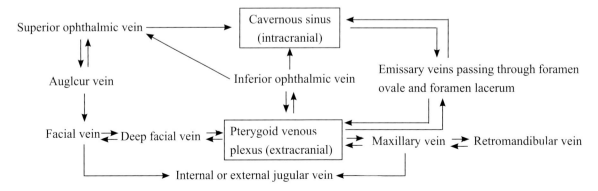

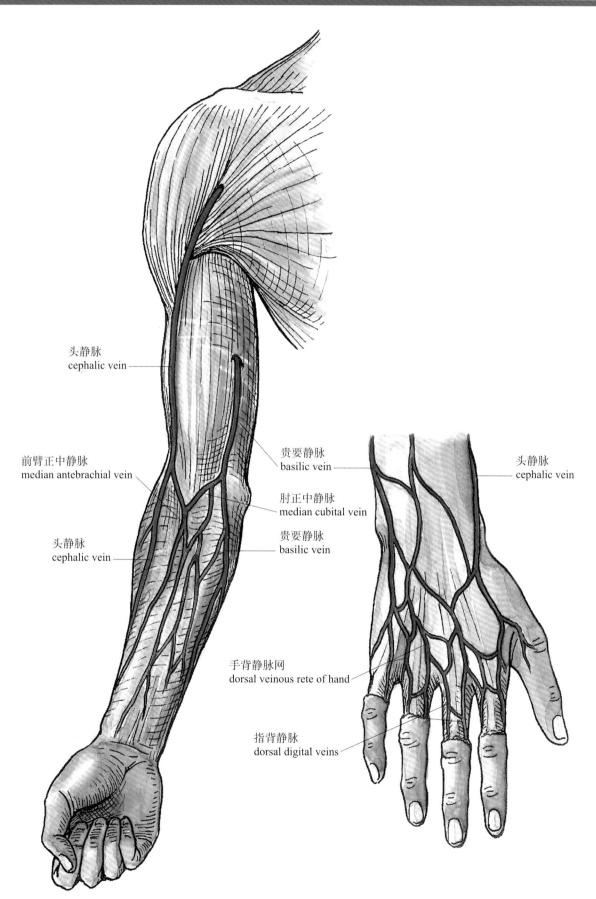

头静脉
cephalic vein

前臂正中静脉
median antebrachial vein

头静脉
cephalic vein

贵要静脉
basilic vein

肘正中静脉
median cubital vein

贵要静脉
basilic vein

头静脉
cephalic vein

手背静脉网
dorsal veinous rete of hand

指背静脉
dorsal digital veins

图 9-55　上肢浅静脉（模式图）
Superficial veins of upper limb (diagram)

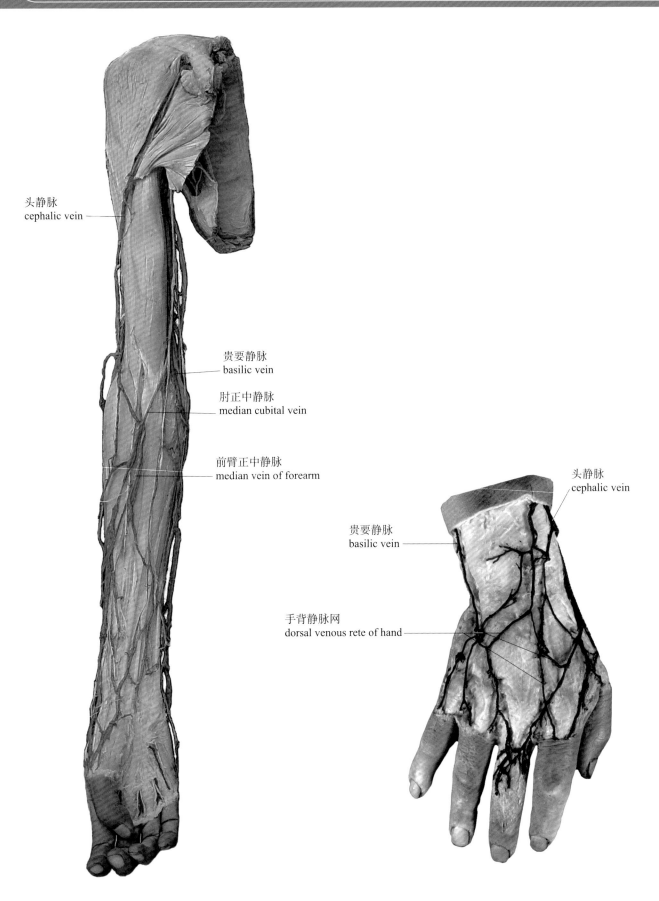

头静脉
cephalic vein

贵要静脉
basilic vein

肘正中静脉
median cubital vein

前臂正中静脉
median vein of forearm

头静脉
cephalic vein

贵要静脉
basilic vein

手背静脉网
dorsal venous rete of hand

图 9-56　上肢浅静脉
Superficial veins of upper limb

图 9-57　手背静脉网
Dorsal venous rete of hand

下腔静脉系的血液流注

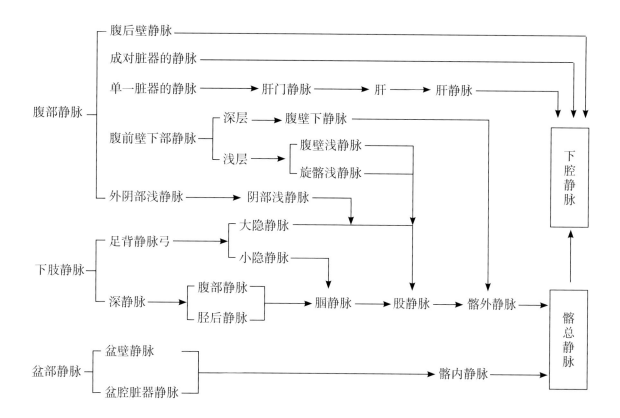

The venous drainage of the inferior vena cava system

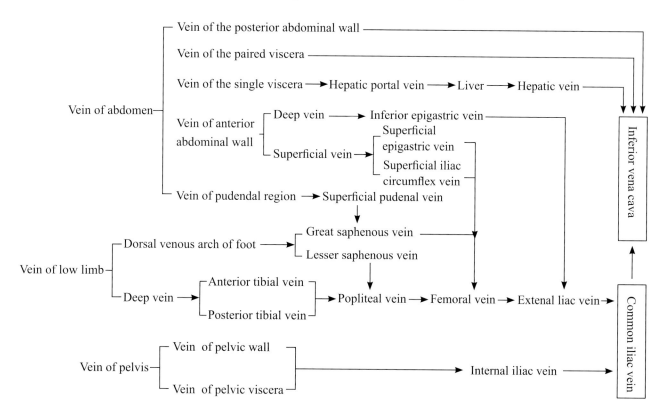

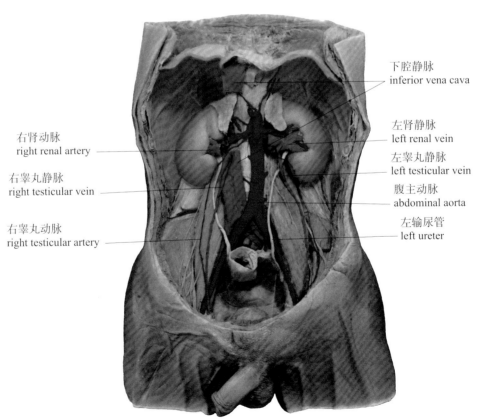

右颈内静脉
right internal jugular vein

右锁骨下静脉
right subclavian vein

右头臂静脉
right brachiocephalic vein

奇静脉
azygos vein

右肋间后静脉
right posterior intercostal veins

左颈内静脉
left internal jugular vein

左锁骨下静脉
left subclavian vein

左头臂静脉
left brachiocephalic vein

上腔静脉
superior vena cava

半奇静脉
hemiazygos vein

图 9–58　奇静脉、半奇静脉
Azygos vein and hemiazygos vein

下腔静脉
inferior vena cava

右肾动脉
right renal artery

右睾丸静脉
right testicular vein

右睾丸动脉
right testicular artery

左肾静脉
left renal vein

左睾丸静脉
left testicular vein

腹主动脉
abdominal aorta

左输尿管
left ureter

图 9–59　腹后壁的静脉
Veins of posterior abdominal wall

1. 在大隐静脉管腔内，有9~10对静脉瓣，呈袋状，可保证血液向心回流。

2. 大隐静脉曲张是常见的下肢静脉病理改变。其曲张静脉的瓣膜呈瘤样扩张，皮下可见变色迂曲血管。损伤使下肢浅静脉与深静脉汇合处的瓣膜失去"单向阀门"的作用，出现下肢血液回流障碍、静脉血液倒流、大隐静脉瘀血，造成静脉迂曲、扩张。

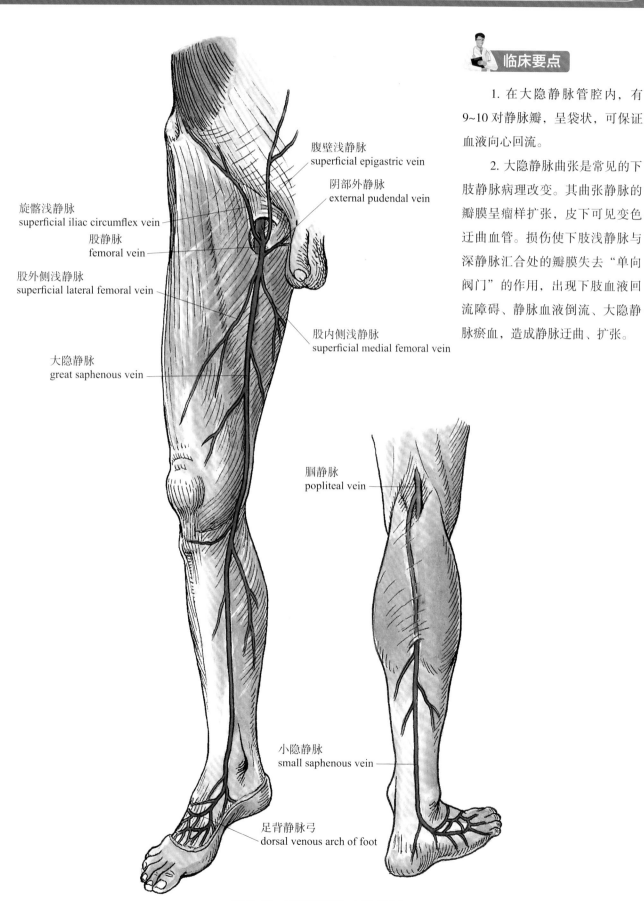

腹壁浅静脉
superficial epigastric vein

阴部外静脉
external pudendal vein

旋髂浅静脉
superficial iliac circumflex vein

股静脉
femoral vein

股外侧浅静脉
superficial lateral femoral vein

股内侧浅静脉
superficial medial femoral vein

大隐静脉
great saphenous vein

腘静脉
popliteal vein

小隐静脉
small saphenous vein

足背静脉弓
dorsal venous arch of foot

图 9-60　下肢浅静脉（模式图）
Superficial veins of lower limb (diagram)

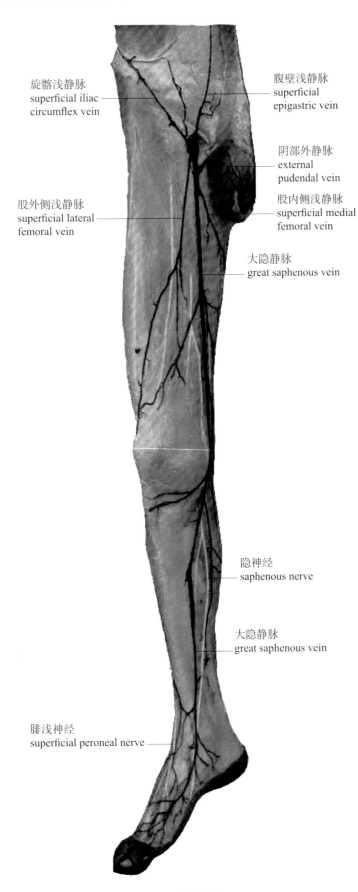

旋髂浅静脉
superficial iliac
circumflex vein

腹壁浅静脉
superficial
epigastric vein

阴部外静脉
external
pudendal vein

股外侧浅静脉
superficial lateral
femoral vein

股内侧浅静脉
superficial medial
femoral vein

大隐静脉
great saphenous vein

隐神经
saphenous nerve

大隐静脉
great saphenous vein

腓浅神经
superficial peroneal nerve

图 9-61　大隐静脉
Great saphenous vein

Key Points of the Clinic

1. Within the great saphenous vein lumen, there are 9 to 10 pairs of venous valves. Usually the two valves face each other in a pouch shape to ensure a return of blood to the heart.

2. Varicosis of great saphenous vein is a common pathological change of lower extremity vein. The valve of its varicose vein is tumor like dilate, subcutaneous visible discoloration tortuous vessels. The valve injury makes the valve at the confluence of superficial vein and deep vein of lower limb lose the function of "one-way valve", the lower limb blood backflow disorder, venous blood backflow, great saphenous vein stasis, make the vein tortuosity, expansion.

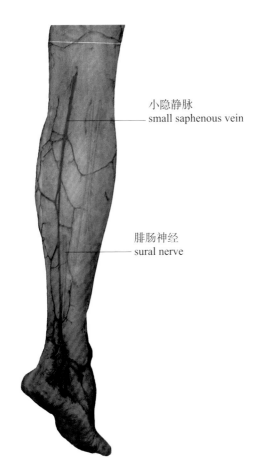

小隐静脉
small saphenous vein

腓肠神经
sural nerve

图 9-62　小隐静脉
Small saphenous vein

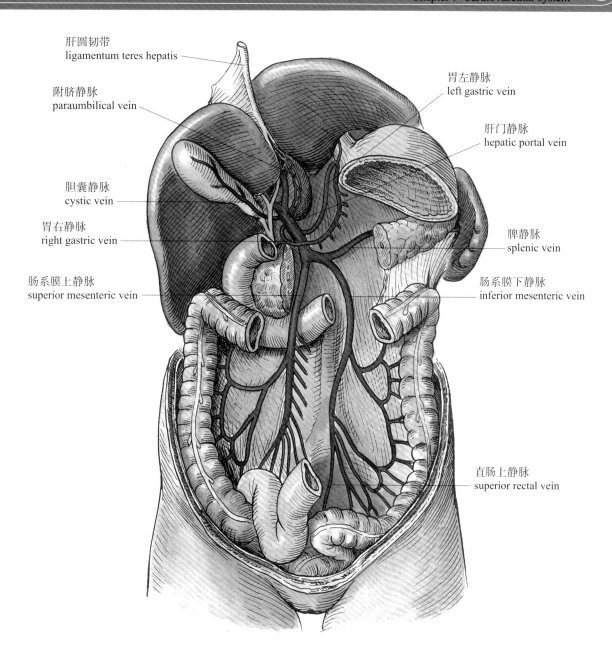

肝圆韧带
ligamentum teres hepatis

附脐静脉
paraumbilical vein

胆囊静脉
cystic vein

胃右静脉
right gastric vein

肠系膜上静脉
superior mesenteric vein

胃左静脉
left gastric vein

肝门静脉
hepatic portal vein

脾静脉
splenic vein

肠系膜下静脉
inferior mesenteric vein

直肠上静脉
superior rectal vein

图 9-63　肝门静脉及其属支
Hepatic portal vein and its tributaries

门静脉与腔静脉吻合

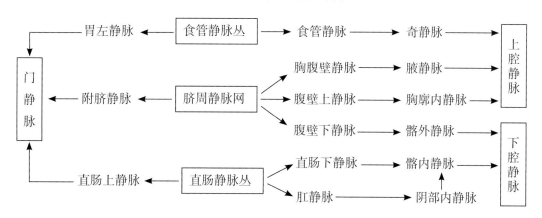

胃左静脉 ← 食管静脉丛 → 食管静脉 → 奇静脉 → 上腔静脉

门静脉 ← 附脐静脉 ← 脐周静脉网 → 胸腹壁静脉 → 腋静脉 → 上腔静脉

脐周静脉网 → 腹壁上静脉 → 胸廓内静脉 → 上腔静脉

脐周静脉网 → 腹壁下静脉 → 髂外静脉 → 下腔静脉

直肠上静脉 ← 直肠静脉丛 → 直肠下静脉 → 髂内静脉 → 下腔静脉

直肠静脉丛 → 肛静脉 → 阴部内静脉

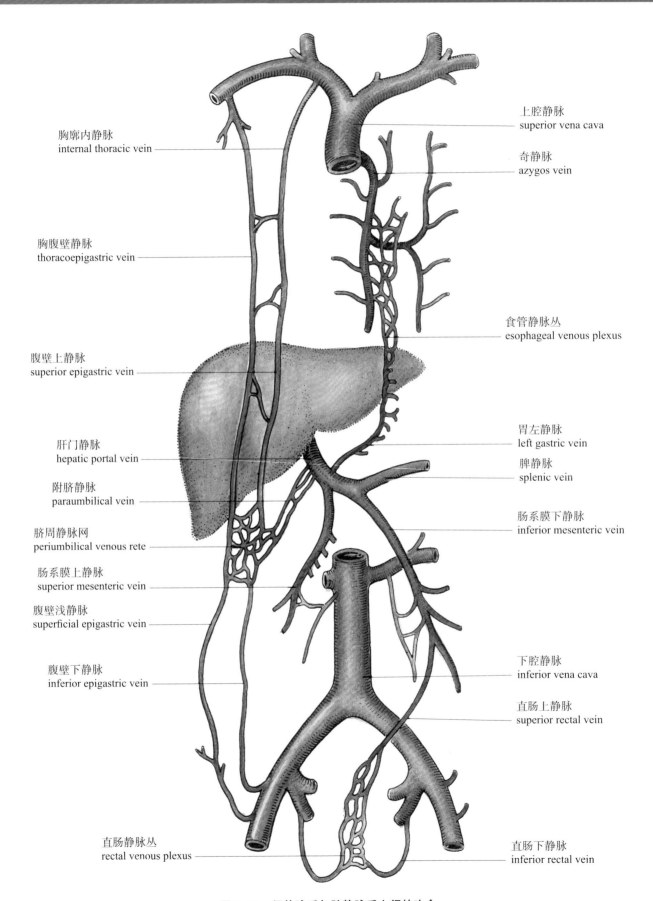

胸廓内静脉
internal thoracic vein

胸腹壁静脉
thoracoepigastric vein

腹壁上静脉
superior epigastric vein

肝门静脉
hepatic portal vein

附脐静脉
paraumbilical vein

脐周静脉网
periumbilical venous rete

肠系膜上静脉
superior mesenteric vein

腹壁浅静脉
superficial epigastric vein

腹壁下静脉
inferior epigastric vein

直肠静脉丛
rectal venous plexus

上腔静脉
superior vena cava

奇静脉
azygos vein

食管静脉丛
esophageal venous plexus

胃左静脉
left gastric vein

脾静脉
splenic vein

肠系膜下静脉
inferior mesenteric vein

下腔静脉
inferior vena cava

直肠上静脉
superior rectal vein

直肠下静脉
inferior rectal vein

图 9-64　门静脉系与腔静脉系之间的吻合
Anastomoses between portal venous system and vena caval system

Anastomoses between the portal vein and the vena cava

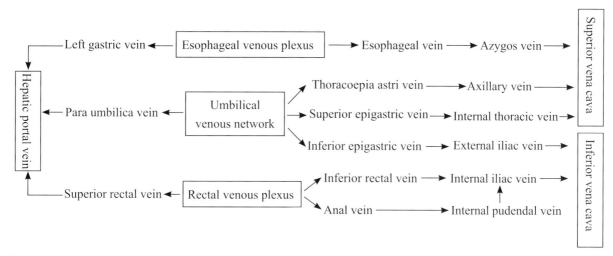

 临床要点

门静脉高压是由门静脉压力持久增高引起的一系列症状。门静脉压力增高后，门静脉属支静脉回流受阻，门-体静脉间的交通支开放，大量门静脉血直接经交通支进入体循环，结果出现静脉曲张，如食管静脉丛、直肠静脉丛和脐周静脉丛曲张，脾肿大和脾功能亢进，肝功能失代偿和腹水等。

Key Points of the Clinic

Portal hypertension is a group of symptoms caused by prolonged increased portal pressure. After the portal vein blood pressure is increased, the tributaries of portal vein reflux are blocked by the venous return, and the communicating branches between the portal vein and the vena cava are open. a large number of portal vein blood enters the systemic circulation directly through the communicating branches. The result appears the varicose veins, such as esophageal vein plexus, rectal vein plexus, and periumbilical vein plexus, splenomegaly and hypersplenism, liver dysfunction and ascites and so on.

第十章 淋巴系统

Chapter 10 Lymphatic system

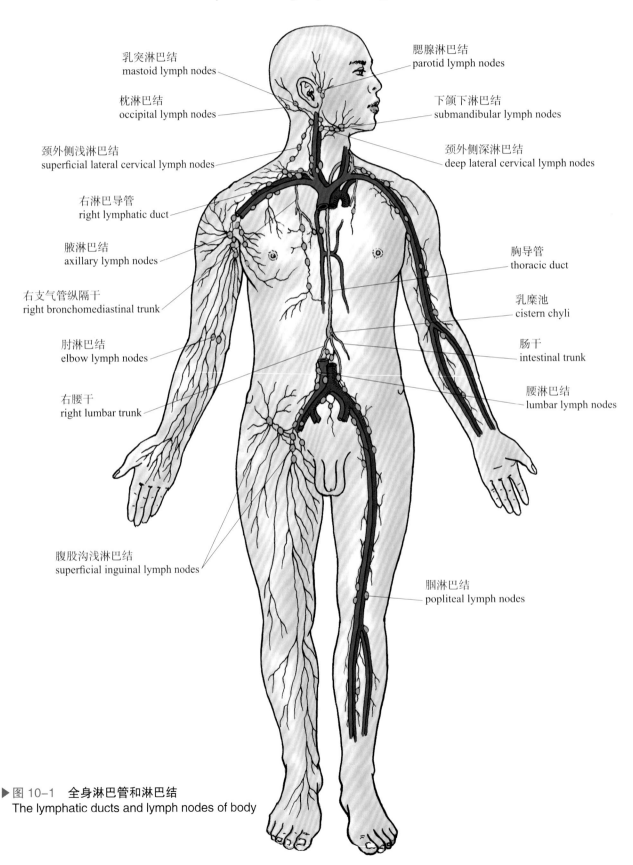

乳突淋巴结
mastoid lymph nodes

枕淋巴结
occipital lymph nodes

颈外侧浅淋巴结
superficial lateral cervical lymph nodes

右淋巴导管
right lymphatic duct

腋淋巴结
axillary lymph nodes

右支气管纵隔干
right bronchomediastinal trunk

肘淋巴结
elbow lymph nodes

右腰干
right lumbar trunk

腹股沟浅淋巴结
superficial inguinal lymph nodes

腮腺淋巴结
parotid lymph nodes

下颌下淋巴结
submandibular lymph nodes

颈外侧深淋巴结
deep lateral cervical lymph nodes

胸导管
thoracic duct

乳糜池
cistern chyli

肠干
intestinal trunk

腰淋巴结
lumbar lymph nodes

腘淋巴结
popliteal lymph nodes

▶图 10-1 全身淋巴管和淋巴结
The lymphatic ducts and lymph nodes of body

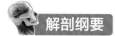 解剖纲要

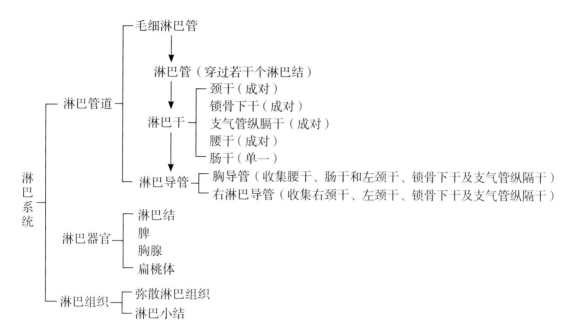

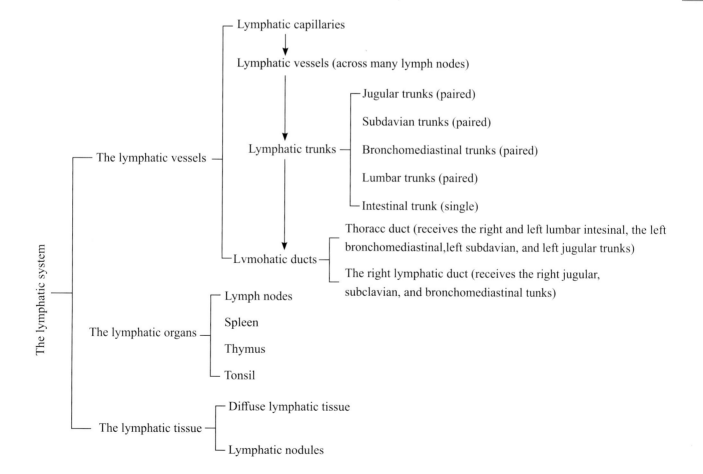 Anatomical Outline

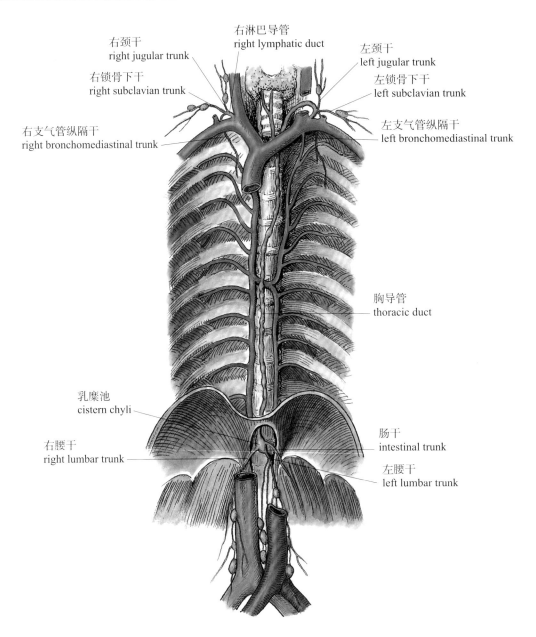

右颈干
right jugular trunk

右淋巴导管
right lymphatic duct

左颈干
left jugular trunk

右锁骨下干
right subclavian trunk

左锁骨下干
left subclavian trunk

右支气管纵隔干
right bronchomediastinal trunk

左支气管纵隔干
left bronchomediastinal trunk

胸导管
thoracic duct

乳糜池
cistern chyli

肠干
intestinal trunk

右腰干
right lumbar trunk

左腰干
left lumbar trunk

图 10-2　胸导管（模式图）
Thoracic duct (diagram)

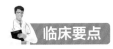　临床要点

胸导管的临床解剖要点

1. 胸导管起始处的膨大称乳糜池，因接收从肠干输入的乳糜微粒，故得名。由此向上，胸导管内的淋巴液呈乳白色，而非无色透明。

2. 胸导管常发出较细的侧支注入奇静脉和肋间后静脉，故手术误将胸导管末段结扎后，一般不会引起严重的淋巴淤积。

3. 胸导管上段与左纵隔胸膜相邻，下段与右纵隔胸膜相邻。若上段损伤合并胸膜破裂常引起左侧乳糜胸；下段损伤常引起右侧乳糜胸。

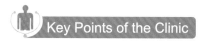 Key Points of the Clinic

The clinic anatomic key points of thoracic duct

1. Dilatation at the beginning of the thoracic duct is called cisterna chyli, which is named for receiving chylous particles from the intestinal trunk. Upward from the thoracic duct, the lymphatic fluid in the thoracic duct is milky white, not colorless and transparent.

2. The thoracic duct often gives off the finer collateral branches, by which the lymph is drained into the azygos vein and the posterior intercostal veins. Therefore, the operation generally will not cause serious lymph accumulation after ligation of the thoracic duct by mistake.

3. The upper segment of the thoracic duct is adjacent to the left mediastinal pleura, and the lower segment is adjacent to the right mediastinal pleura. If the injury in the upper part of the duct combined with pleural rupture often cause left chylothorax; the injury in the lower part of the duct often causes right chylothorax.

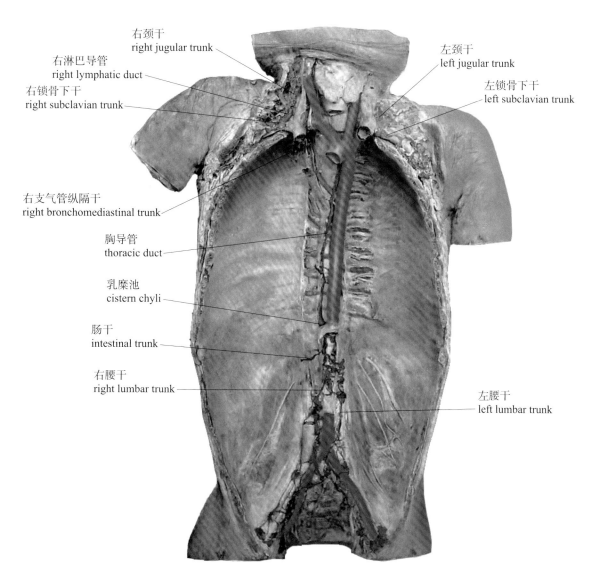

右颈干
right jugular trunk

右淋巴导管
right lymphatic duct

右锁骨下干
right subclavian trunk

左颈干
left jugular trunk

左锁骨下干
left subclavian trunk

右支气管纵隔干
right bronchomediastinal trunk

胸导管
thoracic duct

乳糜池
cistern chyli

肠干
intestinal trunk

右腰干
right lumbar trunk

左腰干
left lumbar trunk

图 10-3　胸导管
Thoracic duct

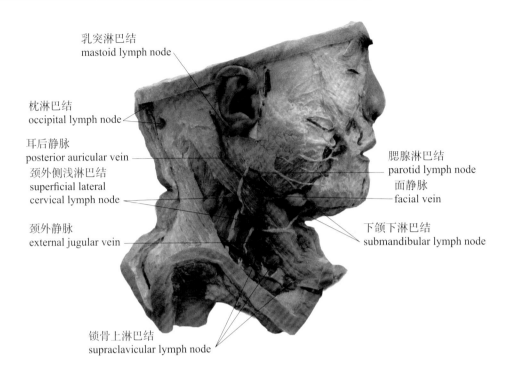

乳突淋巴结
mastoid lymph node

枕淋巴结
occipital lymph node

耳后静脉
posterior auricular vein

颈外侧浅淋巴结
superficial lateral
cervical lymph node

颈外静脉
external jugular vein

腮腺淋巴结
parotid lymph node

面静脉
facial vein

下颌下淋巴结
submandibular lymph node

锁骨上淋巴结
supraclavicular lymph node

图 10-4　颈淋巴结
The lymph nodes of neck

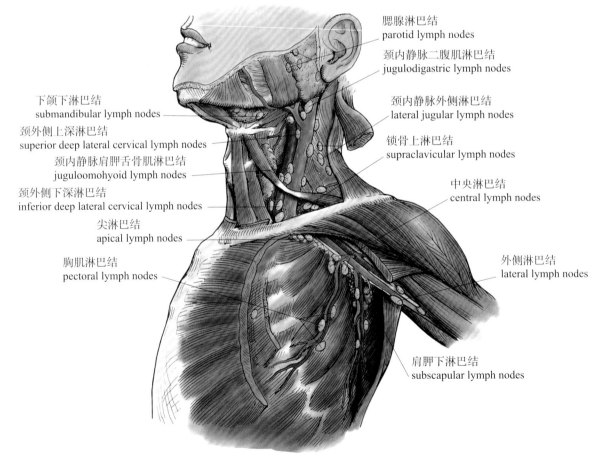

腮腺淋巴结
parotid lymph nodes

颈内静脉二腹肌淋巴结
jugulodigastric lymph nodes

下颌下淋巴结
submandibular lymph nodes

颈外侧上深淋巴结
superior deep lateral cervical lymph nodes

颈内静脉肩胛舌骨肌淋巴结
juguloomohyoid lymph nodes

颈外侧下深淋巴结
inferior deep lateral cervical lymph nodes

尖淋巴结
apical lymph nodes

胸肌淋巴结
pectoral lymph nodes

颈内静脉外侧淋巴结
lateral jugular lymph nodes

锁骨上淋巴结
supraclavicular lymph nodes

中央淋巴结
central lymph nodes

外侧淋巴结
lateral lymph nodes

肩胛下淋巴结
subscapular lymph nodes

图 10-5　颈深部及腋窝淋巴结（模式图）
Deep lymph nodes of neck and axillary（diagram）

上肢淋巴结

分群	位置	收容范围	输出管注入淋巴结或干
滑车上淋巴结	肱骨内上髁上方	手尺侧半、手掌和前臂	腋淋巴结
外侧淋巴结	腋静脉远侧端	上肢浅淋巴	中央、尖淋巴结
胸肌淋巴结（前群）	胸外侧血管	脐以上胸、腹壁浅层及乳房大部	中央、尖淋巴结
肩胛下淋巴结（后群）	肩胛下血管	项背部浅、深淋巴	中央、尖淋巴结
中央淋巴结	腋窝中央疏松结缔组织	外侧群、前群和后群淋巴结输出管	尖淋巴结
尖淋巴结	腋静脉近侧端	上述各群	锁骨下干

The lymph nodes of the upper limb

Groups	Location	Region of the lymphatic drainage	Efferent ducts drain into lymph nodes or trunk
Supratrochlear lymph nodes	Above medial epicondyle of humerus	Hand ulnar half, palm and forearm	Axillary lymph nodes
Lateral lymph nodes	The distal end of the axillary vein	Superficial lymph of upper limb	Central and apical lymph nodes
Pectoral lymph nodes (anterior group)	Lateral thoracic vessels	Superficial layer of the thoracic, abdominal wall above the umbilicus, majority part of the breast	Central and apical lymph nodes
Subscapular lymph node (posterior group)	Subscapular vessels	Superficial or deep lymph of nape and back	Central and apical lymph nodes
Central lymph nodes	Loose connective tissue in the axillary center	Efferent duct of the lateral group, anterior group, and posterior group lymph nodes	Apical lymph nodes
Apical lymph nodes	Proximal end of the axillary vein	Above groups	Subclavian trunks

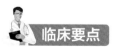 **临床要点**

腋淋巴结群

腋窝淋巴结是上肢最大的淋巴结组群。1/3 以上的乳腺癌患者有腋窝淋巴结转移。患者患病初期即可出现同侧腋窝淋巴结肿大。随着病情发展，淋巴结逐渐融合，并与皮肤和周围组织粘连、固定。晚期可在锁骨上和对侧腋窝出现转移的淋巴结。

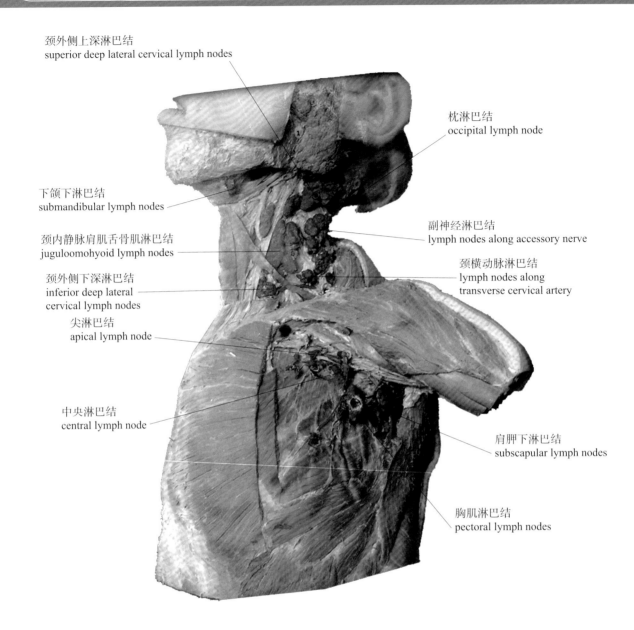

颈外侧上深淋巴结
superior deep lateral cervical lymph nodes

枕淋巴结
occipital lymph node

下颌下淋巴结
submandibular lymph nodes

副神经淋巴结
lymph nodes along accessory nerve

颈内静脉肩肌舌骨肌淋巴结
juguloomohyoid lymph nodes

颈横动脉淋巴结
lymph nodes along transverse cervical artery

颈外侧下深淋巴结
inferior deep lateral cervical lymph nodes

尖淋巴结
apical lymph node

中央淋巴结
central lymph node

肩胛下淋巴结
subscapular lymph nodes

胸肌淋巴结
pectoral lymph nodes

图 10-6　颈深部及腋窝淋巴结
Deep lymph nodes of neck and axillary

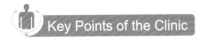 Key Points of the Clinic

Axillary lymph nodes group

Axillary lymph nodes are the largest group of lymph nodes in the upper extremities. More than 1/3 of breast cancer patients have axillary lymph nodes metastasis. In the early stage of the disease, ipsilateral axillary lymph nodes enlargement may occur. As the disease progresses, the lymph nodes gradually fuse each other. lymph nodes become adherent and fixed to the skin and surrounding tissues. Metastatic lymph nodes may appear late in the supraclavicular regin and contralateral axilla.

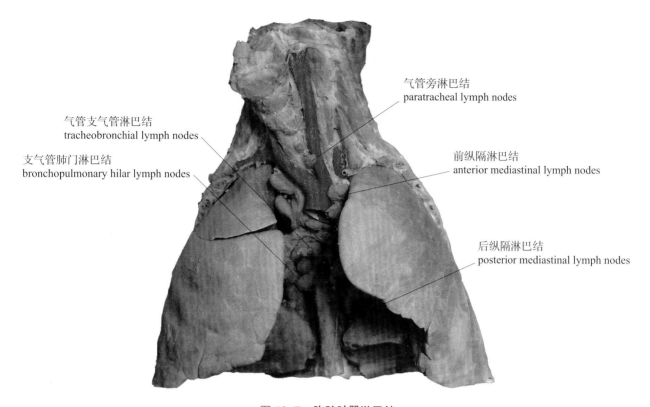

气管支气管淋巴结
tracheobronchial lymph nodes

支气管肺门淋巴结
bronchopulmonary hilar lymph nodes

气管旁淋巴结
paratracheal lymph nodes

前纵隔淋巴结
anterior mediastinal lymph nodes

后纵隔淋巴结
posterior mediastinal lymph nodes

图 10-7 胸腔脏器淋巴结
Lymph nodes of thoracic viscera

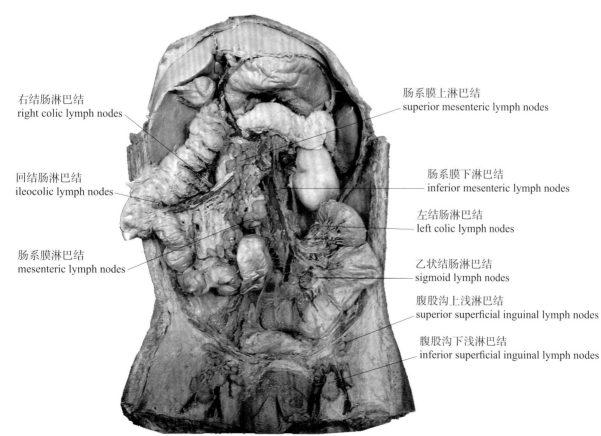

右结肠淋巴结
right colic lymph nodes

回结肠淋巴结
ileocolic lymph nodes

肠系膜淋巴结
mesenteric lymph nodes

肠系膜上淋巴结
superior mesenteric lymph nodes

肠系膜下淋巴结
inferior mesenteric lymph nodes

左结肠淋巴结
left colic lymph nodes

乙状结肠淋巴结
sigmoid lymph nodes

腹股沟上浅淋巴结
superior superficial inguinal lymph nodes

腹股沟下浅淋巴结
inferior superficial inguinal lymph nodes

图 10-8 肠系膜淋巴结
Mesenteric lymph nodes

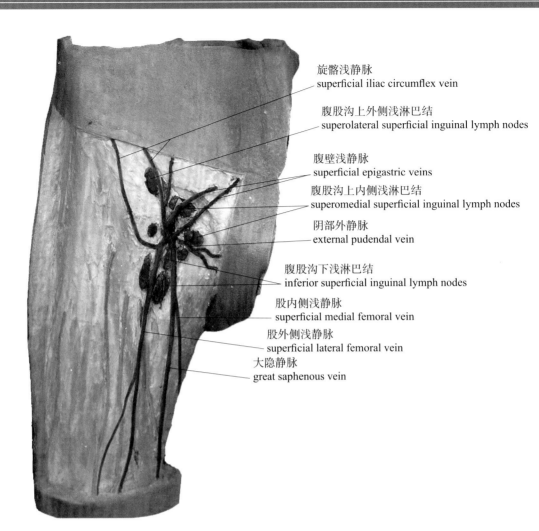

旋髂浅静脉
superficial iliac circumflex vein

腹股沟上外侧浅淋巴结
superolateral superficial inguinal lymph nodes

腹壁浅静脉
superficial epigastric veins

腹股沟上内侧浅淋巴结
superomedial superficial inguinal lymph nodes

阴部外静脉
external pudendal vein

腹股沟下浅淋巴结
inferior superficial inguinal lymph nodes

股内侧浅静脉
superficial medial femoral vein

股外侧浅静脉
superficial lateral femoral vein

大隐静脉
great saphenous vein

图 10-9 腹股沟浅淋巴结
Superficial inguinal lymph nodes

下肢的淋巴结

分群	位置	收容范围	输出管注入
腘淋巴结	沿小隐静脉末端和腘血管排列	足、小腿	腹股沟深淋巴结
腹股沟浅淋巴结	腹股沟韧带下方，分上、下2群，上群与腹股沟韧带平行，下群沿大隐静脉末端排列	上群：腹前外侧壁下部、臀部、会阴和子宫底 下群：下肢浅淋巴管	腹股沟深淋巴结或髂外淋巴结
腹股沟深淋巴结	股静脉周围和股管内	大腿和会阴深部淋巴，腘和腹股沟浅淋巴结的输出	髂外淋巴结

The lymph nodes of the lower limb

Groups	Location	Region of the lymphatic drainage	Drainage of the efferent duct
Popliteal lymph nodes	Along the end of the small saphenous vein and the popliteal vessels	Foot, crus	Deep inguinal lymph nodes
Superficial inguinal lymph nodes	Below the inguinal ligament, there are two groups. The upper group is parallel to the inguinal ligament, and the lower group are arranged along the end of the great saphenous vein	Upper group: lower anterior lateral abdominal wall, hips, perineum, and uterine bottom. Lower group: superficial lymph drainage of the lower limbs	Deep inguinal lymph nodes or external iliac lymph nodes
Deep inguinal lymph nodes	Around the femoral vein and inside the femoral canal	Deep lymph of the thigh and perineum, superficial lymph of popliteal and inguinal nodes	External iliac lymph nodes

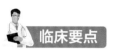 临床要点

腹股沟淋巴结群

腹股沟淋巴结主要引流下肢、下腹壁和会阴部的淋巴。腹股沟淋巴结肿大常提示其引流淋巴的组织器官出现了病变，以便进一步诊断和治疗。

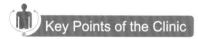 Key Points of the Clinic

Inguinal lymph nodes group

The inguinal lymph nodes mainly drain the lower limbs, the lower abdominal wall and the lymph nodes of the perineum. The inguinal lymphadenopathy often indicates a lesion in the tissues and organs around the lymph nodes for further diagnosis and treatment.

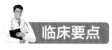 临床要点

脾破裂：脾质软而脆，是腹腔内最容易受损伤的器官。当受外力作用脾脏容易损伤破裂。

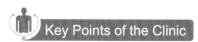 Key Points of the Clinic

Spleen rupture: spleen is soft and brittle, and is the most vulnerable organ in the abdominal cavity. The spleen is easily damaged and ruptured when subjected to the external force.

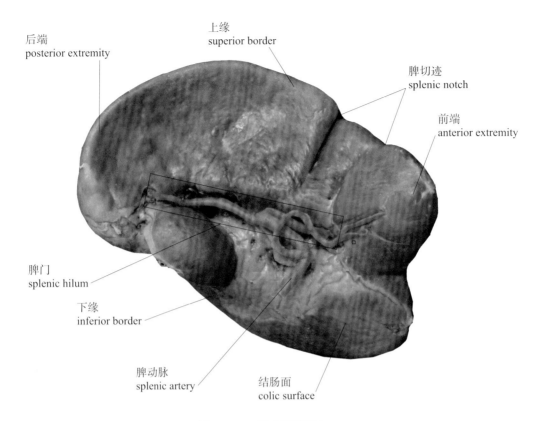

后端
posterior extremity

上缘
superior border

脾切迹
splenic notch

前端
anterior extremity

脾门
splenic hilum

下缘
inferior border

脾动脉
splenic artery

结肠面
colic surface

图 10-10　脾（脏面观）
Spleen (visceral surface view)

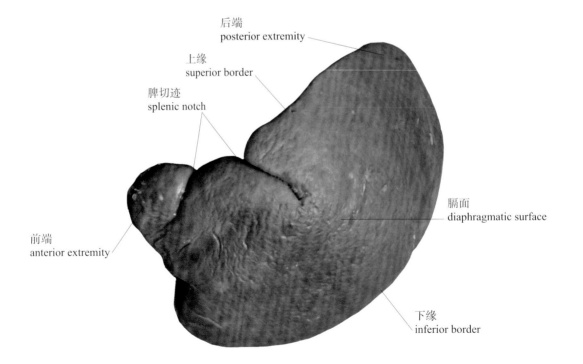

后端
posterior extremity

上缘
superior border

脾切迹
splenic notch

膈面
diaphragmatic surface

前端
anterior extremity

下缘
inferior border

图 10-11　脾（膈面观）
Spleen (diaphragmatic surface view)

第四篇
感觉器

Part 4 Sensory Organs

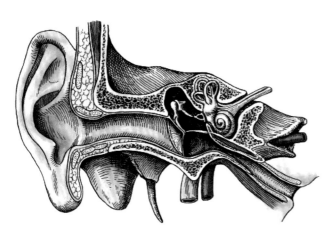

第十一章 视器

Chapter 11 Visual organ

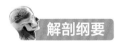 解剖纲要

视器的构成：视器由眼球和眼副器构成。眼球包括眼球壁和眼球内容物。眼球壁由 3 层组成，从外向内依次是纤维膜（角膜和巩膜）、血管膜（虹膜、睫状体和脉络膜）和视网膜。眼副器包括眼睑、结膜、泪器、眼球外肌等。

Anatomical Outline

Constitution of visual organ: Visual organ is composed of eyeball and accessory organs of eye. The eyeball includes the wall of eyeball and the contents. The wall of eyeball consists of three tunics, from outside inwards, which are the fibrous tunic (cornea and sclera), the vascular tunic (iris, ciliary body and choroid) and the retina. The accessory organs of eye include eyelid/palpebrae, conjunctiva, lacrimal apparatus, extraocular muscles and so on.

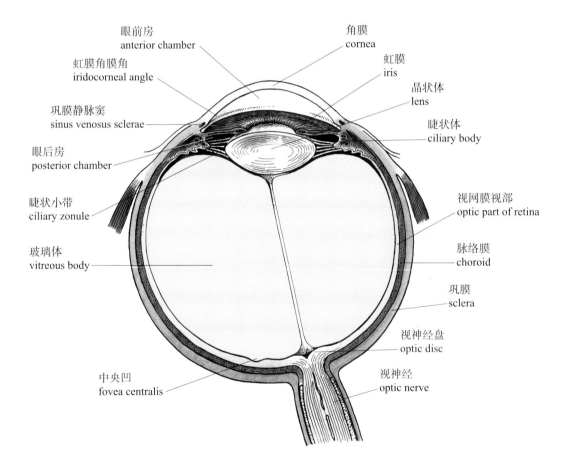

图 11-1 眼球水平切面
Horizontal section of eyeball

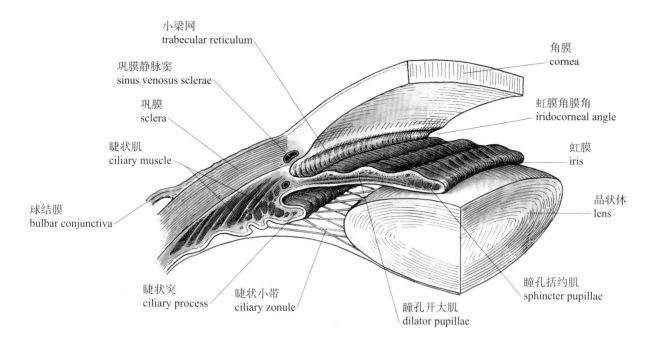

图 11-2 眼球前部切面
Section of anterior part of eyeball

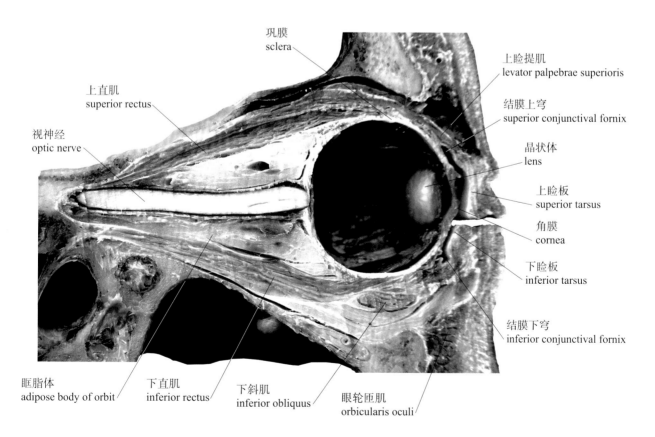

图 11-3 眶腔和眼球的矢状切面
Sagittal section of orbital cavity and eyeball

第四篇 感觉器
Part 4 Sensory Organs

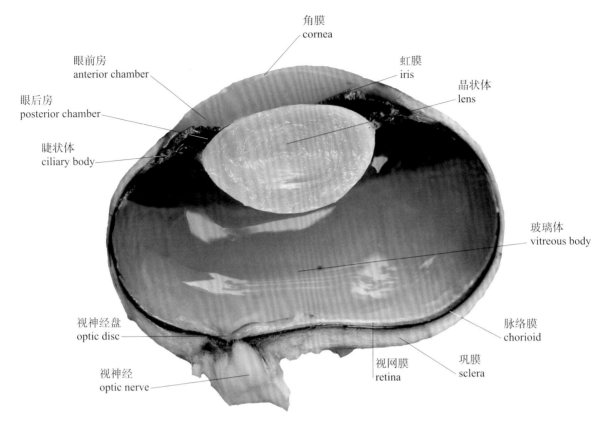

角膜
cornea

虹膜
iris

晶状体
lens

眼前房
anterior chamber

眼后房
posterior chamber

睫状体
ciliary body

玻璃体
vitreous body

视神经盘
optic disc

视神经
optic nerve

视网膜
retina

巩膜
sclera

脉络膜
chorioid

图 11-4　眼球矢状切面
Sagittal section of eyeball

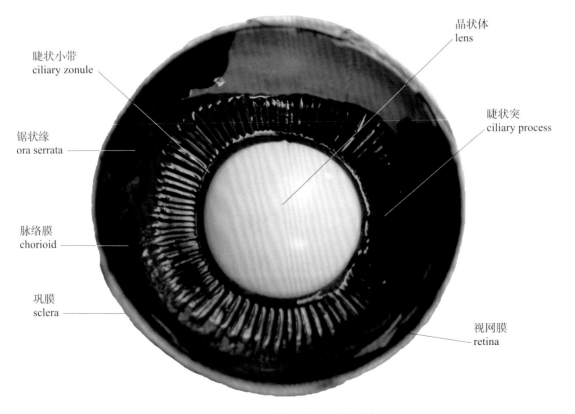

晶状体
lens

睫状小带
ciliary zonule

睫状突
ciliary process

锯状缘
ora serrata

脉络膜
chorioid

巩膜
sclera

视网膜
retina

图 11-5　眼球前半部（后面观）
Anterior part of the eyeball (posterior view)

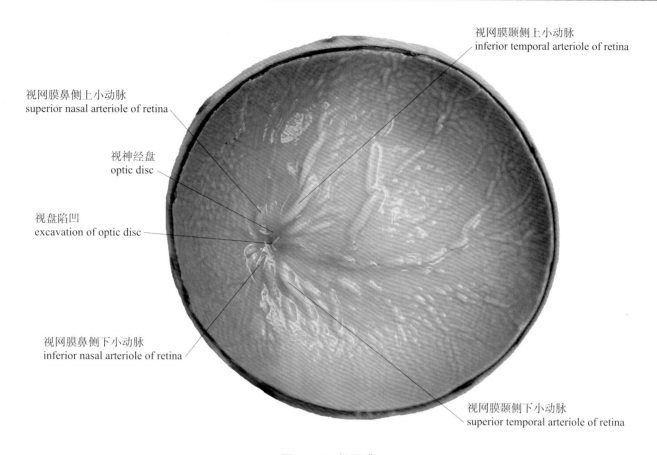

图 11-6 视网膜
Retina

视网膜颞侧上小动脉
inferior temporal arteriole of retina

视网膜鼻侧上小动脉
superior nasal arteriole of retina

视神经盘
optic disc

视盘陷凹
excavation of optic disc

视网膜鼻侧下小动脉
inferior nasal arteriole of retina

视网膜颞侧下小动脉
superior temporal arteriole of retina

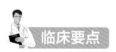 临床要点

1. 视网膜脱离：视网膜视部分为两层，外层是色素上皮层，内层是神经层，是视网膜的固有结构，两层之间有一潜在性间隙，是临床上造成视网膜脱离的解剖学基础。

2. 白内障：晶状体位于虹膜和玻璃体之间，呈双凸透镜状。由于老化、疾病或创伤使晶状体变混浊，称为白内障。此时光线被混浊晶状体阻扰无法投射在视网膜上，导致视物模糊，常见于糖尿病并发症患者或老年人。

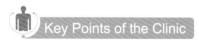 Key Points of the Clinic

1. The retinal detachment：The optic part of retina consists of two layers. The outer layer is the pigment epithelium, and the inner one is the nervous layer which is the inherent structure of the retina. There is a potential gap between the two layers, which is the anatomical basis of the retinal detachment in clinical.

2. Cataract：The lens is located between iris and vitreous, showing a double convex lens. The lens becomes turbid due to aging, disease or trauma, called cataract. At this time, the incoming light is blocked by the turbid lens and cannot be projected on the retina, resulting in blurred vision. It is common in patients with diabetic complications or the elderly.

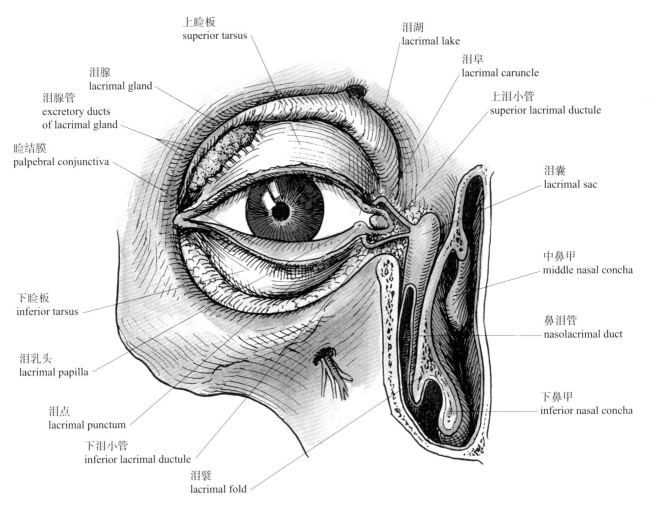

上睑板
superior tarsus

泪湖
lacrimal lake

泪腺
lacrimal gland

泪阜
lacrimal caruncle

泪腺管
excretory ducts
of lacrimal gland

上泪小管
superior lacrimal ductule

睑结膜
palpebral conjunctiva

泪囊
lacrimal sac

中鼻甲
middle nasal concha

下睑板
inferior tarsus

鼻泪管
nasolacrimal duct

泪乳头
lacrimal papilla

下鼻甲
inferior nasal concha

泪点
lacrimal punctum

下泪小管
inferior lacrimal ductule

泪襞
lacrimal fold

图 11-7　泪器（模式图）
Lacrimal apparatus (diagram)

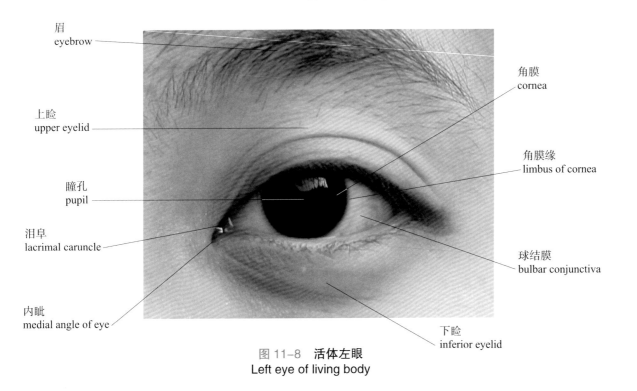

眉
eyebrow

角膜
cornea

上睑
upper eyelid

角膜缘
limbus of cornea

瞳孔
pupil

泪阜
lacrimal caruncle

球结膜
bulbar conjunctiva

内眦
medial angle of eye

下睑
inferior eyelid

图 11-8　活体左眼
Left eye of living body

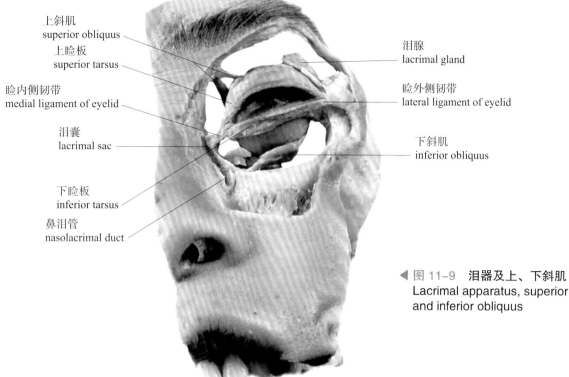

上斜肌
superior obliquus

上睑板
superior tarsus

睑内侧韧带
medial ligament of eyelid

泪囊
lacrimal sac

下睑板
inferior tarsus

鼻泪管
nasolacrimal duct

泪腺
lacrimal gland

睑外侧韧带
lateral ligament of eyelid

下斜肌
inferior obliquus

◀ 图 11-9 泪器及上、下斜肌
Lacrimal apparatus, superior and inferior obliquus

解剖纲要

泪器组成
- 泪腺：位于泪腺窝内，分泌泪液，排泄管开口于结膜上穹
- 泪道：由泪点、泪小管、泪囊和鼻泪管组成，最终开口于下鼻道

Anatomical Outline

Constitution of lacrimal apparatus
- Lacrimal gland：It lies in the fossa of lacrimal gland, secretes tears and its excretory ducts open into the superior fornix of the conjunctival
- Lacrimal passages：It consists of lacrimal punctum, lacrimal ductule, lacrimal sac and nasolacrimal duct, and finally opens into inferior nasal meatus

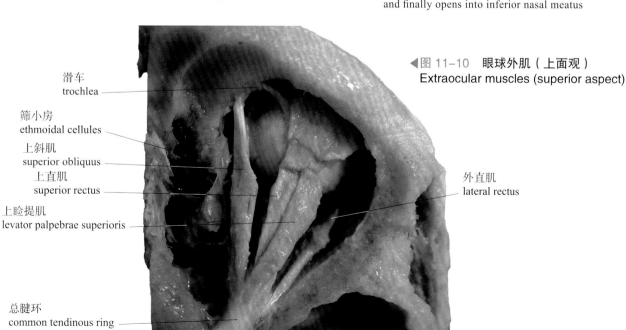

◀ 图 11-10 眼球外肌（上面观）
Extraocular muscles (superior aspect)

滑车
trochlea

筛小房
ethmoidal cellules

上斜肌
superior obliquus

上直肌
superior rectus

上睑提肌
levator palpebrae superioris

外直肌
lateral rectus

总腱环
common tendinous ring

Part 4 Sensory Organs
第四篇 感觉器

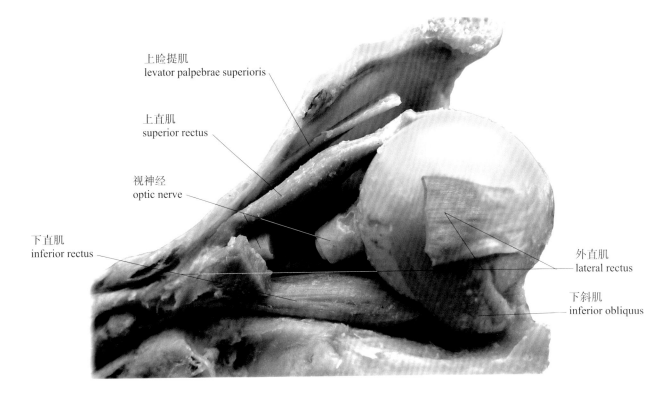

图 11-11　眼球外肌（外侧面观）
Extraocular muscles (lateral view)

上睑提肌
levator palpebrae superioris

上直肌
superior rectus

视神经
optic nerve

下直肌
inferior rectus

外直肌
lateral rectus

下斜肌
inferior obliquus

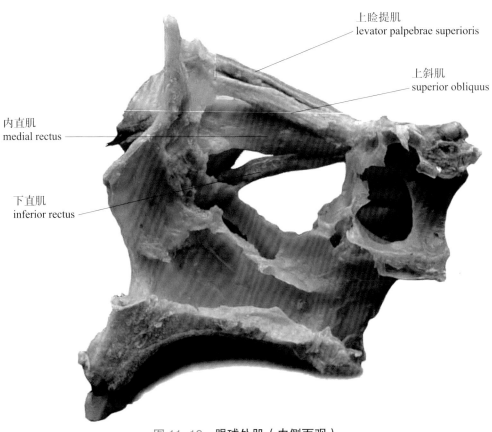

图 11-12　眼球外肌（内侧面观）
Extraocular muscles (medial view)

上睑提肌
levator palpebrae superioris

上斜肌
superior obliquus

内直肌
medial rectus

下直肌
inferior rectus

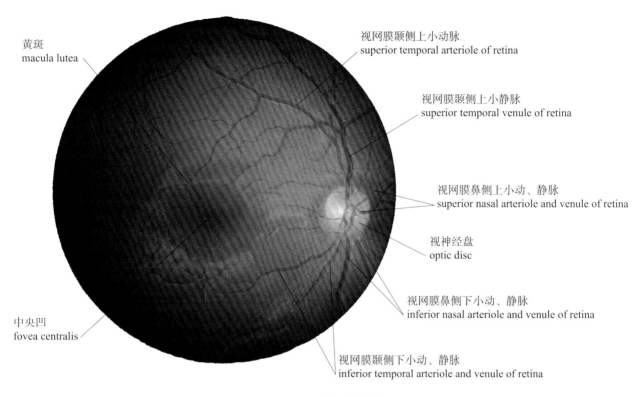

黄斑
macula lutea

视网膜颞侧上小动脉
superior temporal arteriole of retina

视网膜颞侧上小静脉
superior temporal venule of retina

视网膜鼻侧上小动、静脉
superior nasal arteriole and venule of retina

视神经盘
optic disc

视网膜鼻侧下小动、静脉
inferior nasal arteriole and venule of retina

中央凹
fovea centralis

视网膜颞侧下小动、静脉
inferior temporal arteriole and venule of retina

图 11-13　眼底（右侧）
Fundus of the eye (right side)

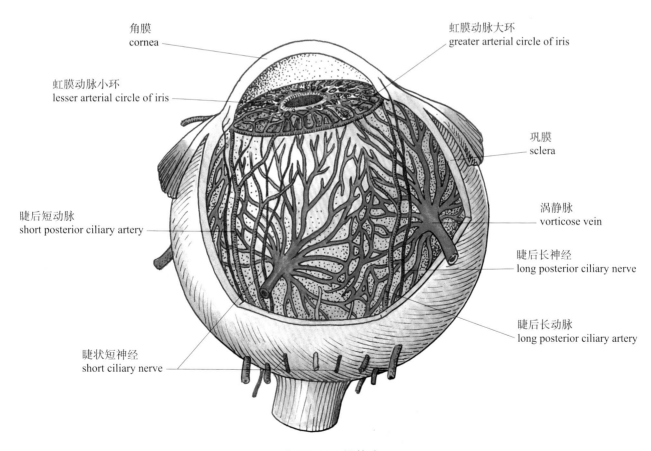

角膜
cornea

虹膜动脉大环
greater arterial circle of iris

虹膜动脉小环
lesser arterial circle of iris

巩膜
sclera

睫后短动脉
short posterior ciliary artery

涡静脉
vorticose vein

睫后长神经
long posterior ciliary nerve

睫后长动脉
long posterior ciliary artery

睫状短神经
short ciliary nerve

图 11-14　涡静脉
Vorticose vein

Part 4 Sensory Organs　第四篇　感觉器

第十二章 前庭蜗器

Chapter 12 Vestibulocochlear organ

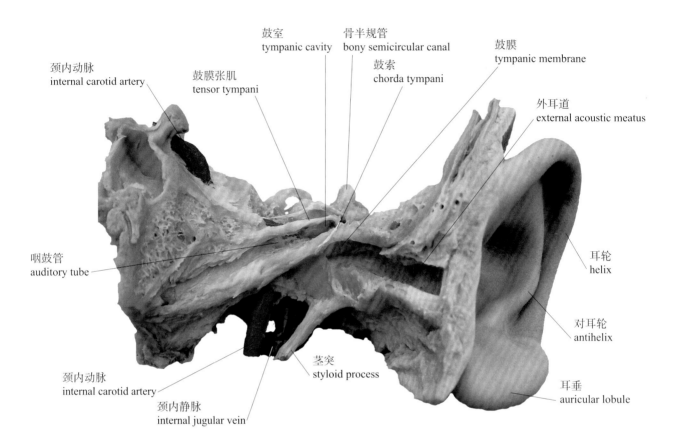

颈内动脉
internal carotid artery

鼓膜张肌
tensor tympani

鼓室
tympanic cavity

骨半规管
bony semicircular canal

鼓索
chorda tympani

鼓膜
tympanic membrane

外耳道
external acoustic meatus

咽鼓管
auditory tube

耳轮
helix

对耳轮
antihelix

颈内动脉
internal carotid artery

茎突
styloid process

颈内静脉
internal jugular vein

耳垂
auricular lobule

图 12-1 前庭蜗器
Vestibulocochlear organ

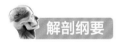 解剖纲要

　　前庭蜗器的组成：前庭蜗器包括外耳、中耳和内耳。外耳由耳郭、外耳道和鼓膜组成；中耳由鼓室、咽鼓管、乳突窦和乳突小房组成；内耳由骨迷路和膜迷路两部分组成。骨迷路由耳蜗、前庭和骨半规管构成；膜迷路由蜗管、球囊、椭圆囊和膜半规管构成。

Anatomical Outline

The composition of vestibulocochlear organ: The vestibulocochlear organ includes external ear, middle ear and internal ear. The external ear consists of the auricle, external acoustic meatus and tympanic membrane; The middle ear consists of tympanic cavity, auditory tube, mastoid antrum and mastoid cells; The internal ear consists of the bony labyrinth and membranous labyrinth. The bony labyrinth is composed of the cochlea, vestibule and bony semicircular canal, while the membranous labyrinth is composed of the cochlear duct, saccule, utricle and membranous semicircular ducts.

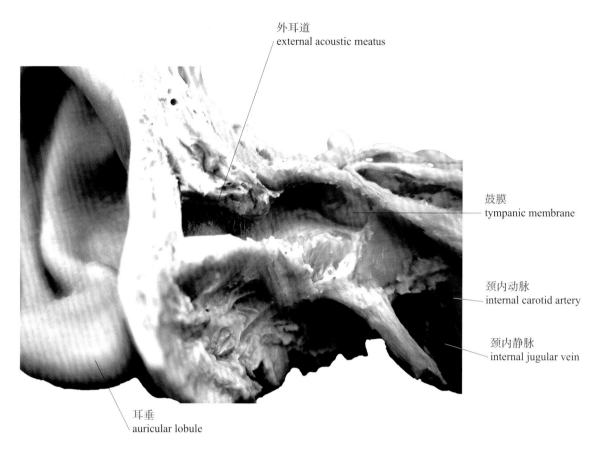

外耳道
external acoustic meatus

鼓膜
tympanic membrane

颈内动脉
internal carotid artery

颈内静脉
internal jugular vein

耳垂
auricular lobule

图 12-2 外耳
External ear

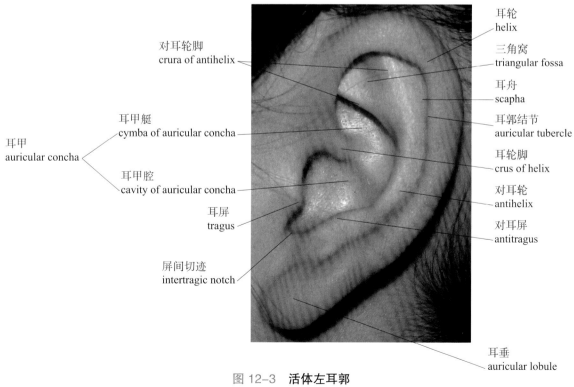

耳轮
helix

三角窝
triangular fossa

耳舟
scapha

耳郭结节
auricular tubercle

耳轮脚
crus of helix

对耳轮
antihelix

对耳屏
antitragus

对耳轮脚
crura of antihelix

耳甲艇
cymba of auricular concha

耳甲
auricular concha

耳甲腔
cavity of auricular concha

耳屏
tragus

屏间切迹
intertragic notch

耳垂
auricular lobule

图 12-3 活体左耳郭
Left auricle of living body

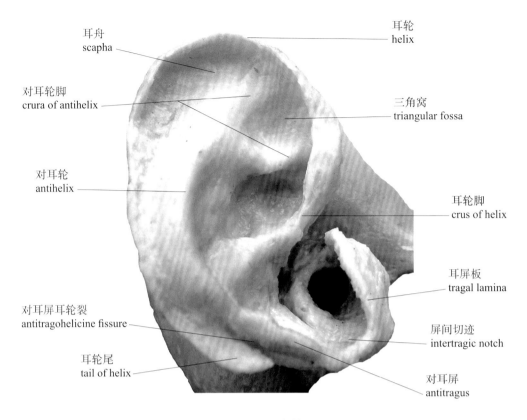

耳舟
scapha

耳轮
helix

对耳轮脚
crura of antihelix

三角窝
triangular fossa

对耳轮
antihelix

耳轮脚
crus of helix

耳屏板
tragal lamina

对耳屏耳轮裂
antitragohelicine fissure

屏间切迹
intertragic notch

耳轮尾
tail of helix

对耳屏
antitragus

图 12-4　耳郭软骨
Auricular cartilage

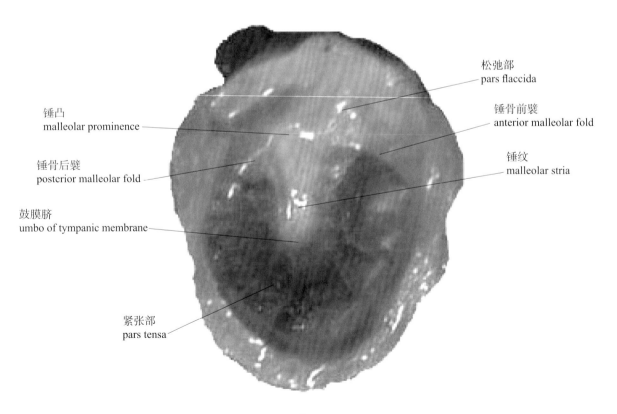

松弛部
pars flaccida

锤凸
malleolar prominence

锤骨前襞
anterior malleolar fold

锤骨后襞
posterior malleolar fold

锤纹
malleolar stria

鼓膜脐
umbo of tympanic membrane

紧张部
pars tensa

图 12-5　鼓膜（外侧面观）
Tympanic membrane (lateral view)

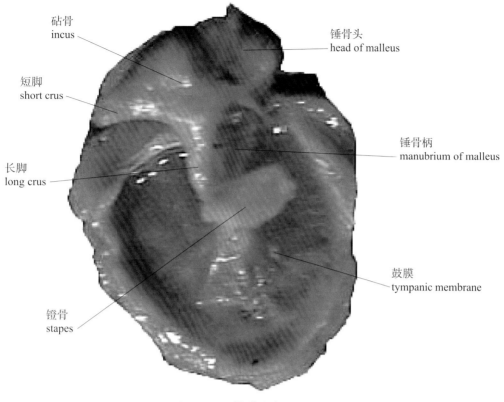

砧骨
incus

锤骨头
head of malleus

短脚
short crus

长脚
long crus

锤骨柄
manubrium of malleus

鼓膜
tympanic membrane

镫骨
stapes

图 12-6　鼓膜（内侧面观）
Tympanic membrane (medial view)

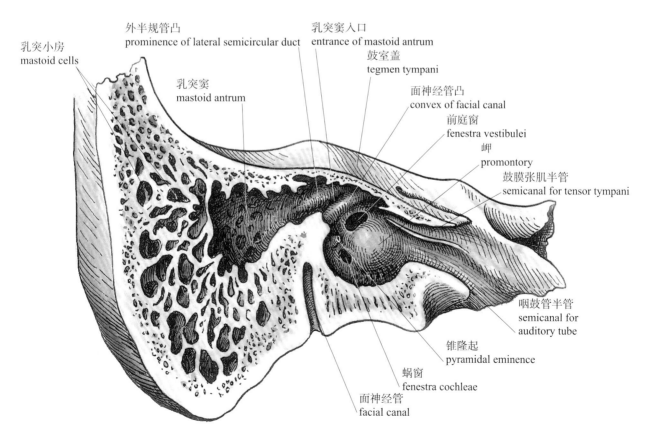

乳突小房
mastoid cells

外半规管凸
prominence of lateral semicircular duct

乳突窦入口
entrance of mastoid antrum

鼓室盖
tegmen tympani

乳突窦
mastoid antrum

面神经管凸
convex of facial canal

前庭窗
fenestra vestibulei

岬
promontory

鼓膜张肌半管
semicanal for tensor tympani

咽鼓管半管
semicanal for
auditory tube

锥隆起
pyramidal eminence

蜗窗
fenestra cochleae

面神经管
facial canal

图 12-7　鼓室内侧壁（模式图）
Medial wall of tympanic cavity (diagram)

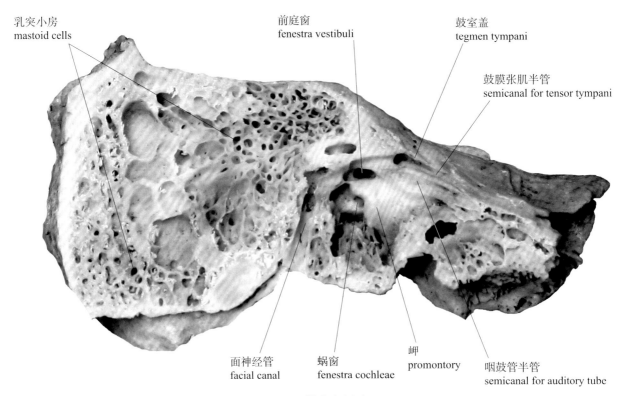

乳突小房
mastoid cells

前庭窗
fenestra vestibuli

鼓室盖
tegmen tympani

鼓膜张肌半管
semicanal for tensor tympani

面神经管
facial canal

蜗窗
fenestra cochleae

岬
promontory

咽鼓管半管
semicanal for auditory tube

图 12-8　鼓室内侧壁
Medial wall of tympanic cavity

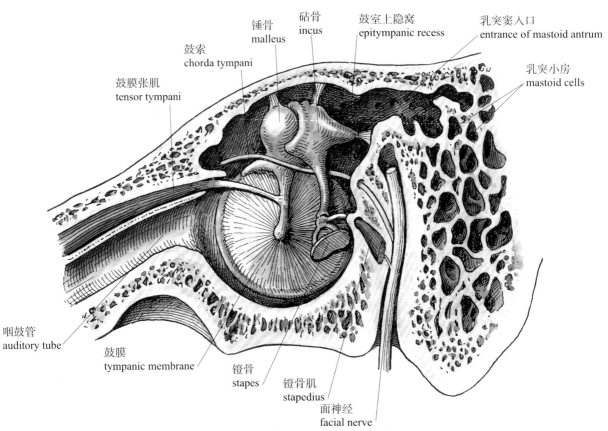

锤骨
malleus

砧骨
incus

鼓室上隐窝
epitympanic recess

乳突窦入口
entrance of mastoid antrum

鼓索
chorda tympani

乳突小房
mastoid cells

鼓膜张肌
tensor tympani

咽鼓管
auditory tube

鼓膜
tympanic membrane

镫骨
stapes

镫骨肌
stapedius

面神经
facial nerve

图 12-9　鼓室外侧壁（模式图）
Lateral wall of tympanic cavity (diagram)

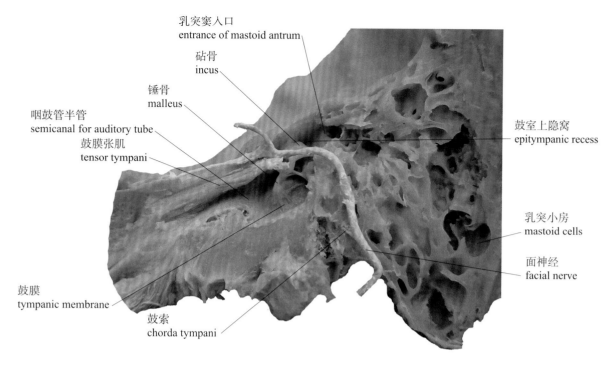

乳突窦入口
entrance of mastoid antrum

砧骨
incus

锤骨
malleus

咽鼓管半管
semicanal for auditory tube
鼓膜张肌
tensor tympani

鼓室上隐窝
epitympanic recess

乳突小房
mastoid cells

面神经
facial nerve

鼓膜
tympanic membrane

鼓索
chorda tympani

图 12-10　鼓室外侧壁
Lateral wall of tympanic cavity

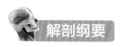解剖纲要

鼓室壁的构成及其特点

构成	特点
上壁（盖壁）	由颞骨岩部鼓室盖构成
下壁（颈静脉壁）	为一层薄骨板，分隔鼓室与颈静脉窝内的颈静脉球
前壁（颈动脉壁）	借薄骨板分隔鼓室与颈内动脉，其上有咽鼓管的开口
后壁（乳突壁）	上部有乳突窦入口、乳突窦、乳突小房；入口下方有锥隆起
外侧壁（鼓膜壁）	由鼓膜和鼓室上隐窝组成
内侧壁（迷路壁）	中部圆形隆起称岬，其后上方有前庭窗，后下方有蜗窗

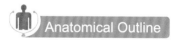Anatomical Outline

The composition of tympanic wall and its characteristics

Composition	Characteristics
Superior wall (tegmental wall)	It's made up of the tegmen tympani of petrous part of the temporal bone
Inferior wall (jugular wall)	A thin bony plate, separating the tympanic cavity from the jugular bulb which is in jugular fossa
Anterior wall (carotid wall)	To separate the tympanic cavity from the internal carotid artery by a thin bony plate. There is an opening of the auditory tube on it
Posterior wall (mastoid wall)	The upper part has an entrance to the mastoia sinus, mastoid antrum, mastoid cells; There is a pyramidal eminence below the entrance
Lateral wall (membranous wall)	It is composed of tympanic membrane and epitympanic recess
Medial wall (labyrinthine wall)	In the middle of it, there is a round protuberance called the promontory with a fenestra vestibuli above and a fenestra cochleae below

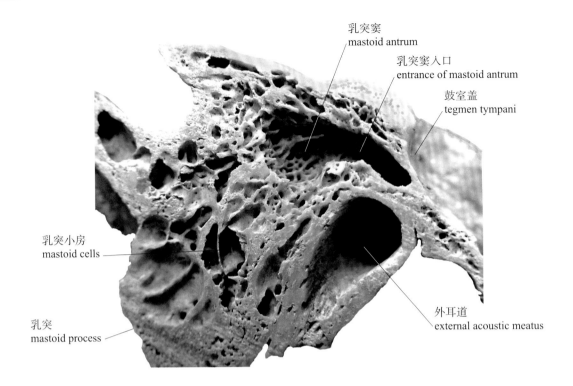

乳突窦
mastoid antrum

乳突窦入口
entrance of mastoid antrum

鼓室盖
tegmen tympani

乳突小房
mastoid cells

外耳道
external acoustic meatus

乳突
mastoid process

图 12-11　乳突窦
Mastoid antrum

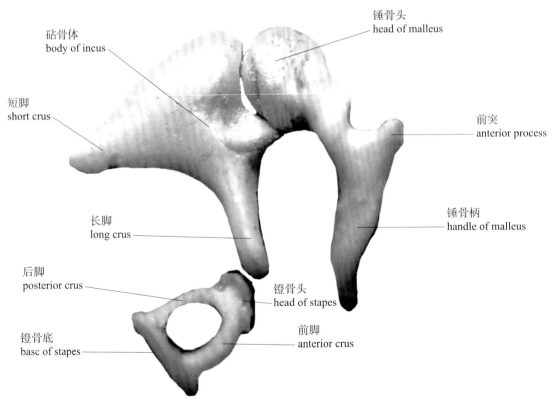

砧骨体
body of incus

锤骨头
head of malleus

短脚
short crus

前突
anterior process

长脚
long crus

锤骨柄
handle of malleus

后脚
posterior crus

镫骨头
head of stapes

镫骨底
basc of stapes

前脚
anterior crus

图 12-12　听小骨
Auditory ossicles

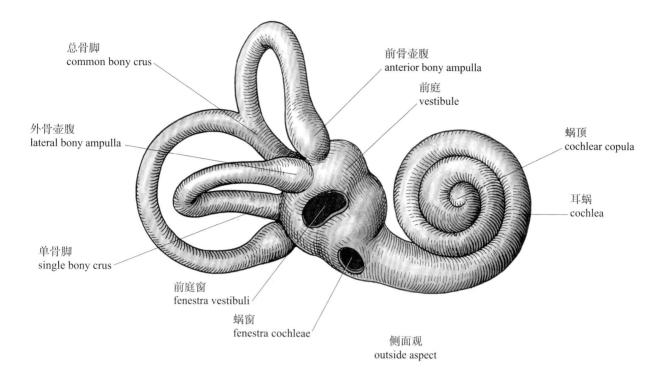

总骨脚
common bony crus

前骨壶腹
anterior bony ampulla

前庭
vestibule

外骨壶腹
lateral bony ampulla

蜗顶
cochlear copula

耳蜗
cochlea

单骨脚
single bony crus

前庭窗
fenestra vestibuli

蜗窗
fenestra cochleae

侧面观
outside aspect

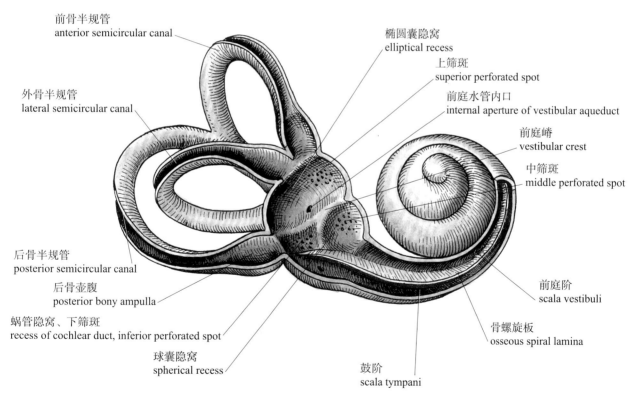

前骨半规管
anterior semicircular canal

椭圆囊隐窝
elliptical recess

上筛斑
superior perforated spot

外骨半规管
lateral semicircular canal

前庭水管内口
internal aperture of vestibular aqueduct

前庭嵴
vestibular crest

中筛斑
middle perforated spot

后骨半规管
posterior semicircular canal

后骨壶腹
posterior bony ampulla

蜗管隐窝、下筛斑
recess of cochlear duct, inferior perforated spot

球囊隐窝
spherical recess

前庭阶
scala vestibuli

骨螺旋板
osseous spiral lamina

鼓阶
scala tympani

内面观
Inside aspect

图 12-13 骨迷路模式图
Diagram of bony labyrinth

第四篇 感觉器 Part 4 Sensory Organs

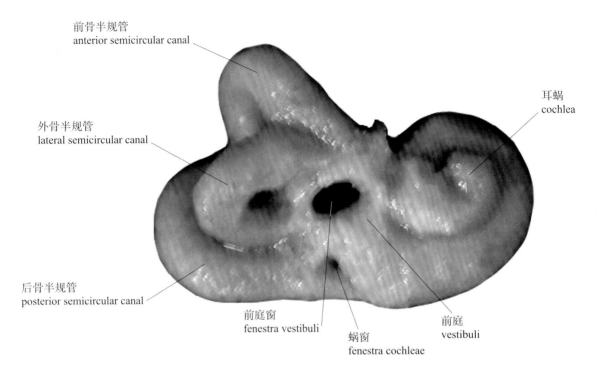

前骨半规管
anterior semicircular canal

外骨半规管
lateral semicircular canal

后骨半规管
posterior semicircular canal

耳蜗
cochlea

前庭窗
fenestra vestibuli

蜗窗
fenestra cochleae

前庭
vestibuli

图 12-14　右耳骨迷路
Bony labyrinth of right ear

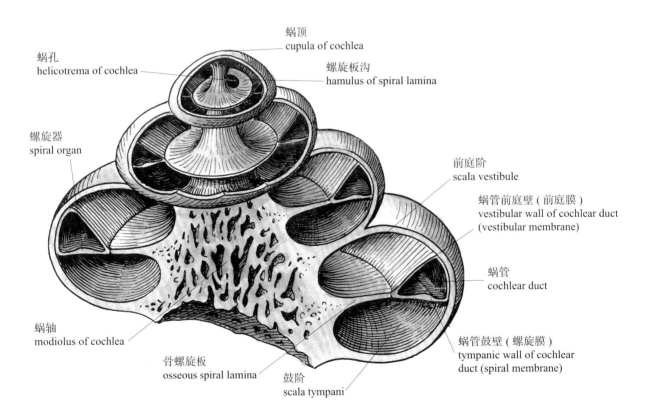

蜗顶
cupula of cochlea

蜗孔
helicotrema of cochlea

螺旋板沟
hamulus of spiral lamina

螺旋器
spiral organ

前庭阶
scala vestibule

蜗管前庭壁 (前庭膜)
vestibular wall of cochlear duct
(vestibular membrane)

蜗管
cochlear duct

蜗轴
modiolus of cochlea

骨螺旋板
osseous spiral lamina

鼓阶
scala tympani

蜗管鼓壁 (螺旋膜)
tympanic wall of cochlear
duct (spiral membrane)

图 12-15　耳蜗切面
Section of cochlea

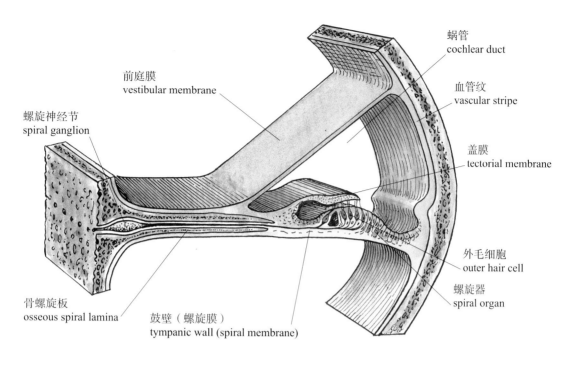

前庭膜
vestibular membrane

蜗管
cochlear duct

血管纹
vascular stripe

盖膜
tectorial membrane

螺旋神经节
spiral ganglion

外毛细胞
outer hair cell

螺旋器
spiral organ

骨螺旋板
osseous spiral lamina

鼓壁（螺旋膜）
tympanic wall (spiral membrane)

图 12-16　**蜗管横切面**
Cross section of cochlear duct

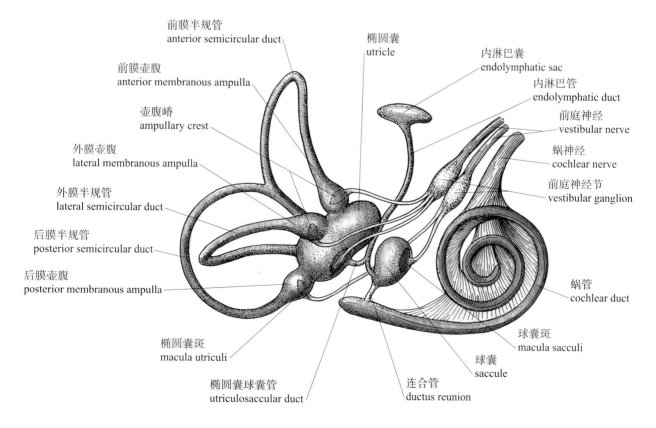

前膜半规管
anterior semicircular duct

椭圆囊
utricle

内淋巴囊
endolymphatic sac

前膜壶腹
anterior membranous ampulla

内淋巴管
endolymphatic duct

壶腹嵴
ampullary crest

前庭神经
vestibular nerve

外膜壶腹
lateral membranous ampulla

蜗神经
cochlear nerve

外膜半规管
lateral semicircular duct

前庭神经节
vestibular ganglion

后膜半规管
posterior semicircular duct

蜗管
cochlear duct

后膜壶腹
posterior membranous ampulla

椭圆囊斑
macula utriculi

球囊斑
macula sacculi

椭圆囊球囊管
utriculosaccular duct

连合管
ductus reunion

球囊
saccule

图 12-17　**膜迷路**
Membranous labyrinth

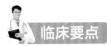

临床要点

1. 中耳炎。咽鼓管是沟通鼓室与鼻咽部的通道，感冒后咽部、鼻部的炎症向咽鼓管蔓延至中耳可诱发中耳炎，好发于儿童。若治疗不及时，病情加重可导致鼓膜穿孔、听力下降等。

2. 梅尼埃病。内耳由骨迷路和膜迷路构成。骨迷路和膜迷路之间的腔隙被外淋巴液填充，膜迷路内充满内淋巴液，且内、外淋巴液互不相通。梅尼埃病病因不明，以膜迷路积水为基本病理特征，是以反复发作的旋转性眩晕、耳聋、耳鸣和耳胀满感为主要症状的内耳疾病。

Key Points of the Clinic

1. Otitis Media.The pharyngolympanic auditory tube is the channel of communication between tympanic cavity and nasopharynx. Resulting from a cold, inflammation of pharynx and nose spread to auditory tube can induce otitis media. It often occurs in children easily. If the treatment is not timely, the disease can lead to tympanic membrane perforation, hearing loss and so on.

2. Meniere's Disease.The inner ear consists of bony labyrinth and membranous labyrinth. The space between the bony labyrinth and the membranous labyrinth is filled with perilymph, the membranous labyrinth is filled with endolymph. The perilymph and endolymph do not communicate with each other. Meniere's disease is an internal ear disease with unknown etiology, with labyrinthine hydrops of the membranous labyrinth as the basic pathological feature and recurrent episodes of rotational vertigo, deafness, tinnitus and ear fullness as the main symptoms.

第五篇
神经与
内分泌系统

Part 5 Nervous and Endocrine System

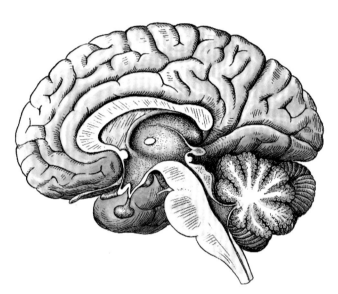

第十三章 中枢神经系统
Chapter 13 Central nervous system

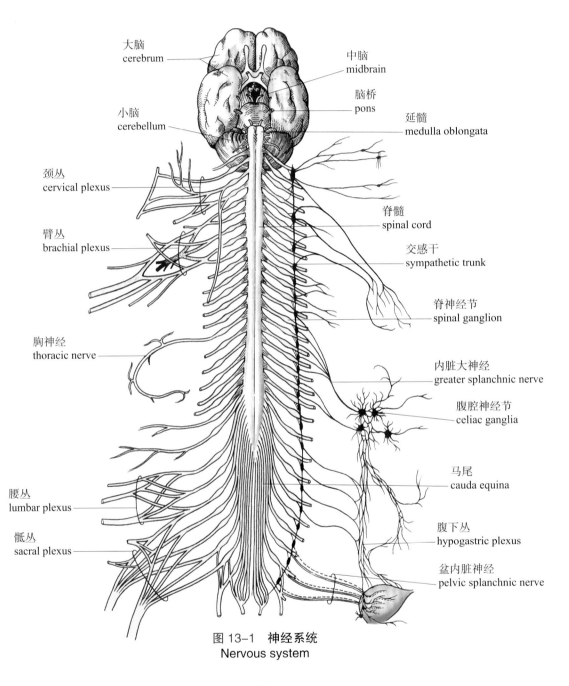

大脑
cerebrum

中脑
midbrain

脑桥
pons

小脑
cerebellum

延髓
medulla oblongata

颈丛
cervical plexus

脊髓
spinal cord

臂丛
brachial plexus

交感干
sympathetic trunk

脊神经节
spinal ganglion

胸神经
thoracic nerve

内脏大神经
greater splanchnic nerve

腹腔神经节
celiac ganglia

马尾
cauda equina

腰丛
lumbar plexus

腹下丛
hypogastric plexus

骶丛
sacral plexus

盆内脏神经
pelvic splanchnic nerve

图 13-1　神经系统
Nervous system

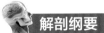 解剖纲要

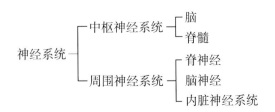

神经系统 ┬ 中枢神经系统 ┬ 脑
　　　　│　　　　　　└ 脊髓
　　　　└ 周围神经系统 ┬ 脊神经
　　　　　　　　　　　├ 脑神经
　　　　　　　　　　　└ 内脏神经系统

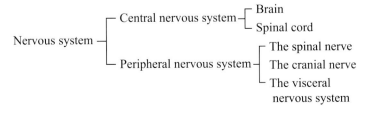 Anatomical Outline

Nervous system ┬ Central nervous system ┬ Brain
　　　　　　　│　　　　　　　　　　　└ Spinal cord
　　　　　　　└ Peripheral nervous system ┬ The spinal nerve
　　　　　　　　　　　　　　　　　　　├ The cranial nerve
　　　　　　　　　　　　　　　　　　　└ The visceral nervous system

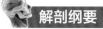 解剖纲要

中枢神经系统 ─┬─ 脑 ─┬─ 端脑
　　　　　　　　　├─ 间脑
　　　　　　　　　├─ 中脑 ─┐
　　　　　　　　　├─ 脑桥 ─┼─ 脑干
　　　　　　　　　├─ 延髓 ─┘
　　　　　　　　　└─ 小脑
　　　　　　　└─ 脊髓

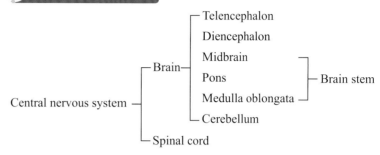 Anatomical Outline

Central nervous system ─┬─ Brain ─┬─ Telencephalon
　　　　　　　　　　　　　　　├─ Diencephalon
　　　　　　　　　　　　　　　├─ Midbrain ─┐
　　　　　　　　　　　　　　　├─ Pons ─────┼─ Brain stem
　　　　　　　　　　　　　　　├─ Medulla oblongata ─┘
　　　　　　　　　　　　　　　└─ Cerebellum
　　　　　　　　　　　└─ Spinal cord

第一节　脊髓　Section 1　Spinal cord

解剖纲要

脊髓的外形 ─┬─ 前后略扁的圆柱状
　　　　　　├─ 两个膨大 ─┬─ 颈膨大：$C_4 \sim T_1$ 脊髓节段，与臂丛的相应脊神经相连，其功能与上肢运动和感觉相关
　　　　　　│　　　　　　└─ 腰骶膨大：$L_1 \sim S_3$ 脊髓节段，与组成腰、骶丛的脊神经相连，其功能与下肢运动和感觉相关
　　　　　　├─ 六条沟裂 ─┬─ 前正中裂
　　　　　　│　　　　　　├─ 后正中沟
　　　　　　│　　　　　　├─ 前外侧沟：脊神经前根根丝附着处
　　　　　　│　　　　　　└─ 后外侧沟：脊神经后根根丝附着处
　　　　　　├─ 上端：在枕骨大孔处与延髓相连
　　　　　　└─ 下端：呈圆锥状，称脊髓圆锥，其下借终丝连于尾骨，终丝周围有马尾

Anatomical Outline

External feature of spinal cord ─┬─ Flattened cylindrical structure
　├─ Two enlargements ─┬─ Cervical enlargement: C_4-T_1 spinal segment, it is connected with the corresponding spinal nerve of the brachial plexus, and its function is related to upper limb movement and sensation
　│　　　　　　　　　　└─ Lumbosacral enlargement: L_1-S_3 spinal segment, it is connected with the corresponding spinal nerve of the lumbar and sacral plexuses, and its function is related to lower limb movement and sensation
　├─ Six fissures and sulci ─┬─ Anterior median fissure
　│　　　　　　　　　　　　　├─ Posterior median sulcus
　│　　　　　　　　　　　　　├─ Anterolateral sulcus: filaments of anterior roots attachment
　│　　　　　　　　　　　　　└─ Posterolateral sulcus: filaments of posterior roots attachment
　├─ Superior: continues with medulla oblongata at the level of foramen magnum
　└─ Inferior: forms conical termination known as conus medullaris. Its lower end connects with coccyx by filum terminale. Cauda equine surrounds the filum terminale

第五篇　神经与内分泌系统　Part 5 Nervous and Endocrine System

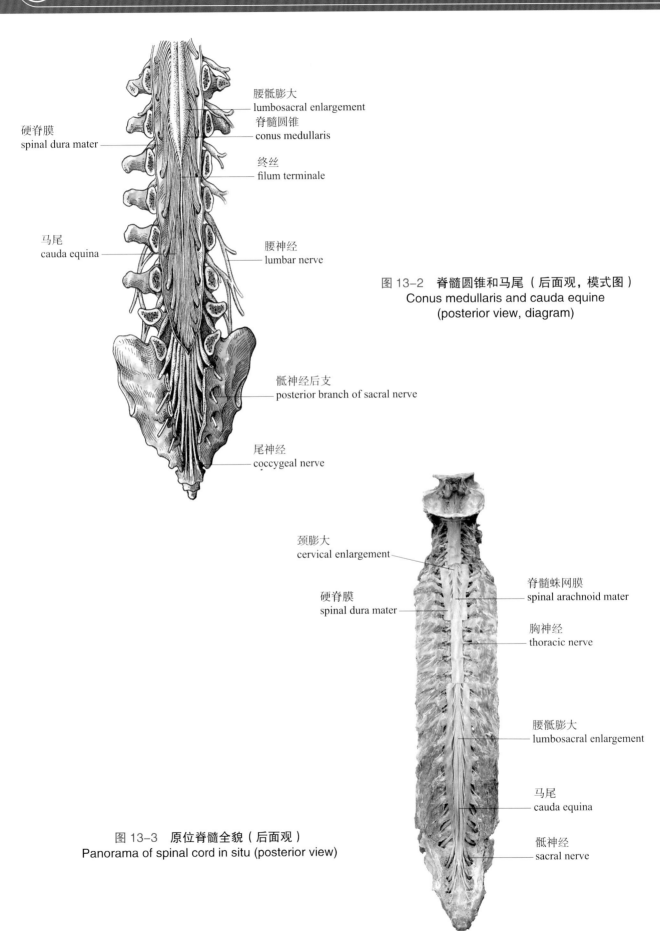

硬脊膜
spinal dura mater

马尾
cauda equina

腰骶膨大
lumbosacral enlargement

脊髓圆锥
conus medullaris

终丝
filum terminale

腰神经
lumbar nerve

骶神经后支
posterior branch of sacral nerve

尾神经
coccygeal nerve

图 13-2　脊髓圆锥和马尾（后面观，模式图）
Conus medullaris and cauda equine
(posterior view, diagram)

颈膨大
cervical enlargement

硬脊膜
spinal dura mater

脊髓蛛网膜
spinal arachnoid mater

胸神经
thoracic nerve

腰骶膨大
lumbosacral enlargement

马尾
cauda equina

骶神经
sacral nerve

图 13-3　原位脊髓全貌（后面观）
Panorama of spinal cord in situ (posterior view)

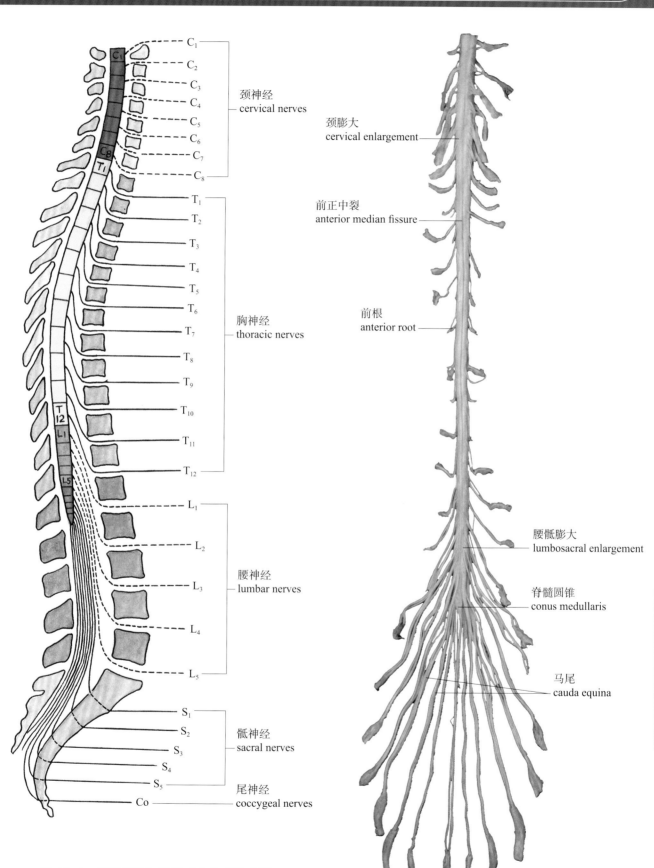

图 13-4　脊髓节段与椎骨对应关系模式图
Diagram showing the relation of the segments of the
spinal cord to the vertebrae

图 13-5　脊髓（后面观）
Spinal cord (posterior view)

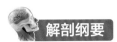

解剖纲要

脊髓节段与椎骨对应关系

脊髓节段	椎骨
上颈髓节 (C_1~C_4)	与同序数颈椎相对应
下颈髓节 (C_5~C_8) 和上胸髓节 (T_1~T_4)	比同序数椎骨高一个椎体高度
中胸髓节 (T_5~T_8)	比同序数椎骨高两个椎体高度
下胸髓节 (T_9~T_{12})	比同序数椎骨高三个椎体高度
腰髓节 (L_1~L_5)	平对第 10~12 胸椎高度
骶、尾髓节	平对第 1 腰椎高度

 Anatomical Outline

Corresponding relationship between spinal segment and vertebra

Spinal segment	Vertebra
Upper cervical segments (C_1-C_4)	Corresponding to the same ordinal cervicall vertebra
Lower cervical and upper thoracic segments (C_5-C_8, T_1-T_4)	One vertebra height higher in number than corresponding vertebra
Middle thoracic segments (T_5-T_8)	Two vertebra heights higher in number than corresponding vertebra
Lower thoracic segments (T_9-T_{12})	Three vertebra heights higher in number than corresponding vertebra
Lumbar segments (L_1-L_5)	Level with the the 10th-12th thoracic vertebrae
Sacral and coccygeal segments	Level with the 1st lumbar vertebra

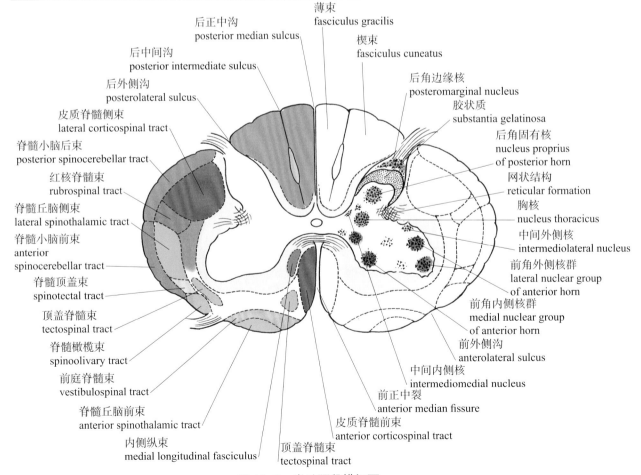

图 13-6　脊髓颈段横切面
Transverse section through cervical segment of the spinal cord

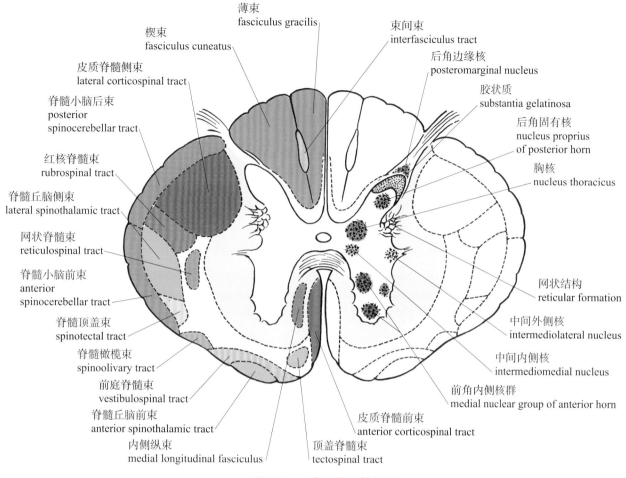

薄束
fasciculus gracilis

楔束
fasciculus cuneatus

皮质脊髓侧束
lateral corticospinal tract

脊髓小脑后束
posterior
spinocerebellar tract

红核脊髓束
rubrospinal tract

脊髓丘脑侧束
lateral spinothalamic tract

网状脊髓束
reticulospinal tract

脊髓小脑前束
anterior
spinocerebellar tract

脊髓顶盖束
spinotectal tract

脊髓橄榄束
spinoolivary tract

前庭脊髓束
vestibulospinal tract

脊髓丘脑前束
anterior spinothalamic tract

内侧纵束
medial longitudinal fasciculus

束间束
interfasciculus tract

后角边缘核
posteromarginal nucleus

胶状质
substantia gelatinosa

后角固有核
nucleus proprius
of posterior horn

胸核
nucleus thoracicus

网状结构
reticular formation

中间外侧核
intermediolateral nucleus

中间内侧核
intermediomedial nucleus

前角内侧核群
medial nuclear group of anterior horn

皮质脊髓前束
anterior corticospinal tract

顶盖脊髓束
tectospinal tract

图 13-7　脊髓胸段横切面
Transverse section through thoracic segment of the spinal cord

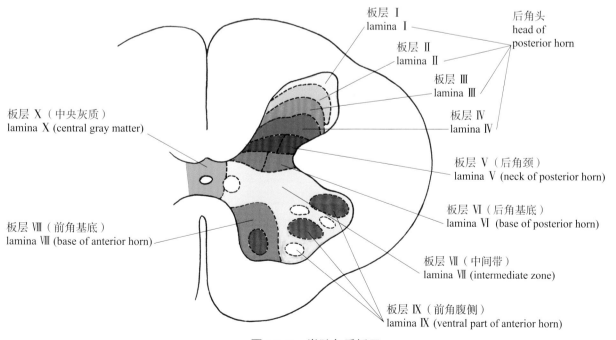

板层 Ⅰ
lamina Ⅰ

后角头
head of
posterior horn

板层 Ⅱ
lamina Ⅱ

板层 Ⅲ
lamina Ⅲ

板层 Ⅳ
lamina Ⅳ

板层 Ⅹ（中央灰质）
lamina Ⅹ (central gray matter)

板层 Ⅴ（后角颈）
lamina Ⅴ (neck of posterior horn)

板层 Ⅵ（后角基底）
lamina Ⅵ (base of posterior horn)

板层 Ⅷ（前角基底）
lamina Ⅷ (base of anterior horn)

板层 Ⅶ（中间带）
lamina Ⅶ (intermediate zone)

板层 Ⅸ（前角腹侧）
lamina Ⅸ (ventral part of anterior horn)

图 13-8　脊髓灰质板层
Laminas of gray matter of the spinal cord

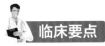临床要点

外伤致脊髓突然完全横断后，出现损伤平面以下全部感觉和运动丧失，反射消失，这种状态称为脊髓休克。一般数周至数月后各种反射可逐渐恢复，但恢复后的深反射和肌张力比正常时高，而损伤平面以下的感觉和随意运动不能恢复。

Key Points of the Clinic

After the spinal cord is suddenly and completely transected by trauma, all of sensory and motor loss occurs below the injury plane, and reflexes will be lost. This state refers to spinal shock. After a few weeks to a few months, the reflexes can be gradually restored, but both the deep reflexes and muscle tones are higher than normal condition, and the feeling and voluntary movement below the injury plane cannot be restored.

第二节　脑干　Section 2　Brain stem

脑干外形特征

位置	腹侧面	背侧面	相连脑神经
延髓	前正中裂，锥体交叉，锥体，橄榄	构成菱形窝的下半部，后正中沟，薄束结节，楔束结节，小脑下脚（绳状体）	Ⅸ、Ⅹ、Ⅺ、Ⅻ
脑桥	基底部，基底沟，小脑中脚（桥臂）	构成菱形窝的上半部，小脑上脚（结合臂），上髓帆	Ⅴ、Ⅵ、Ⅶ、Ⅷ
中脑	大脑脚底，脚间窝	上丘、上丘臂、下丘、下丘臂	Ⅲ、Ⅳ

External features of the brain stem

Position	Ventral surface	Dorsal surface	Connected cranial nerves
Medulla oblongata	Anterior median fissure, decussation of pyramid, pyramid, olive	Lower half of the rhomboid fossa, posterior median sulcus, gracile tubercle, cuneate tubercle, inferior cerebellar peduncle (restiform body)	Ⅸ、Ⅹ、Ⅺ、Ⅻ
Pons	Basilar part, basilar sulcus, middle cerebellar peduncle (brachium pontis)	Upper half of the rhomboid fossa, superior cerebellar peduncle (brachium conjunctivum), superior medullary velum	Ⅴ、Ⅵ、Ⅶ、Ⅷ
Midbrain	Crus cerebri, interpeduncular fossa	Superior colliculus, brachium of superior colliculus, inferior colliculus, brachium of inferior colliculus	Ⅲ、Ⅳ

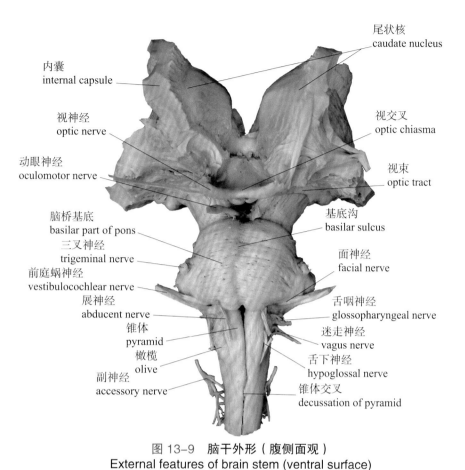

尾状核
caudate nucleus

内囊
internal capsule

视交叉
optic chiasma

视神经
optic nerve

视束
optic tract

动眼神经
oculomotor nerve

脑桥基底
basilar part of pons

基底沟
basilar sulcus

三叉神经
trigeminal nerve

面神经
facial nerve

前庭蜗神经
vestibulocochlear nerve

展神经
abducent nerve

舌咽神经
glossopharyngeal nerve

锥体
pyramid

迷走神经
vagus nerve

橄榄
olive

舌下神经
hypoglossal nerve

副神经
accessory nerve

锥体交叉
decussation of pyramid

图 13-9　脑干外形（腹侧面观）
External features of brain stem (ventral surface)

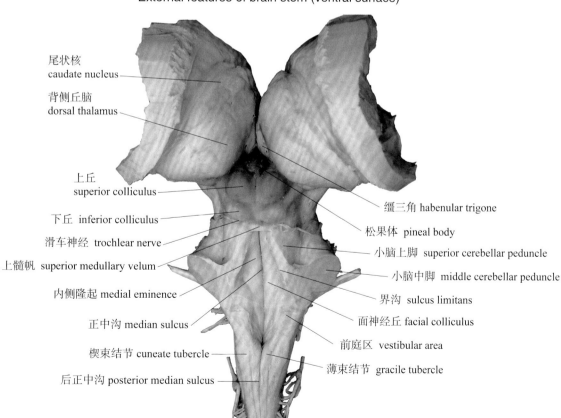

尾状核
caudate nucleus

背侧丘脑
dorsal thalamus

上丘
superior colliculus

缰三角 habenular trigone

下丘 inferior colliculus

松果体 pineal body

滑车神经 trochlear nerve

小脑上脚 superior cerebellar peduncle

上髓帆 superior medullary velum

小脑中脚 middle cerebellar peduncle

内侧隆起 medial eminence

界沟 sulcus limitans

正中沟 median sulcus

面神经丘 facial colliculus

楔束结节 cuneate tubercle

前庭区 vestibular area

后正中沟 posterior median sulcus

薄束结节 gracile tubercle

图 13-10　脑干外形（背侧面观）
External features of brain stem (dorsal surface)

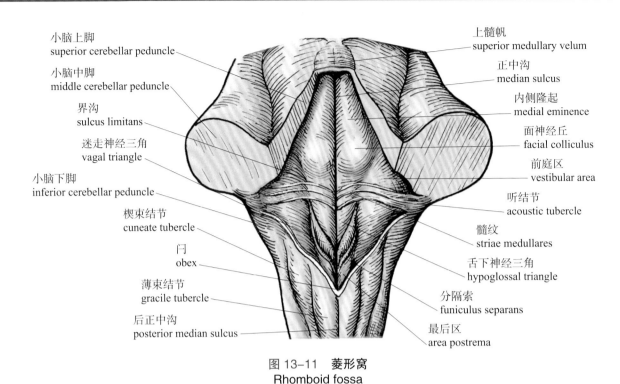

小脑上脚
superior cerebellar peduncle

小脑中脚
middle cerebellar peduncle

界沟
sulcus limitans

迷走神经三角
vagal triangle

小脑下脚
inferior cerebellar peduncle

楔束结节
cuneate tubercle

闩
obex

薄束结节
gracile tubercle

后正中沟
posterior median sulcus

上髓帆
superior medullary velum

正中沟
median sulcus

内侧隆起
medial eminence

面神经丘
facial colliculus

前庭区
vestibular area

听结节
acoustic tubercle

髓纹
striae medullares

舌下神经三角
hypoglossal triangle

分隔索
funiculus separans

最后区
area postrema

图 13-11 菱形窝
Rhomboid fossa

动眼神经副核
accessory nucleus of oculomotor nerve

动眼神经核
nucleus of oculomotor nerve

滑车神经核
trochlear nucleus

三叉神经运动核
motor nucleus of trigeminal nerve

展神经核
nucleus of abducent nerve

面神经核
nucleus of facial nerve

上泌涎核
superior salivatory nucleus

下泌涎核
inferior salivatory nucleus

疑核
nucleus ambiguus

迷走神经背核
dorsal nucleus of vagus nerve

舌下神经核
hypoglossal nucleus

三叉神经中脑核
mesencephalic nucleus of trigeminal nerve

三叉神经脑桥核
pontine nucleus of trigeminal nerve

前庭神经核
vestibular nuclei

蜗神经核
cochlear nuclei

孤束核
solitary tract nucleus

三叉神经脊束核
spinal nucleus of trigeminal nerve

副神经核
nucleus of accessory nerve

图 13-12 脑神经核模式图（背面投影图）
Diagram of the nuclei of cranial nerve (dorsal surface projection)

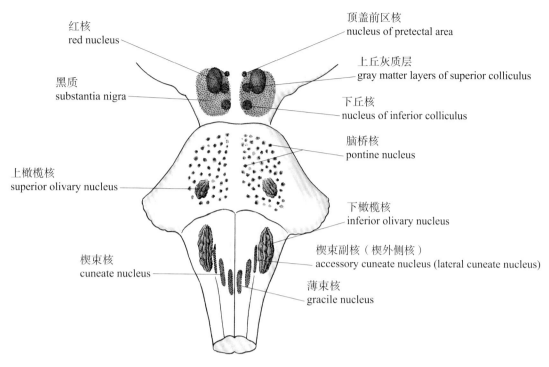

图 13-13　脑干内非脑神经核模式图（前面投影图）
Diagram of the non-cranial nerve nuclei in brain stem (anterior surface projection)

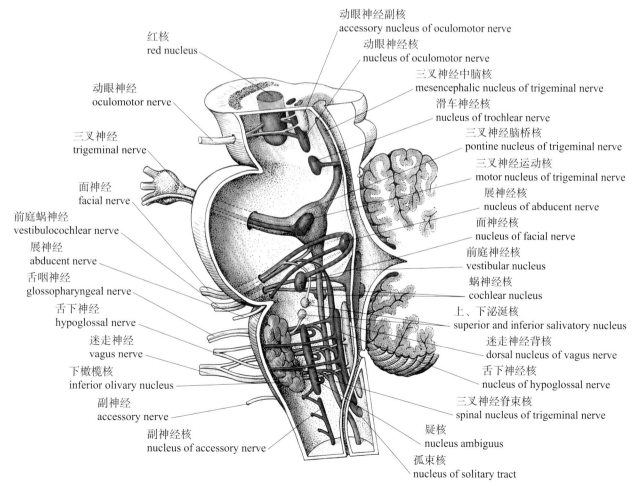

图 13-14　脑神经核模式图（内侧面观）
Diagram of the nuclei of cranial nerve (medial view)

脑神经核位置、性质及相连脑神经

位置	名称	性质	相连的脑神经
中脑	动眼神经核	一般躯体运动核	Ⅲ
	动眼神经副核	一般内脏运动核	
	滑车神经核	一般躯体运动核	Ⅳ
	三叉神经中脑核	一般躯体感觉核	Ⅴ
脑桥	展神经核	一般躯体运动核	Ⅵ
	三叉神经运动核	特殊内脏运动核	Ⅴ
	三叉神经脑桥核	一般躯体感觉核	
	面神经核	特殊内脏运动核	Ⅶ
	上泌涎核	一般内脏运动核	
	蜗神经核	特殊躯体感觉核	Ⅷ
	前庭神经核	特殊躯体感觉核	
延髓	三叉神经脊束核	一般躯体感觉核	Ⅴ，Ⅶ，Ⅸ，Ⅹ
	下泌涎核	一般内脏运动核	Ⅸ
	疑核	特殊内脏运动核	Ⅸ，Ⅹ，Ⅺ
	孤束核	一般和特殊内脏感觉核	Ⅶ，Ⅸ，Ⅹ
	迷走神经背核	一般内脏运动核	Ⅹ
	副神经核	特殊内脏运动核	Ⅺ
	舌下神经核	一般躯体运动核	Ⅻ

Position, characters of the nuclei of cranial nerve and connected cranial nerves

Position	Name	Character	Connected cranial nerves
Midbrain	Nucleus of oculomotor nerve	General somatic motor nucleus	Ⅲ
	Accessory nucleus of oculomotor nerve	General visceral motor nucleus	
	Nucleus of trochlear nerve	General somatic motor nucleus	Ⅳ
	Mesencephalic nucleus of trigeminal nerve	General somatic sensory nucleus	Ⅴ
Pons	Nucleus of abducent nerve	General somatic motor nucleus	Ⅵ
	Motor nucleus of trigeminal nerve	Special visceral motor nucleus	Ⅴ
	Pontine nucleus of trigeminal nerve	General somatic sensory nucleus	
	Nucleus of facial nerve	Special visceral motor nucleus	Ⅶ
	Superior salivatory nucleus	General visceral motor nucleus	
	Cochlear nucleus	Special visceral sensory nucleus	Ⅷ
	Vestibular nucleus	Special visceral sensory nucleus	
Medulla oblongata	Spinal nucleus of trigeminal nerve	General somatic sensory nucleus	Ⅴ，Ⅶ，Ⅸ，Ⅹ
	Inferior salivatory nucleus	General visceral motor nucleus	Ⅸ
	Nucleus ambiguus	Special visceral motor nucleus	Ⅸ，Ⅹ，Ⅺ
	Nucleus of solitary tract	General and special visceral sensory nucleus	Ⅶ，Ⅸ，Ⅹ
	Dorsal nucleus of vagus nerve	General visceral motor nucleus	Ⅹ
	Nucleus of accessory nerve	Special visceral motor nucleus	Ⅺ
	Nucleus of hypoglossal nerve	General somatic motor nucleus	Ⅻ

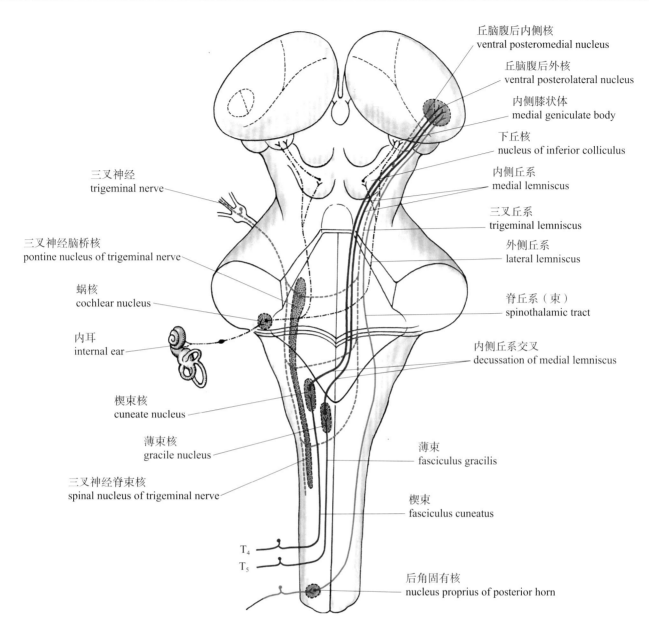

丘脑腹后内侧核
ventral posteromedial nucleus

丘脑腹后外核
ventral posterolateral nucleus

内侧膝状体
medial geniculate body

下丘核
nucleus of inferior colliculus

内侧丘系
medial lemniscus

三叉丘系
trigeminal lemniscus

外侧丘系
lateral lemniscus

脊丘系（束）
spinothalamic tract

内侧丘系交叉
decussation of medial lemniscus

薄束
fasciculus gracilis

楔束
fasciculus cuneatus

后角固有核
nucleus proprius of posterior horn

三叉神经
trigeminal nerve

三叉神经脑桥核
pontine nucleus of trigeminal nerve

蜗核
cochlear nucleus

内耳
internal ear

楔束核
cuneate nucleus

薄束核
gracile nucleus

三叉神经脊束核
spinal nucleus of trigeminal nerve

T₄
T₅

图 13–15　脑干内四个长上行传导束模式图
Diagram of four long ascending pathways in brain stem

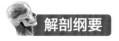解剖纲要

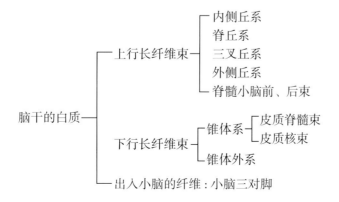

脑干的白质
├─ 上行长纤维束
│   ├─ 内侧丘系
│   ├─ 脊丘系
│   ├─ 三叉丘系
│   ├─ 外侧丘系
│   └─ 脊髓小脑前、后束
├─ 下行长纤维束
│   ├─ 锥体系 ── 皮质脊髓束 / 皮质核束
│   └─ 锥体外系
└─ 出入小脑的纤维：小脑三对脚

Anatomical Outline

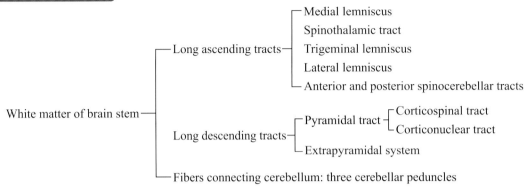

White matter of brain stem
- Long ascending tracts
  - Medial lemniscus
  - Spinothalamic tract
  - Trigeminal lemniscus
  - Lateral lemniscus
  - Anterior and posterior spinocerebellar tracts
- Long descending tracts
  - Pyramidal tract
    - Corticospinal tract
    - Corticonuclear tract
  - Extrapyramidal system
- Fibers connecting cerebellum: three cerebellar peduncles

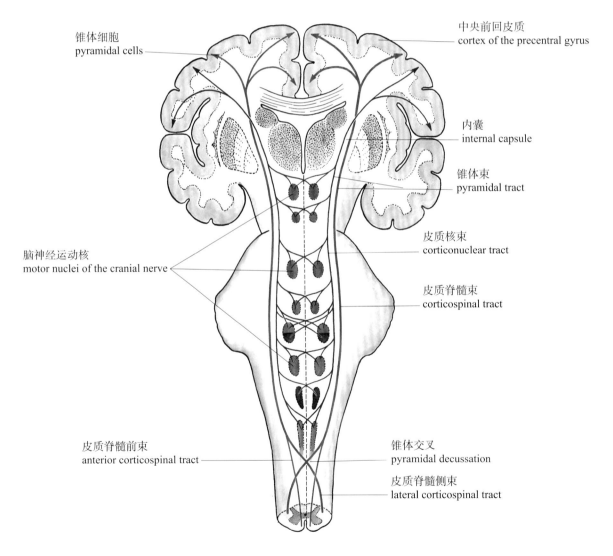

图 13-16　脑干内主要下行传导束模式图
Diagram of main descending pathways in brain stem

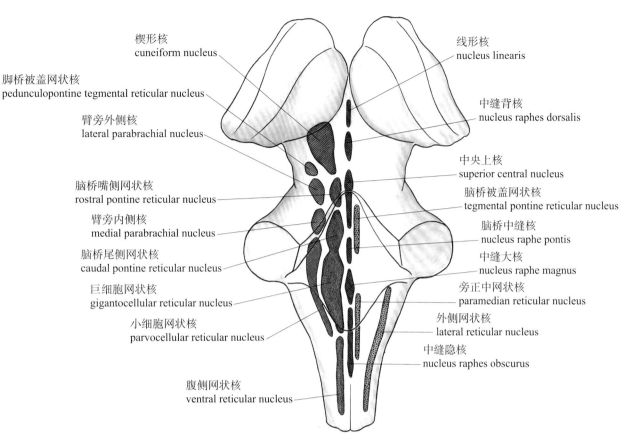

图 13-17　脑干网状结构核团模式图（背面投影图）
Diagram of the nuclei of reticular formation in brain stem (dorsal surface projection)

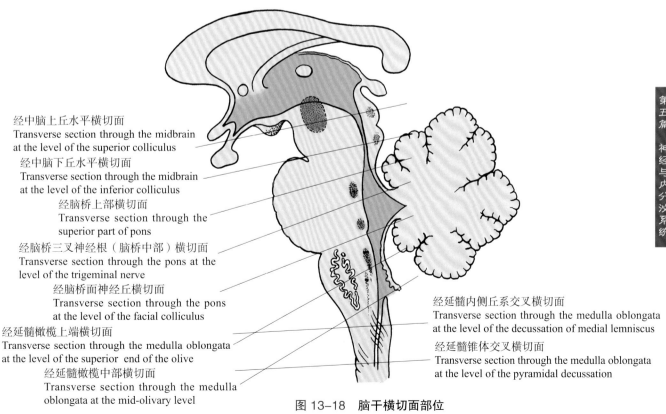

图 13-18　脑干横切面部位
Location of transverse section of brain stem

第五篇　神经与内分泌系统
Part 5 Nervous and Endocrine System

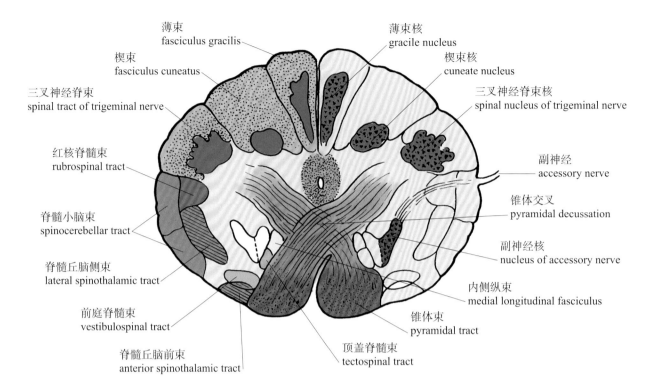

图 13-19 经延髓锥体交叉横切面
Transverse section through the medulla oblongata at the level of pyramidal decussation

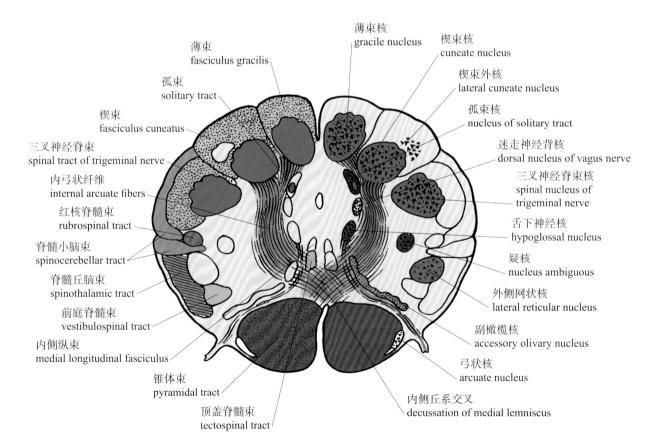

图 13-20 经延髓内侧丘系交叉横切面
Transverse section through the medulla oblongata at the level of the decussation of medial lemniscus

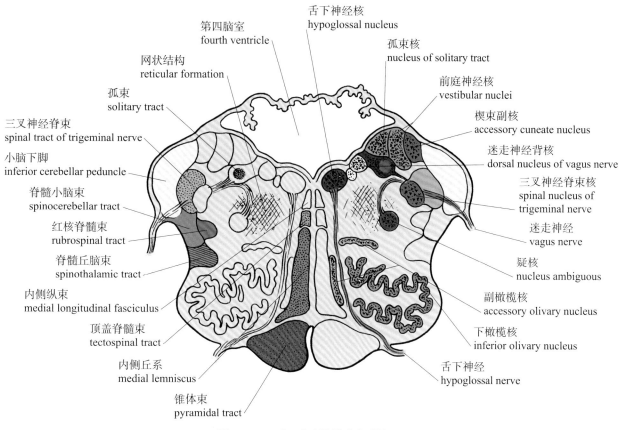

图 13-21　经延髓橄榄中部横切面
Transverse section through the medulla oblongata at the mid-olivary level

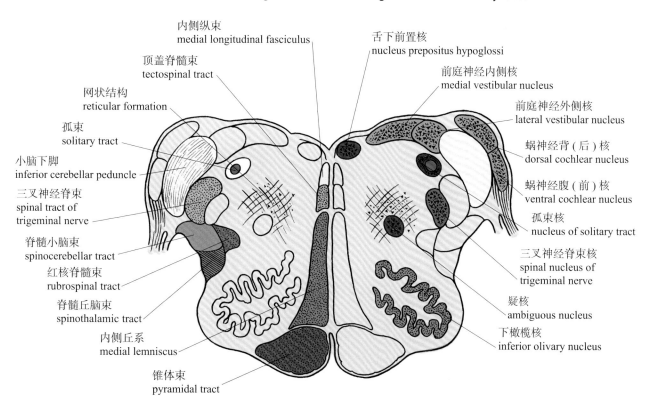

图 13-22　经延髓橄榄上端横切面
Transverse section through the medulla oblongata at the level of the superior end of the olive

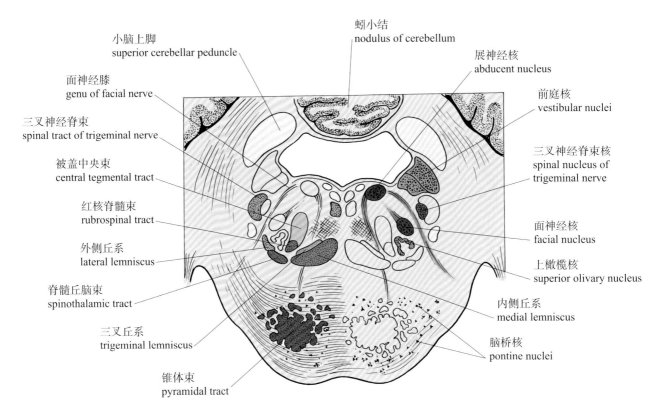

小脑上脚
superior cerebellar peduncle

蚓小结
nodulus of cerebellum

展神经核
abducent nucleus

面神经膝
genu of facial nerve

前庭核
vestibular nuclei

三叉神经脊束
spinal tract of trigeminal nerve

三叉神经脊束核
spinal nucleus of
trigeminal nerve

被盖中央束
central tegmental tract

红核脊髓束
rubrospinal tract

面神经核
facial nucleus

外侧丘系
lateral lemniscus

上橄榄核
superior olivary nucleus

脊髓丘脑束
spinothalamic tract

内侧丘系
medial lemniscus

三叉丘系
trigeminal lemniscus

脑桥核
pontine nuclei

锥体束
pyramidal tract

图 13-23　经脑桥面神经丘横切面
Transverse section through the pons at the level of the facial colliculus

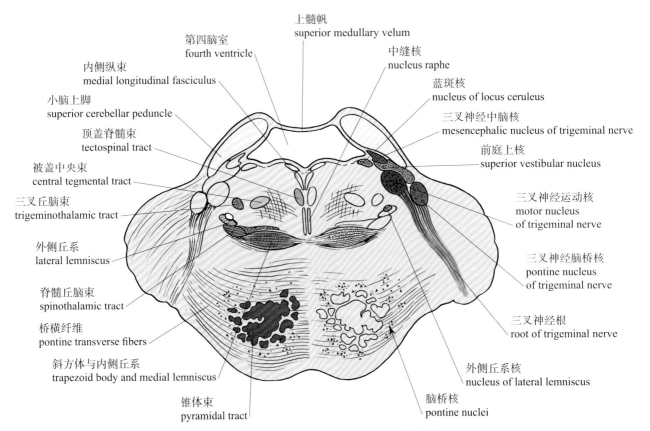

第四脑室
fourth ventricle

上髓帆
superior medullary velum

中缝核
nucleus raphe

内侧纵束
medial longitudinal fasciculus

蓝斑核
nucleus of locus ceruleus

小脑上脚
superior cerebellar peduncle

三叉神经中脑核
mesencephalic nucleus of trigeminal nerve

顶盖脊髓束
tectospinal tract

前庭上核
superior vestibular nucleus

被盖中央束
central tegmental tract

三叉神经运动核
motor nucleus
of trigeminal nerve

三叉丘脑束
trigeminothalamic tract

外侧丘系
lateral lemniscus

三叉神经脑桥核
pontine nucleus
of trigeminal nerve

脊髓丘脑束
spinothalamic tract

桥横纤维
pontine transverse fibers

三叉神经根
root of trigeminal nerve

斜方体与内侧丘系
trapezoid body and medial lemniscus

外侧丘系核
nucleus of lateral lemniscus

锥体束
pyramidal tract

脑桥核
pontine nuclei

图 13-24　经脑桥三叉神经根（脑桥中部）横切面
Transverse section through the pons at the level of the trigeminal nerve

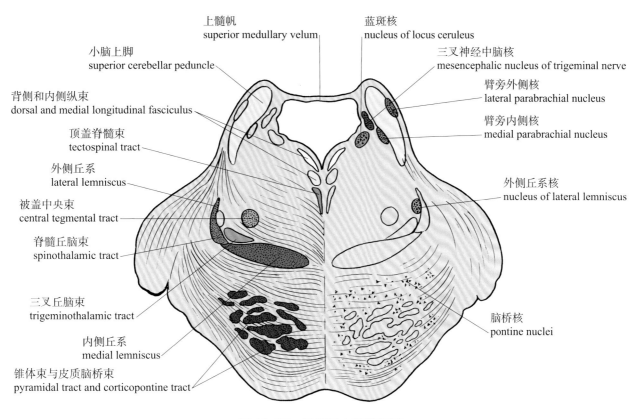

上髓帆
superior medullary velum

蓝斑核
nucleus of locus ceruleus

小脑上脚
superior cerebellar peduncle

三叉神经中脑核
mesencephalic nucleus of trigeminal nerve

背侧和内侧纵束
dorsal and medial longitudinal fasciculus

臂旁外侧核
lateral parabrachial nucleus

顶盖脊髓束
tectospinal tract

臂旁内侧核
medial parabrachial nucleus

外侧丘系
lateral lemniscus

被盖中央束
central tegmental tract

外侧丘系核
nucleus of lateral lemniscus

脊髓丘脑束
spinothalamic tract

三叉丘脑束
trigeminothalamic tract

内侧丘系
medial lemniscus

脑桥核
pontine nuclei

锥体束与皮质脑桥束
pyramidal tract and corticopontine tract

图 13-25　经脑桥上部横切面
Transverse section through the superior part of pons

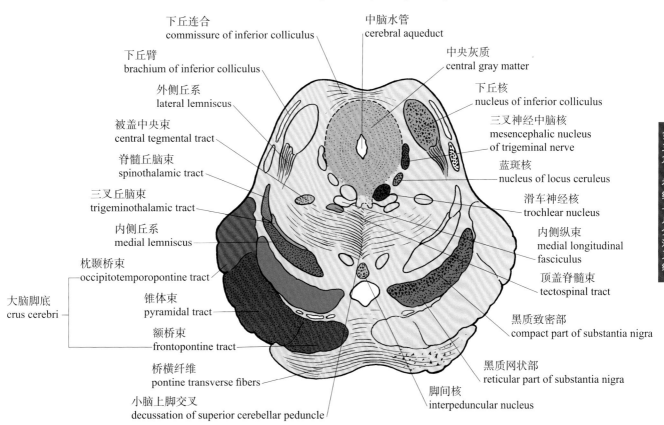

下丘连合
commissure of inferior colliculus

中脑水管
cerebral aqueduct

下丘臂
brachium of inferior colliculus

中央灰质
central gray matter

外侧丘系
lateral lemniscus

下丘核
nucleus of inferior colliculus

被盖中央束
central tegmental tract

三叉神经中脑核
mesencephalic nucleus
of trigeminal nerve

脊髓丘脑束
spinothalamic tract

蓝斑核
nucleus of locus ceruleus

三叉丘脑束
trigeminothalamic tract

滑车神经核
trochlear nucleus

内侧丘系
medial lemniscus

内侧纵束
medial longitudinal
fasciculus

枕颞桥束
occipitotemporopontine tract

顶盖脊髓束
tectospinal tract

大脑脚底
crus cerebri

锥体束
pyramidal tract

黑质致密部
compact part of substantia nigra

额桥束
frontopontine tract

黑质网状部
reticular part of substantia nigra

桥横纤维
pontine transverse fibers

脚间核
interpeduncular nucleus

小脑上脚交叉
decussation of superior cerebellar peduncle

图 13-26　经中脑下丘水平横切面
Transverse section through the midbrain at the level of the inferior colliculus

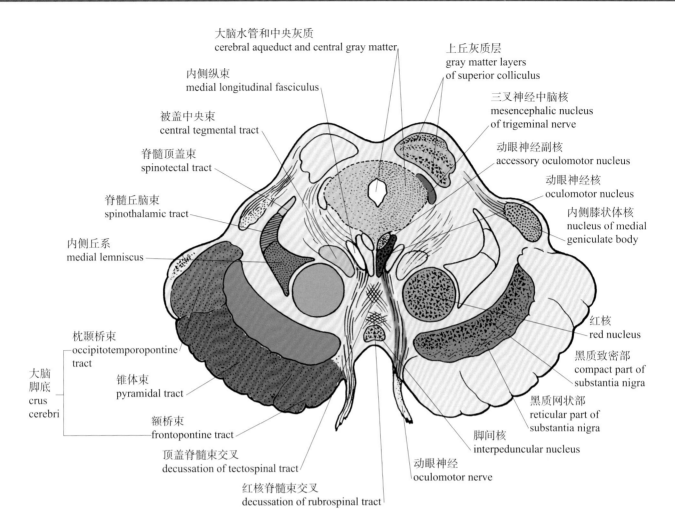

大脑水管和中央灰质
cerebral aqueduct and central gray matter

上丘灰质层
gray matter layers
of superior colliculus

内侧纵束
medial longitudinal fasciculus

三叉神经中脑核
mesencephalic nucleus
of trigeminal nerve

被盖中央束
central tegmental tract

动眼神经副核
accessory oculomotor nucleus

脊髓顶盖束
spinotectal tract

动眼神经核
oculomotor nucleus

脊髓丘脑束
spinothalamic tract

内侧膝状体核
nucleus of medial
geniculate body

内侧丘系
medial lemniscus

枕颞桥束
occipitotemporopontine
tract

红核
red nucleus

大脑
脚底
crus
cerebri

锥体束
pyramidal tract

黑质致密部
compact part of
substantia nigra

额桥束
frontopontine tract

黑质网状部
reticular part of
substantia nigra

顶盖脊髓束交叉
decussation of tectospinal tract

脚间核
interpeduncular nucleus

动眼神经
oculomotor nerve

红核脊髓束交叉
decussation of rubrospinal tract

图 13-27　经中脑上丘水平横切面
Transverse section through the midbrain at the level of the superior colliculus

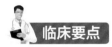 **临床要点**

中脑黑质致密部的神经元合成多巴胺，经黑质–纹状体系统，将多巴胺输送至纹状体。若新纹状体内的多巴胺减少到一定程度（50% 以上）时，可使背侧丘脑向大脑运动皮质发放的兴奋性冲动减少，患者表现为肌肉强直、运动受限、运动减少并出现震颤，称帕金森病，也称震颤麻痹。

Key Points of the Clinic

Neurons in the dense part of the substantia nigra of the midbrain synthesize dopamine, which is transported to the striatum via the substantia nigra-striatum system. If the amount of dopamine in the neostriatum is reduced to a certain degree (more than 50%), the excitatory impulses from the dorsal thalamus to the motor cortex of the brain will be reduced. The symptoms of the patient are muscle rigidity, restricted movement, decreased movement and tremor, which are called Parkinson disease or tremor paralysis.

第三节 小脑 Section 3 Cerebellum

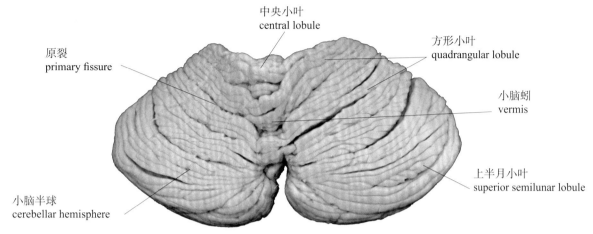

图 13-28 小脑（上面观）
Cerebellum (superior view)

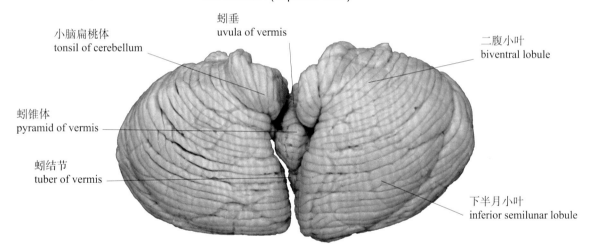

图 13-29 小脑（下面观）
Cerebellum (inferior view)

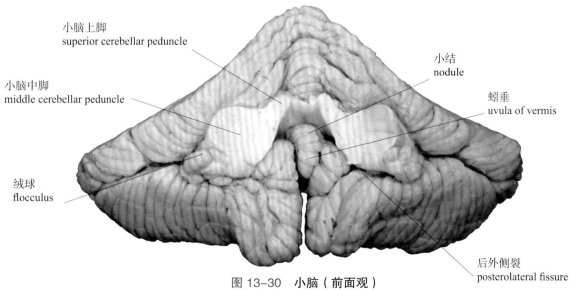

图 13-30 小脑（前面观）
Cerebellum (anterior view)

第五篇 神经与内分泌系统
Part 5 Nervous and Endocrine System

解剖纲要

小脑形态学分叶

分叶	组成
小脑前叶	原裂以前的小脑半球和蚓部
小脑后叶	原裂以后的小脑半球
绒球小结叶	绒球、绒球脚和蚓小结

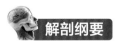 Anatomical Outline

The morphological lobes of cerebellum

Lobe	Formation
The anterior lobe of cerebellum	The cerebellar hemisphere in front of the primordial fissure, and vermis
The posterior lobe of cerebellum	The cerebellar hemisphere behind the primary fissure
The flocculonodular lobe	Flocculus, floccular peduncle and nodule

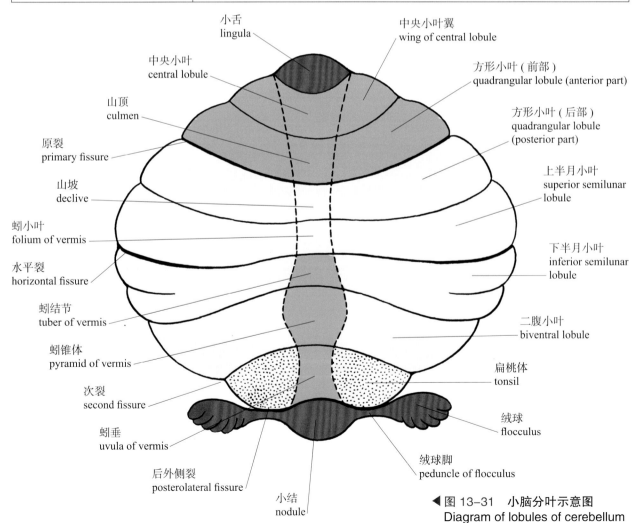

◀ 图 13-31　小脑分叶示意图
Diagram of lobules of cerebellum

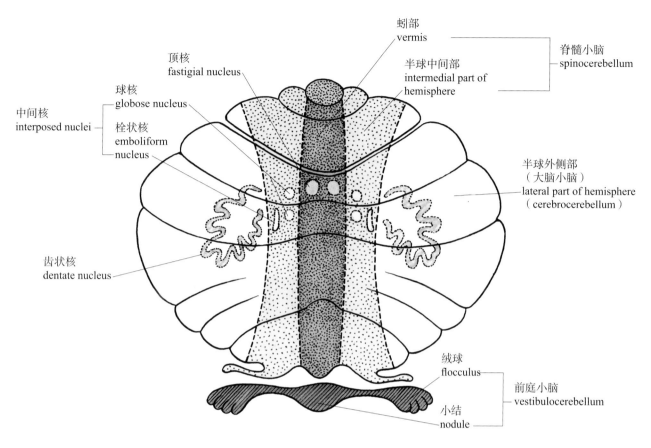

图 13-32 小脑的功能分叶示意图
Diagram of functional lobules of cerebellum

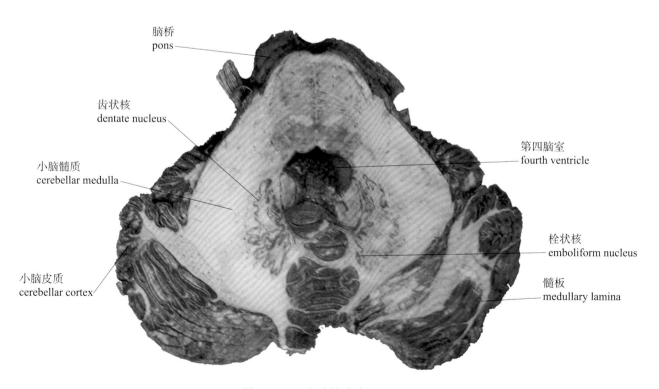

图 13-33 小脑核（水平切面）
Cerebellar nuclei (horizontal section)

第五篇 神经与内分泌系统
Part 5 Nervous and Endocrine System

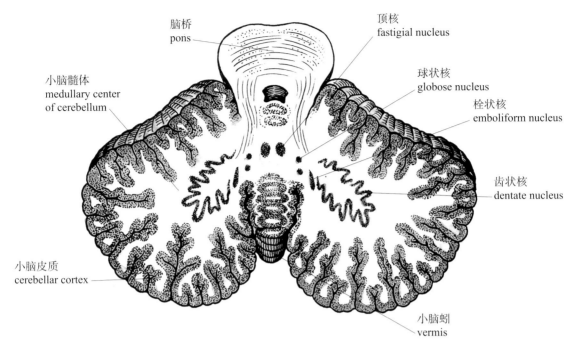

图 13-34　小脑核模式图（水平切面）
Diagram of cerebellar nuclei (horizontal section)

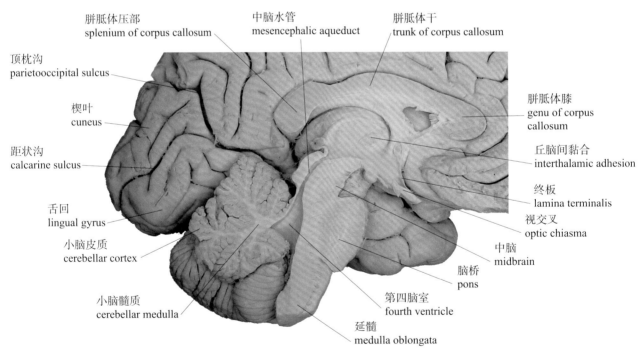

图 13-35　小脑及脑干（正中矢状切面）
Cerebellum and brain stem (median sagittal section)

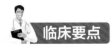 临床要点

小脑损伤后的典型症状：

原小脑综合征：平衡失调，眼球震颤。

新小脑综合征：共济失调，肌张力低下，运动性震颤等。

 Key Points of the Clinic

Typical symptoms after cerebellar injury：

Archicerebellar syndrome: balance disorder, nystagmus.

Neocerebellar syndrome: ataxia, hypotonia, kinetic tremor, etc.

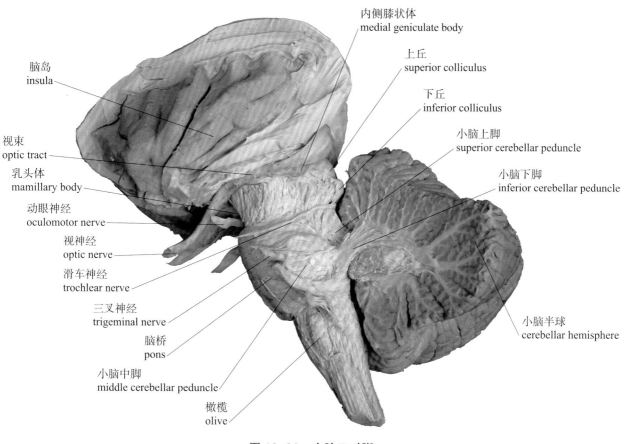

脑岛
insula

内侧膝状体
medial geniculate body

上丘
superior colliculus

下丘
inferior colliculus

小脑上脚
superior cerebellar peduncle

小脑下脚
inferior cerebellar peduncle

视束
optic tract

乳头体
mamillary body

动眼神经
oculomotor nerve

视神经
optic nerve

滑车神经
trochlear nerve

三叉神经
trigeminal nerve

脑桥
pons

小脑中脚
middle cerebellar peduncle

橄榄
olive

小脑半球
cerebellar hemisphere

图 13-36　小脑三对脚
Three pairs of cerebellar peduncle

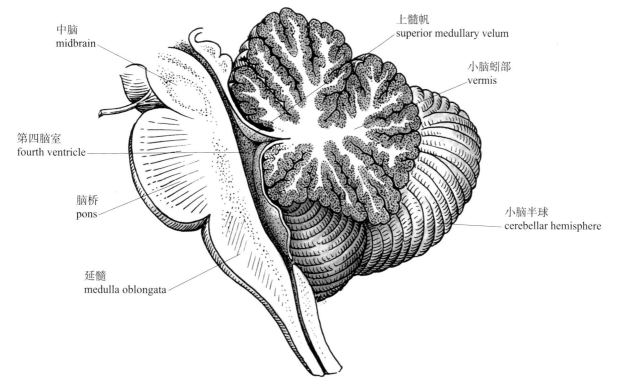

中脑
midbrain

上髓帆
superior medullary velum

小脑蚓部
vermis

第四脑室
fourth ventricle

脑桥
pons

延髓
medulla oblongata

小脑半球
cerebellar hemisphere

图 13-37　小脑及脑干矢状切面模式图
Diagram of sagittal section of the cerebellum and brain stem

第四节 间脑 Section 4 Diencephalon

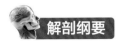解剖纲要

间脑
- 背侧丘脑：一对椭圆形灰质团块
- 上丘脑：松果体、缰三角、缰连合、丘脑髓纹和后连合
- 下丘脑：终板、视交叉、视束、灰结节、乳头体、漏斗、垂体
- 后丘脑：内侧膝状体、外侧膝状体
- 底丘脑：底丘脑核

Anatomical Outline

Dinencephalon
- Dorsal thalamus: a pair of oval gray masses
- Epithalamus: pineal body, habenular trigone, habenular commissure, medullary stria of thalamus and posterior commissure
- Hypothalamus: lamina terminalis, optic chiasma, optic tract, tuber cinereum, mammillary body, infundibulum, hypophysis
- Metathalamus: medial geniculate body, lateral geniculate body
- Subthalamus: subthalamic nucleus

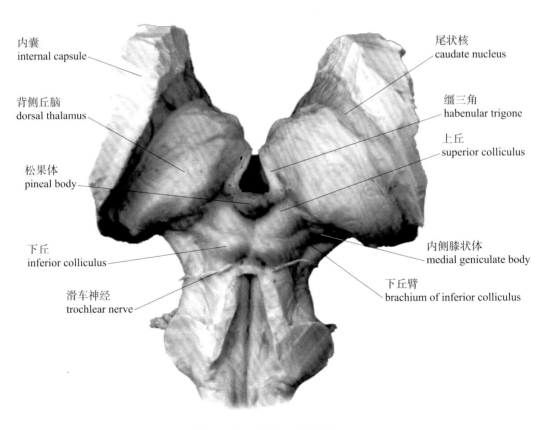

图 13-38　间脑（背面观）
Diencephalon (dorsal surface)

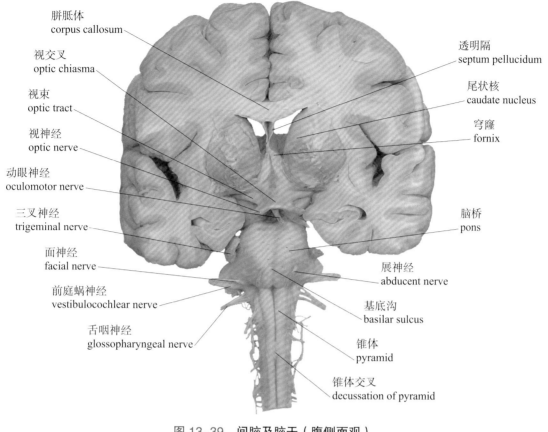

图 13-39　间脑及脑干（腹侧面观）
Diencephalon and brain stem (ventral surface)

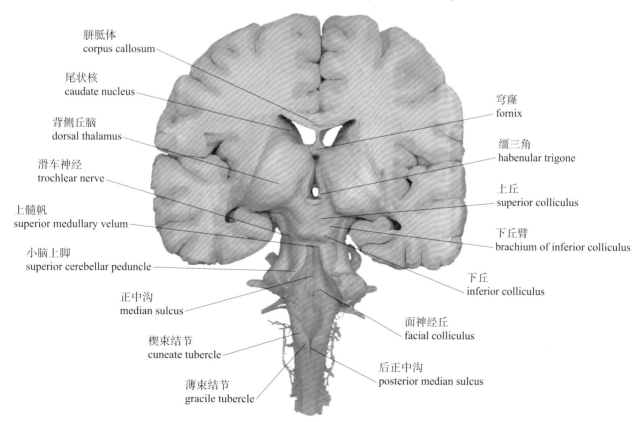

图 13-40　间脑及脑干（背侧面观）
Diencephalon and brain stem (dorsal surface)

第五篇　神经与内分泌系统
Part 5 Nervous and Endocrine System

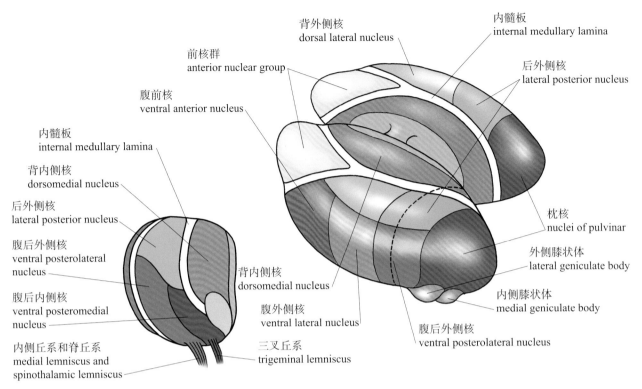

图 13-41　背侧丘脑核群
Nuclear group of dorsal thalamus

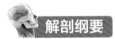 解剖纲要

背侧丘脑以"Y"字形内髓板分为前、内、外侧核群。

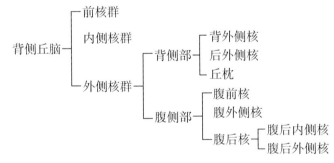

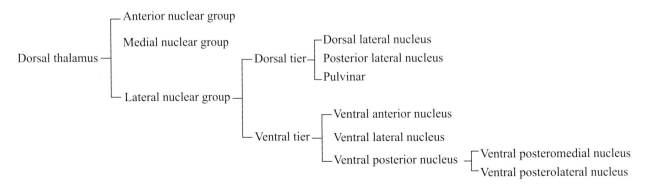 Anatomical Outline

The dorsal thalamus is divided into the anterior, medial and lateral nuclear groups by the "Y"-shaped internal medullary lamina.

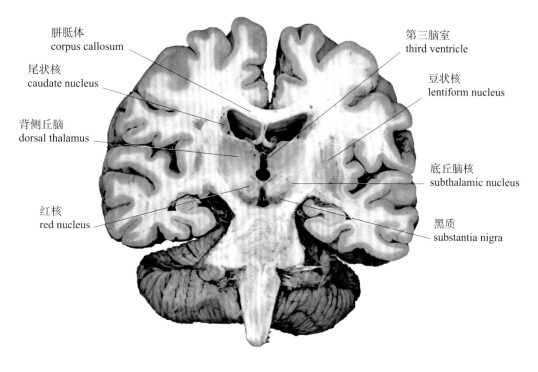

胼胝体 corpus callosum
尾状核 caudate nucleus
背侧丘脑 dorsal thalamus
红核 red nucleus
第三脑室 third ventricle
豆状核 lentiform nucleus
底丘脑核 subthalamic nucleus
黑质 substantia nigra

图 13-42 大脑冠状切面（示意背侧丘脑）
Coronal section of the brain (showing dorsal thalamus)

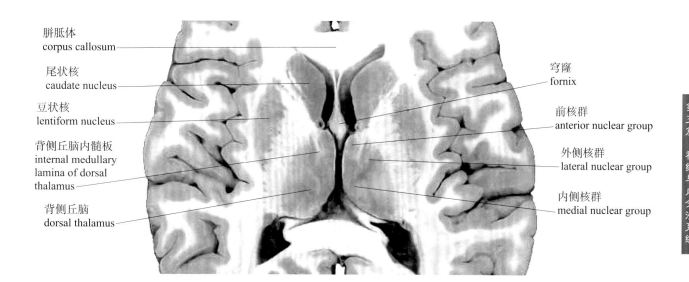

胼胝体 corpus callosum
尾状核 caudate nucleus
豆状核 lentiform nucleus
背侧丘脑内髓板 internal medullary lamina of dorsal thalamus
背侧丘脑 dorsal thalamus
穹窿 fornix
前核群 anterior nuclear group
外侧核群 lateral nuclear group
内侧核群 medial nuclear group

图 13-43 大脑水平切面（示意背侧丘脑）
Horizontal section of the brain (showing dorsal thalamus)

第五篇 神经与内分泌系统 Part 5 Nervous and Endocrine System

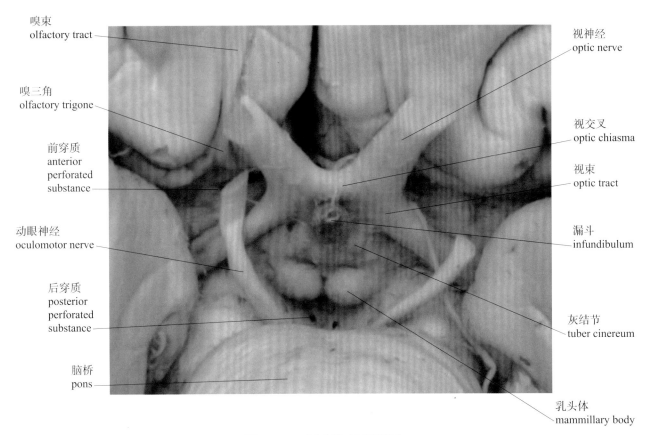

嗅束
olfactory tract

嗅三角
olfactory trigone

前穿质
anterior
perforated
substance

动眼神经
oculomotor nerve

后穿质
posterior
perforated
substance

脑桥
pons

视神经
optic nerve

视交叉
optic chiasma

视束
optic tract

漏斗
infundibulum

灰结节
tuber cinereum

乳头体
mammillary body

图 13-44 下丘脑（下面观）
Hypothalamus (inferior aspect)

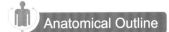 解剖纲要

下丘脑 ┬ 组成：终板、视交叉、视束、灰结节、漏斗、垂体、乳头体
　　　　└ 分区：由前向后分为视前区、视上区、结节区和乳头体区

 Anatomical Outline

Hypothalamus ┬ Formation: lamina terminalis, optic chiasma, optic tracts, tuber cinereum,
　　　　　　　　　　　　funnel, hypophysis, mammillary bodies
　　　　　　　 └ Division: preoptic area, supraoptic area, tuberal area and papillae area (from anterior backward)

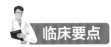 临床要点

先天性或继发性的下丘脑 - 垂体功能异常，可引起下丘脑促性腺激素合成和分泌障碍，从而导致女性闭经。男性出现原发性或继发性下丘脑和垂体病变可引起不育症。

 Key Points of the Clinic

Congenital or secondary dysfunction of hypothalamic-pituitary can cause the hypothalamus gonadotropin releasing hormone (GnRH) synthesis and secretion disorder, leading to amenorrhea in women. For males, primary or secondary hypothalamic and pituitary lesions can cause infertility.

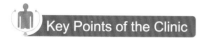 临床要点

1. 背侧丘脑是皮质下感觉的最后中继核，并可感知本体感觉和痛觉。当背侧丘脑受损时，可引起感觉功能障碍和痛觉过敏、自发性疼痛等。

2. 松果体位于上丘脑的后部、胼胝体压部和上丘之间。青春期（16岁）后松果体逐渐钙化，临床影像学上常将其作为颅内定位标志。

Key Points of the Clinic

1. The dorsal thalamus is the last relay nucleus of subcortical sensation, and may perceive proprioception and pain. When the dorsal thalamus is damaged, it can cause sensory dysfunction and hyperalgesia, spontaneous pain, etc.

2. The pineal body is located in the posterior part of the epithalamus and between the splenium of corpus callosum and the superior colliculus. After puberty (16 years old) the pineal body is gradually calcified and can be served as a marker of intracranial localization in clinical imageology.

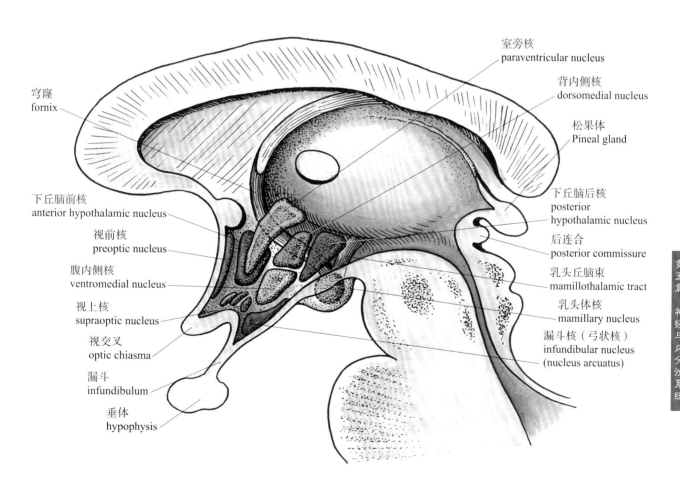

图 13-45 下丘脑核团模式图（矢状切面）
Diagram of hypothalamic nuclei (sagittal section)

第五篇 神经与内分泌系统
Part 5 Nervous and Endocrine System

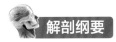

第五节 端脑 Section 5 Telencephalon

端脑区分

端脑以大脑纵裂区分为左、右大脑半球，每一大脑半球又可区分为额叶、顶叶、枕叶、颞叶和岛叶。

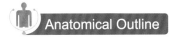

The division of the telencephalon

The telencephalon is divided into left and right cerebral hemispheres by the cerebral longitudinal fissure, and each hemisphere can be divided into frontal lobe, parietal lobe, occipital lobe, temporal lobe and insula lobe.

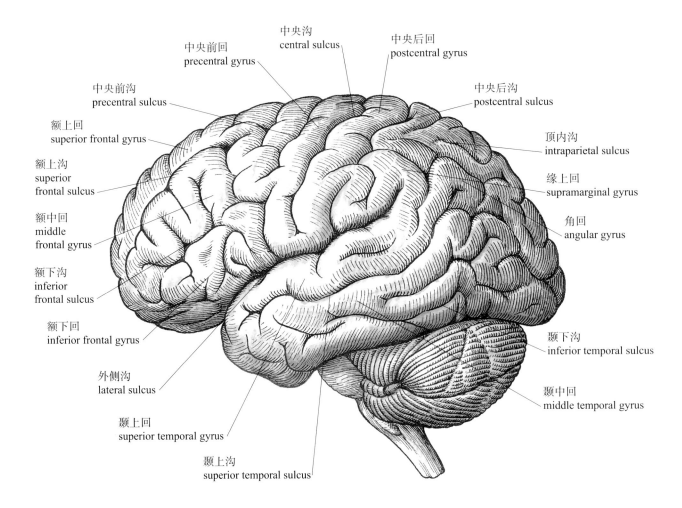

图 13-46 大脑半球上外侧面（模式图）
Superolateral surface of cerebral hemisphere (diagram)

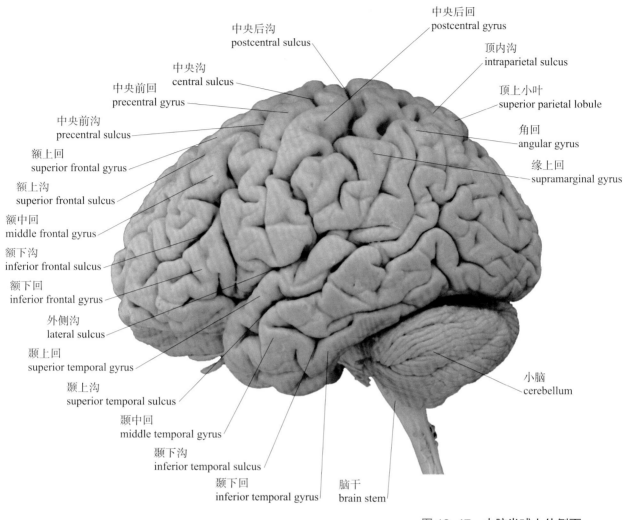

中央后回
postcentral gyrus

中央后沟
postcentral sulcus

顶内沟
intraparietal sulcus

中央沟
central sulcus

顶上小叶
superior parietal lobule

中央前回
precentral gyrus

角回
angular gyrus

中央前沟
precentral sulcus

缘上回
supramarginal gyrus

额上回
superior frontal gyrus

额上沟
superior frontal sulcus

额中回
middle frontal gyrus

额下沟
inferior frontal sulcus

额下回
inferior frontal gyrus

外侧沟
lateral sulcus

颞上回
superior temporal gyrus

小脑
cerebellum

颞上沟
superior temporal sulcus

颞中回
middle temporal gyrus

颞下沟
inferior temporal sulcus

颞下回
inferior temporal gyrus

脑干
brain stem

图 13-47 大脑半球上外侧面
Superolateral surface of cerebral hemisphere

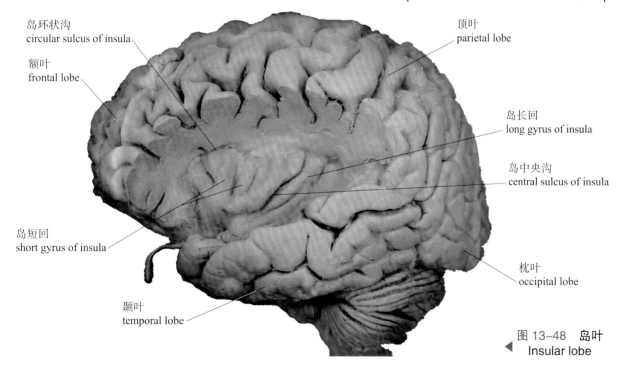

岛环状沟
circular sulcus of insula

顶叶
parietal lobe

额叶
frontal lobe

岛长回
long gyrus of insula

岛中央沟
central sulcus of insula

岛短回
short gyrus of insula

枕叶
occipital lobe

颞叶
temporal lobe

图 13-48 岛叶
Insular lobe

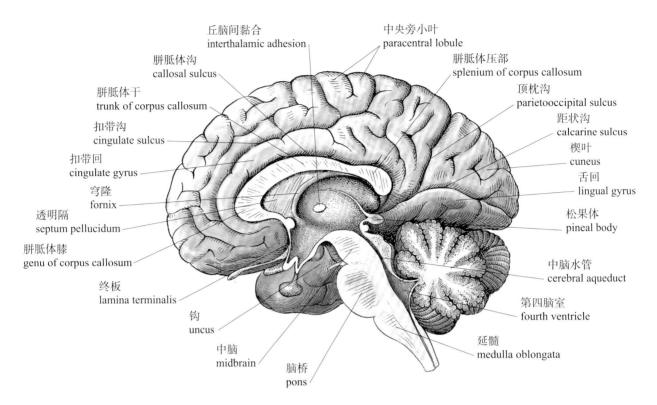

丘脑间黏合
interthalamic adhesion

中央旁小叶
paracentral lobule

胼胝体沟
callosal sulcus

胼胝体压部
splenium of corpus callosum

胼胝体干
trunk of corpus callosum

顶枕沟
parietooccipital sulcus

扣带沟
cingulate sulcus

距状沟
calcarine sulcus

扣带回
cingulate gyrus

楔叶
cuneus

穹隆
fornix

舌回
lingual gyrus

透明隔
septum pellucidum

松果体
pineal body

胼胝体膝
genu of corpus callosum

中脑水管
cerebral aqueduct

终板
lamina terminalis

第四脑室
fourth ventricle

钩
uncus

延髓
medulla oblongata

中脑
midbrain

脑桥
pons

图 13-49　大脑正中矢状切面（模式图）
Median sagittal section of cerebrum (diagram)

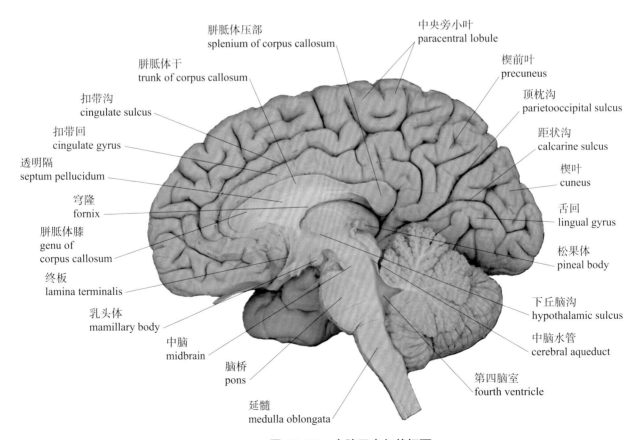

胼胝体压部
splenium of corpus callosum

中央旁小叶
paracentral lobule

胼胝体干
trunk of corpus callosum

楔前叶
precuneus

扣带沟
cingulate sulcus

顶枕沟
parietooccipital sulcus

扣带回
cingulate gyrus

距状沟
calcarine sulcus

透明隔
septum pellucidum

楔叶
cuneus

穹隆
fornix

舌回
lingual gyrus

胼胝体膝
genu of
corpus callosum

松果体
pineal body

终板
lamina terminalis

下丘脑沟
hypothalamic sulcus

乳头体
mamillary body

中脑水管
cerebral aqueduct

中脑
midbrain

第四脑室
fourth ventricle

脑桥
pons

延髓
medulla oblongata

图 13-50　大脑正中矢状切面
Median sagittal section of cerebrum

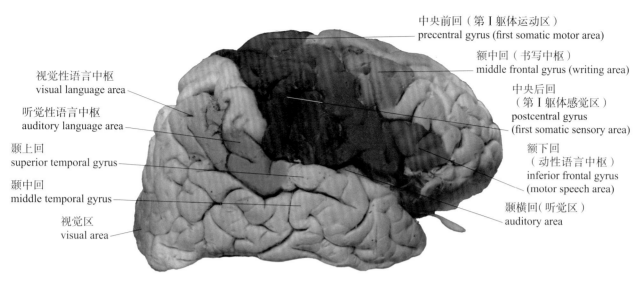

中央前回（第Ⅰ躯体运动区）
precentral gyrus (first somatic motor area)

额中回（书写中枢）
middle frontal gyrus (writing area)

中央后回
（第Ⅰ躯体感觉区）
postcentral gyrus
(first somatic sensory area)

额下回
（动性语言中枢）
inferior frontal gyrus
(motor speech area)

颞横回（听觉区）
auditory area

视觉性语言中枢
visual language area

听觉性语言中枢
auditory language area

颞上回
superior temporal gyrus

颞中回
middle temporal gyrus

视觉区
visual area

图 13-51　大脑半球上外侧面及相关皮质功能区
Superolateral surface of cerebral hemisphere and main functional areas of cerebral cortex

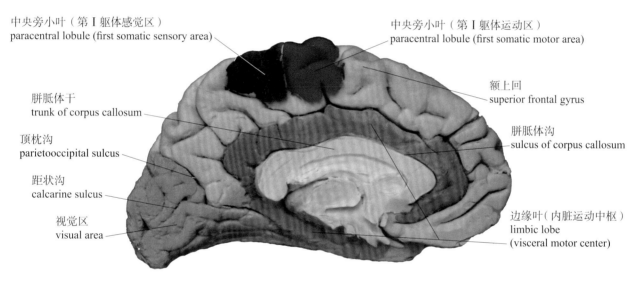

中央旁小叶（第Ⅰ躯体感觉区）
paracentral lobule (first somatic sensory area)

中央旁小叶（第Ⅰ躯体运动区）
paracentral lobule (first somatic motor area)

额上回
superior frontal gyrus

胼胝体干
trunk of corpus callosum

胼胝体沟
sulcus of corpus callosum

顶枕沟
parietooccipital sulcus

距状沟
calcarine sulcus

视觉区
visual area

边缘叶（内脏运动中枢）
limbic lobe
(visceral motor center)

图 13-52　大脑半球内侧面及相关皮质功能区
Medial surface of cerebral hemisphere and main functional areas of cerebral cortex

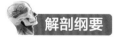 解剖纲要

大脑皮质功能定位区

名称	位置
第1躯体运动区	中央前回、中央旁小叶前部
第1躯体感觉区	中央后回、中央旁小叶后部
视觉区	距状沟上、下的枕叶皮质
听觉区	颞横回
运动性语言中枢	额下回后部
书写中枢	额中回后部
听觉性语言中枢	颞上回后部
视觉性语言中枢	角回

第五篇　神经与内分泌系统　Part 5 Nervous and Endocrine System

Functional localization of the cerebral cortex

Name	Location
First somatic motor area	Precentral gyrus, anterior part of the paracentral lobule
First somatic sensory area	Postcentral gyrus, posterior part of the paracentral lobule
Visual area	Surround the calcarine sulcus of the occipital lobe
Acoustic area	Transverse temporal gyrus
Motor speech area	The posterior portion of the inferior frontal gyrus
Writing area	The posterior portion of the middle frontal gyrus
Auditory language area	The posterior portion of the superior temporal gyrus
Visual language area	Angular gyrus

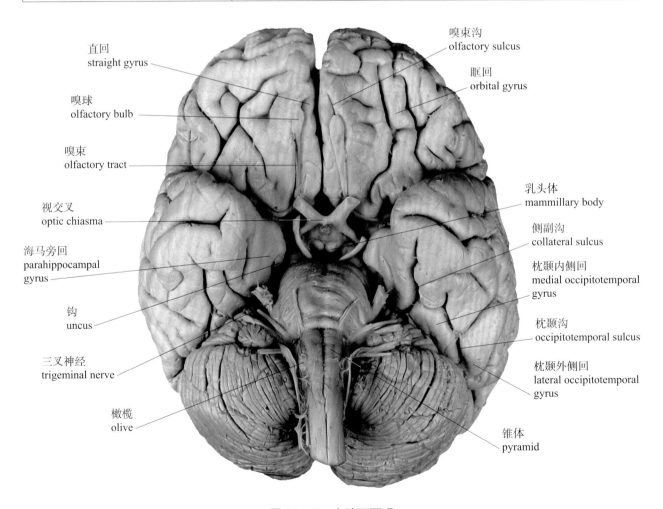

图 13-53　大脑下面观
Inferior surface of cerebrum

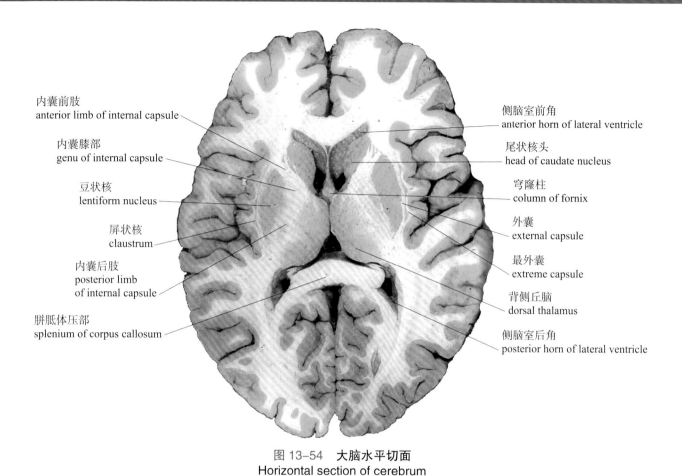

内囊前肢
anterior limb of internal capsule

内囊膝部
genu of internal capsule

豆状核
lentiform nucleus

屏状核
claustrum

内囊后肢
posterior limb
of internal capsule

胼胝体压部
splenium of corpus callosum

侧脑室前角
anterior horn of lateral ventricle

尾状核头
head of caudate nucleus

穹窿柱
column of fornix

外囊
external capsule

最外囊
extreme capsule

背侧丘脑
dorsal thalamus

侧脑室后角
posterior horn of lateral ventricle

图 13-54　大脑水平切面
Horizontal section of cerebrum

胼胝体
corpus callosum

尾状核
caudate nucleus

穹窿
fornix

背侧丘脑
dorsal thalamus

底丘脑核
subthalamic nucleus

红核
red nucleus

黑质
substantia nigra

三叉神经
trigeminal nerve

前庭蜗神经
vestibulocochlear nerve

面神经
facial nerve

内囊
internal capsule

豆状核
lentiform nucleus

岛叶
insular lobe

屏状核
claustrum

侧脑室脉络丛
choroid plexus of
lateral ventricle

舌咽神经
glossopharyngeal nerve

迷走神经
vagus nerve

图 13-55　大脑冠状切面
Coronal section of cerebrum

临床要点

　　临床上，大脑皮质和海马发生变性改变可引起阿尔茨海默病（简称 AD），它是一种以进行性认知功能障碍和记忆力减退为特征的神经系统退行性疾病，是老年痴呆最常见的类型。病理改变主要为大脑皮质弥漫性萎缩（以海马及内侧颞叶较显著）、沟回增宽、脑室扩大、神经元大量减少、星形胶质细胞和小胶质细胞活化，并可见老年斑、神经原纤维缠结等病变。

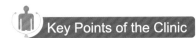 **Key Points of the Clinic**

　　In clinic, the degeneration of the cerebral cortex and hippocampus can cause Alzheimer's disease (AD), which is a neurodegenerative disease characterized by progressive cognitive impairment and memory decline. It is the most common type of dementia in the elderly. The main pathological changes were diffuse atrophy of the cerebral cortex (especially in the hippocampus and medial temporal lobe), widening of sulcus and gyrus, enlargement of ventricles, a large reduction of neurons, activation of astrocytes and microglia, and the appearance of senile plaques and neurofibrillary tangles.

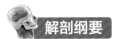 **解剖纲要**

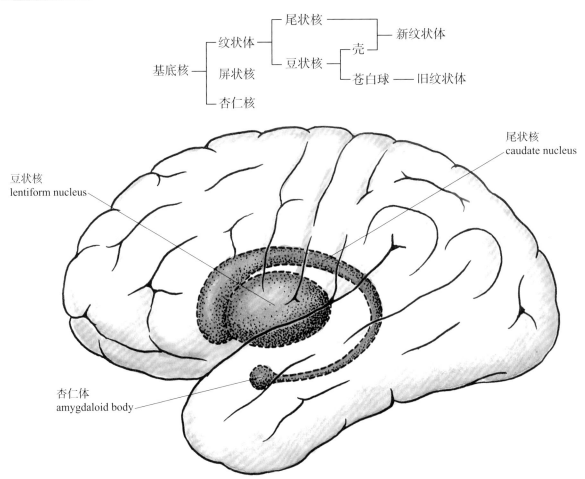

图 13-56　基底核在脑表面投影位置
The projection of basal nuclei on cerebral surface

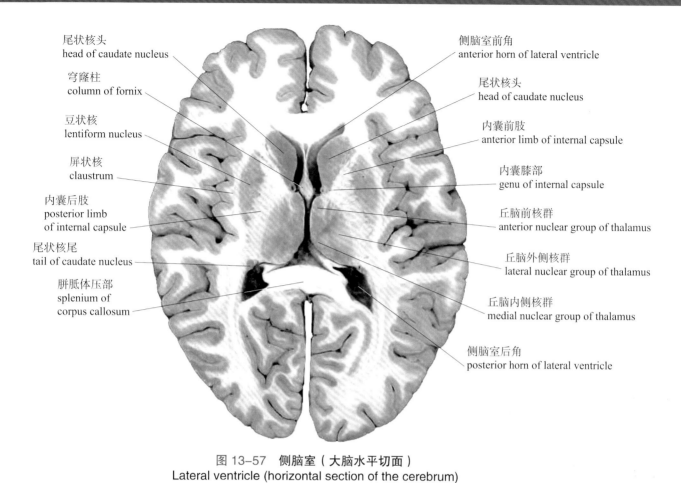

尾状核头
head of caudate nucleus

穹窿柱
column of fornix

豆状核
lentiform nucleus

屏状核
claustrum

内囊后肢
posterior limb
of internal capsule

尾状核尾
tail of caudate nucleus

胼胝体压部
splenium of
corpus callosum

侧脑室前角
anterior horn of lateral ventricle

尾状核头
head of caudate nucleus

内囊前肢
anterior limb of internal capsule

内囊膝部
genu of internal capsule

丘脑前核群
anterior nuclear group of thalamus

丘脑外侧核群
lateral nuclear group of thalamus

丘脑内侧核群
medial nuclear group of thalamus

侧脑室后角
posterior horn of lateral ventricle

图 13-57　侧脑室（大脑水平切面）
Lateral ventricle (horizontal section of the cerebrum)

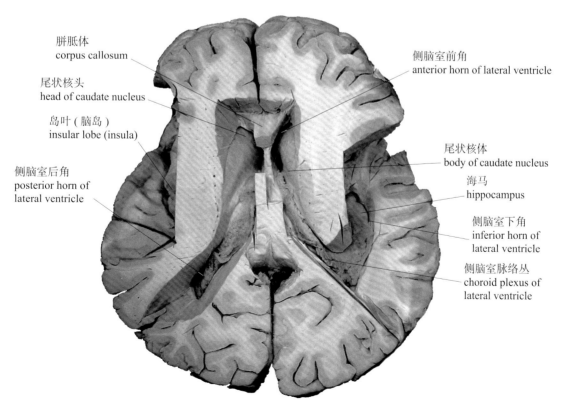

胼胝体
corpus callosum

尾状核头
head of caudate nucleus

岛叶（脑岛）
insular lobe (insula)

侧脑室后角
posterior horn of
lateral ventricle

侧脑室前角
anterior horn of lateral ventricle

尾状核体
body of caudate nucleus

海马
hippocampus

侧脑室下角
inferior horn of
lateral ventricle

侧脑室脉络丛
choroid plexus of
lateral ventricle

图 13-58　侧脑室
Lateral ventricle

Anatomical Outline

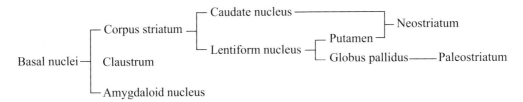

Basal nuclei ─┬─ Corpus striatum ─┬─ Caudate nucleus ──────────────┬─ Neostriatum
　　　　　　　 │　　　　　　　　　 │　　　　　　　　　　　　 ┌─ Putamen ──┘
　　　　　　　 │　　　　　　　　　 └─ Lentiform nucleus ─┤
　　　　　　　 │　　　　　　　　　　　　　　　　　　　　 └─ Globus pallidus ──── Paleostriatum
　　　　　　　 ├─ Claustrum
　　　　　　　 └─ Amygdaloid nucleus

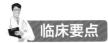 临床要点

　　基底核由尾状核、豆状核、屏状核、杏仁核组成。此外，临床上常将黑质和底丘脑核也列为基底核。临床上基底核损害的主要表现分为两大类：一类是因运动过多而致肌紧张不全的综合征，如亨廷顿病，其病变主要位于纹状体；另一类是因运动过少而致肌紧张过强的综合征，如帕金森病，其病变主要位于黑质。

Key Points of the Clinic

　　Basal nuclei consist of the caudate nucleus, lentiform nucleus, claustrum and amygdaloid nucleus. Besides, substantia nigra and subthalamic nucleus are also involved in its composition. The main clinical manifestations of basal nuclei damage are divided into two types: one is a syndrome with excessive exercises and low muscle tension, such as Huntington's disease, whose lesions are mainly located in the striatum; the other is a syndrome with less exercise and high muscle tension, such as Parkinson's disease, whose lesions are mainly located in the substantia nigra.

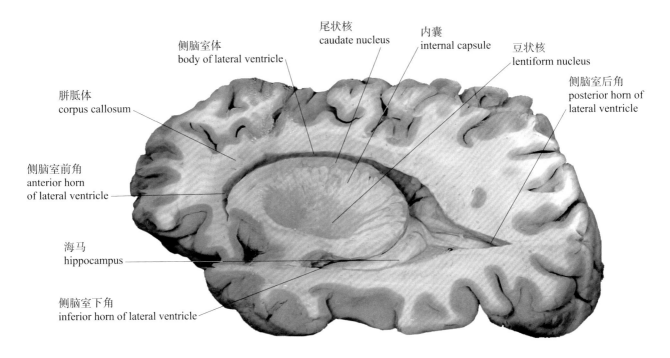

图 13-59　大脑半球斜切面（示侧脑室）
Oblique section of cerebral hemisphere (showing lateral ventricle)

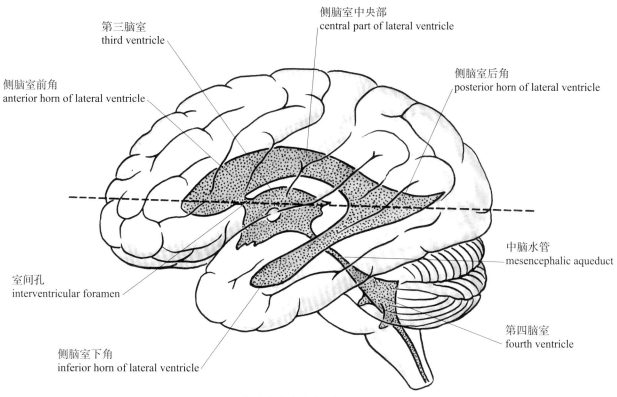

侧脑室在大脑表面投影
The projection of lateral ventricle onlateral cerebral surface

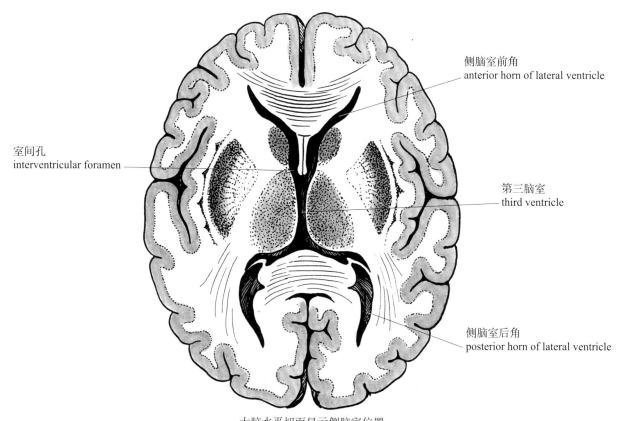

大脑水平切面显示侧脑室位置
Showing location of lateral ventricle of the horizontal section of cerebrum

图 13-60　侧脑室模式图
Diagram of lateral ventricle

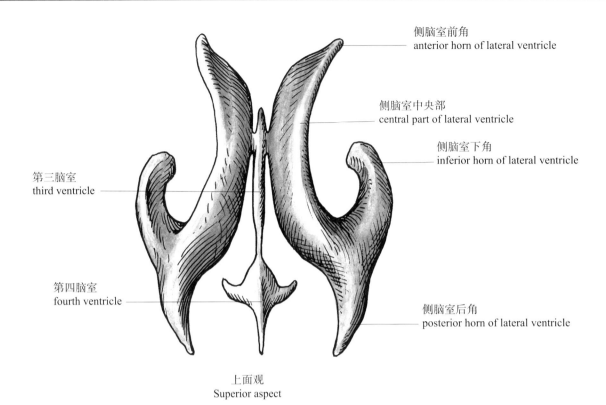

侧脑室前角
anterior horn of lateral ventricle

侧脑室中央部
central part of lateral ventricle

侧脑室下角
inferior horn of lateral ventricle

第三脑室
third ventricle

第四脑室
fourth ventricle

侧脑室后角
posterior horn of lateral ventricle

上面观
Superior aspect

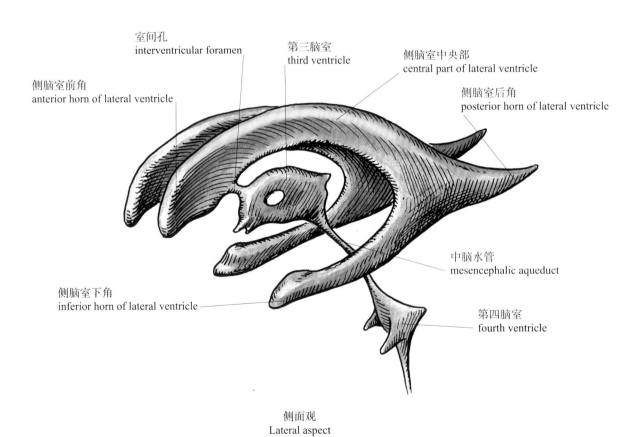

室间孔
interventricular foramen

第三脑室
third ventricle

侧脑室中央部
central part of lateral ventricle

侧脑室前角
anterior horn of lateral ventricle

侧脑室后角
posterior horn of lateral ventricle

中脑水管
mesencephalic aqueduct

侧脑室下角
inferior horn of lateral ventricle

第四脑室
fourth ventricle

侧面观
Lateral aspect

图 13-61　脑室铸型
Cast of the ventricles of brain

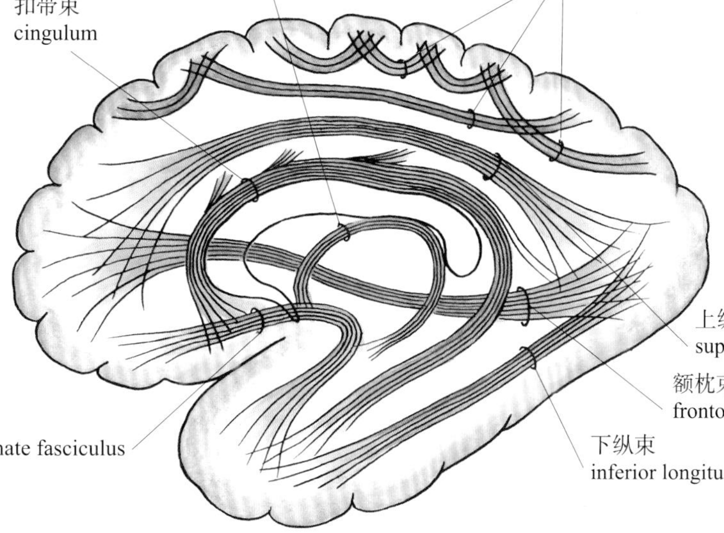

终纹
terminal stria

弓状纤维
arcuate fibers

扣带束
cingulum

上纵束
superior longitudinal fasciculus

额枕束
frontooccipital fasciculus

钩束
uncinate fasciculus

下纵束
inferior longitudinal fasciculus

图 13-62　大脑半球联络纤维
Association fibers of cerebral hemisphere

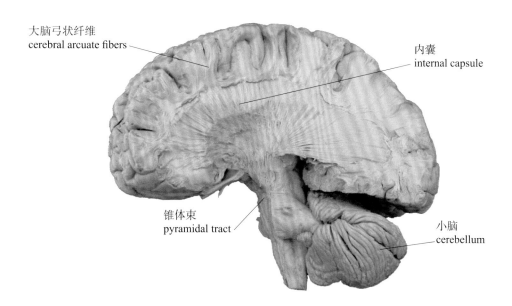

大脑弓状纤维
cerebral arcuate fibers

内囊
internal capsule

锥体束
pyramidal tract

小脑
cerebellum

图 13-63　投射纤维及联络纤维
Projection fibers and association fibers

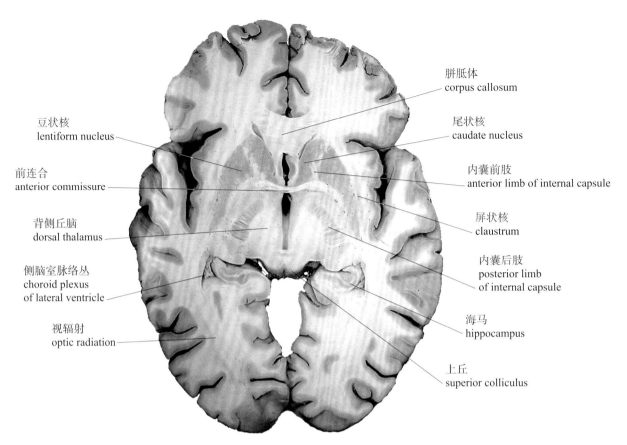

豆状核
lentiform nucleus

前连合
anterior commissure

背侧丘脑
dorsal thalamus

侧脑室脉络丛
choroid plexus
of lateral ventricle

视辐射
optic radiation

胼胝体
corpus callosum

尾状核
caudate nucleus

内囊前肢
anterior limb of internal capsule

屏状核
claustrum

内囊后肢
posterior limb
of internal capsule

海马
hippocampus

上丘
superior colliculus

图 13-64　前连合（脑水平切面）
Anterior commissure (horizontal section of cerebrum)

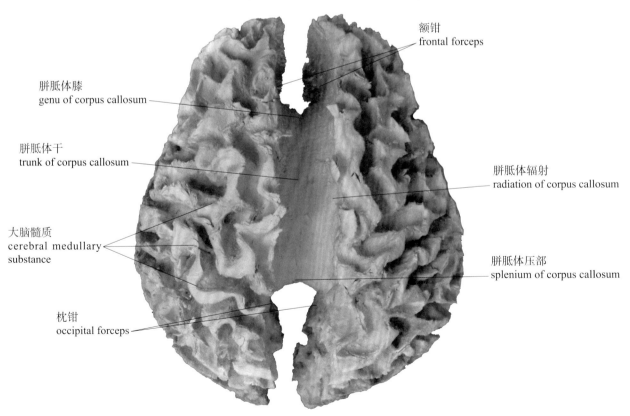

胼胝体膝
genu of corpus callosum

胼胝体干
trunk of corpus callosum

大脑髓质
cerebral medullary
substance

枕钳
occipital forceps

额钳
frontal forceps

胼胝体辐射
radiation of corpus callosum

胼胝体压部
splenium of corpus callosum

图 13-65　大脑髓质（上面观）
Cerebral medullary substance (superior view)

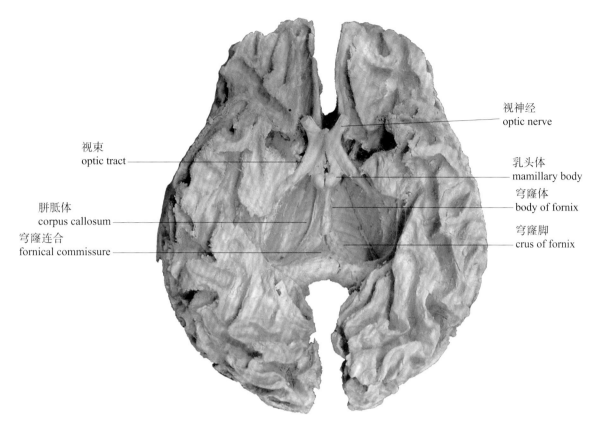

视束
optic tract

胼胝体
corpus callosum

穹窿连合
fornical commissure

视神经
optic nerve

乳头体
mamillary body

穹窿体
body of fornix

穹窿脚
crus of fornix

图 13-66　大脑髓质（底面观）
Cerebral medullary substance (inferior view)

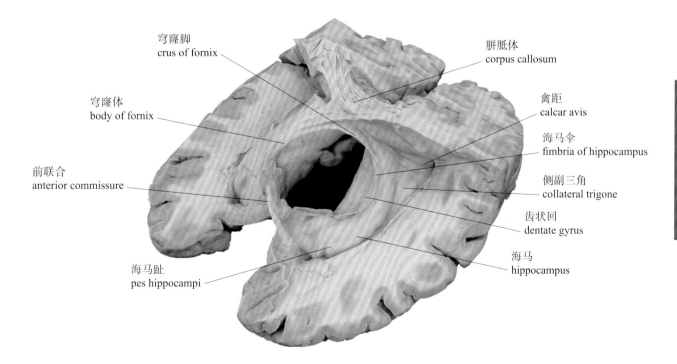

穹窿脚
crus of fornix

穹窿体
body of fornix

前联合
anterior commissure

海马趾
pes hippocampi

胼胝体
corpus callosum

禽距
calcar avis

海马伞
fimbria of hippocampus

侧副三角
collateral trigone

齿状回
dentate gyrus

海马
hippocampus

图 13-67　海马及穹窿
Hippocampus and fornix

第五篇　神经与内分泌系统
Part 5 Nervous and Endocrine System

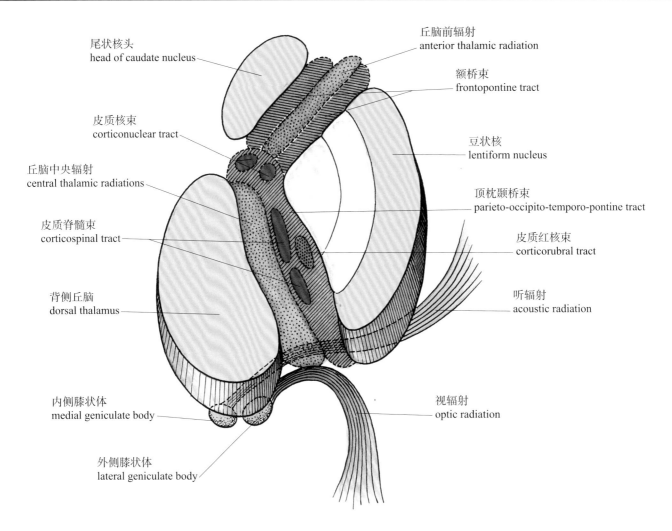

图 13-68 内囊模式图（水平切面）
Diagram of the internal capsule (horizontal section)

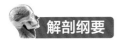 解剖纲要

内囊

内囊位于丘脑、尾状核与豆状核之间，在水平切面上呈向外开放的"V"字形。内囊各部通过的纤维束有：①内囊前肢：位于豆状核与尾状核之间，有额桥束、丘脑前辐射通过。② 内囊膝：前、后肢会合部，有皮质核束通过。③内囊后肢：位于豆状核与丘脑之间，有皮质脊髓束、皮质红核束、丘脑中央辐射、顶枕颞桥束、视辐射、听辐射通过。

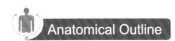 Anatomical Outline

Internal capsule

Internal capsule lies among the thalamus, caudate and lentiform nuclei. It opens outward in the shape of a "V" on horizontal section. Portions of internal capsule and the main fibers passing through them: ① Anterion limb: It lies between

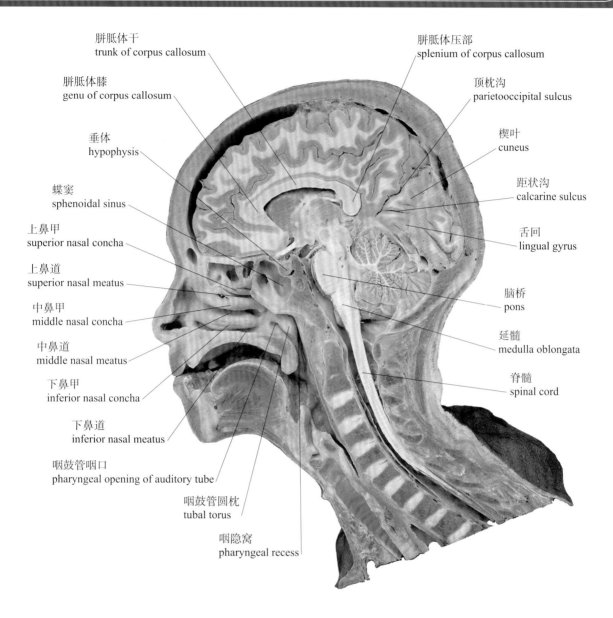

图 13-69 头颈正中矢状切面
Median sagittal section of the head and neck

the lentiform nucleus and the head of the caudate nucleus. The frontopontine tract and anterior thalamic radiation pass through the anterior limb. ② Genu:It lies at the junction of the anterior and posterior limbs and contains the corticonuclear tract. ③ Posterior limb: It lies between the lentiform nucleus and thalamus. There are corticospinal tract, corticorubral tract, central thalamic radiation, parietal-occipital-temporal-pontine tract, optic radiation, and acoustic radiation pass through the posterior limb.

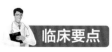 临床要点

临床上当内囊受损时，可出现典型的"三偏症"，即对侧身体感觉丧失（丘脑中央辐射受损），对侧偏瘫（皮质脊髓束、皮质核束受损）及双眼对侧视野同向性偏盲（视辐射受损）。

第五篇 神经与内分泌系统 Part 5 Nervous and Endocrine System

Key Points of the Clinic

When the internal capsule is damaged, the typical symptoms can occur, that is, the loss of contralateral sensation (central thalamic radiation is damaged), contralateral hemiplegia (corticospinal and corticonuclear tracts are damaged) and homonymous hemianopsia of the contralateral visual field of both eyes (visual radiation is damaged).

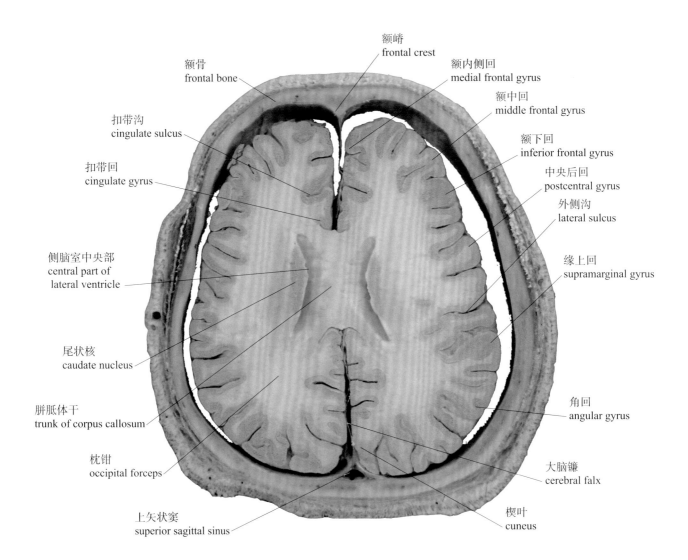

图 13-70　经胼胝体干的脑横切面
Transverse section of brain through the trunk of corpus callosum

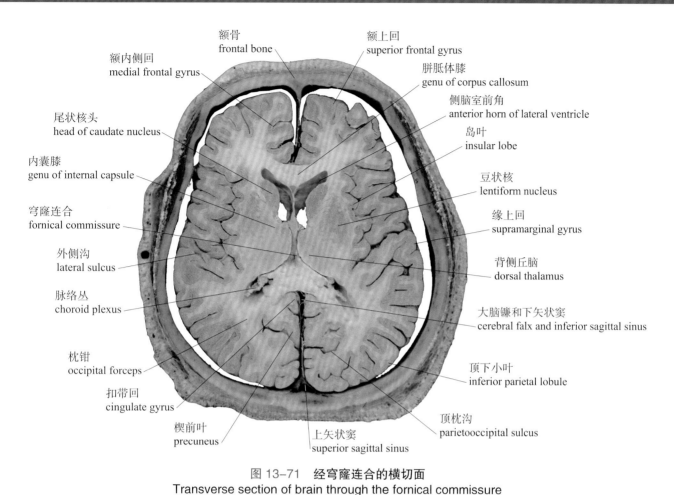

额骨
frontal bone

额上回
superior frontal gyrus

额内侧回
medial frontal gyrus

胼胝体膝
genu of corpus callosum

侧脑室前角
anterior horn of lateral ventricle

尾状核头
head of caudate nucleus

岛叶
insular lobe

内囊膝
genu of internal capsule

豆状核
lentiform nucleus

穹窿连合
fornical commissure

缘上回
supramarginal gyrus

外侧沟
lateral sulcus

背侧丘脑
dorsal thalamus

脉络丛
choroid plexus

大脑镰和下矢状窦
cerebral falx and inferior sagittal sinus

枕钳
occipital forceps

顶下小叶
inferior parietal lobule

扣带回
cingulate gyrus

楔前叶
precuneus

上矢状窦
superior sagittal sinus

顶枕沟
parietooccipital sulcus

图 13-71 经穹窿连合的横切面
Transverse section of brain through the fornical commissure

额窦
frontal sinus

额嵴
frontal crest

额内侧回
medial frontal gyrus

额上回
superior frontal gyrus

侧脑室前角
anterior horn of lateral ventricle

额中回
middle frontal gyrus

内囊前肢
anterior limb of internal capsule

尾状核头
head of caudate nucleus

丘脑间黏合
interthalamic adhesion

屏状核
claustrum

外侧沟
lateral sulcus

第三脑室
third ventricle

豆状核壳
putamen of lentiform nucleus

松果体
pineal body

内囊后肢
posterior limb of internal capsule

海马
hippocampus

背侧丘脑
dorsal thalamus

视辐射
optic radiation

直窦
straight sinus

距状沟
calcarine sulcus

上矢状窦
superior sagittal sinus

图 13-72 经松果体的横切面
Transverse section of brain through the pineal body

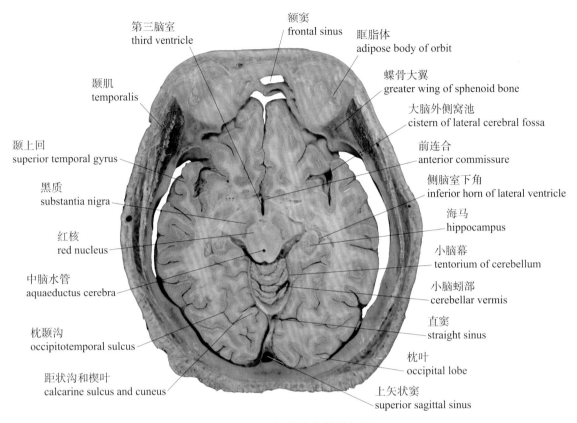

第三脑室
third ventricle

额窦
frontal sinus

眶脂体
adipose body of orbit

颞肌
temporalis

蝶骨大翼
greater wing of sphenoid bone

颞上回
superior temporal gyrus

大脑外侧窝池
cistern of lateral cerebral fossa

黑质
substantia nigra

前连合
anterior commissure

红核
red nucleus

侧脑室下角
inferior horn of lateral ventricle

中脑水管
aquaeductus cerebra

海马
hippocampus

枕颞沟
occipitotemporal sulcus

小脑幕
tentorium of cerebellum

距状沟和楔叶
calcarine sulcus and cuneus

小脑蚓部
cerebellar vermis

直窦
straight sinus

枕叶
occipital lobe

上矢状窦
superior sagittal sinus

图 13-73 经前连合的横切面
Transverse section of brain through the anterior commissure

第六节 脑和脊髓的被膜、血管及脑脊液循环

Section 6 Meninges, blood vessels, and cerebrospinal fluid circulation of brain and spinal cord

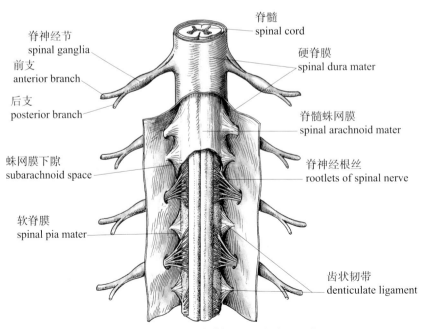

脊神经节
spinal ganglia

脊髓
spinal cord

前支
anterior branch

硬脊膜
spinal dura mater

后支
posterior branch

脊髓蛛网膜
spinal arachnoid mater

蛛网膜下隙
subarachnoid space

脊神经根丝
rootlets of spinal nerve

软脊膜
spinal pia mater

齿状韧带
denticulate ligament

图 13-74 脊髓被膜模式图（前面观）
Diagram of meninges of spinal cord (anterior view)

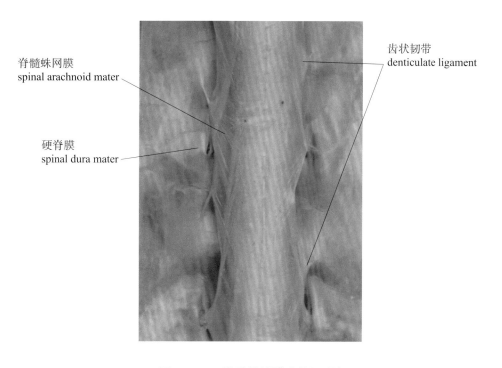

图 13-75　脊髓的被膜（前面观）
Meninges of spinal cord (anterior view)

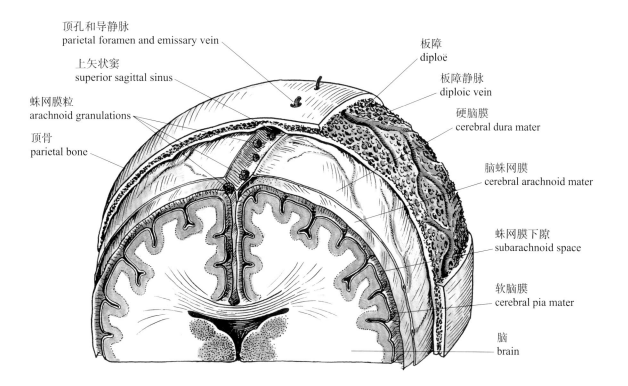

图 13-76　脑的被膜（冠状切面）
Coverings of brain (coronary view)

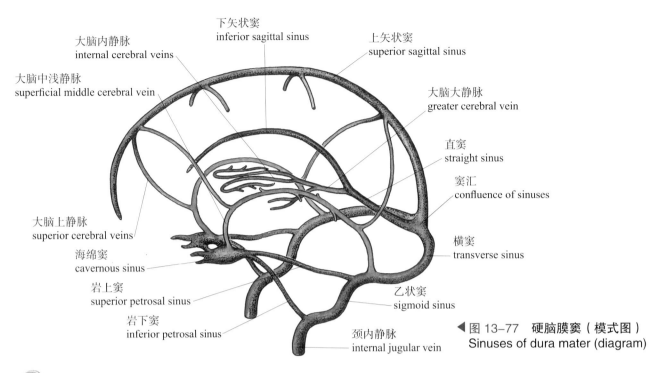

大脑内静脉
internal cerebral veins

下矢状窦
inferior sagittal sinus

上矢状窦
superior sagittal sinus

大脑中浅静脉
superficial middle cerebral vein

大脑大静脉
greater cerebral vein

直窦
straight sinus

窦汇
confluence of sinuses

大脑上静脉
superior cerebral veins

横窦
transverse sinus

海绵窦
cavernous sinus

岩上窦
superior petrosal sinus

乙状窦
sigmoid sinus

岩下窦
inferior petrosal sinus

颈内静脉
internal jugular vein

◀ 图 13-77　硬脑膜窦（模式图）
Sinuses of dura mater (diagram)

解剖纲要

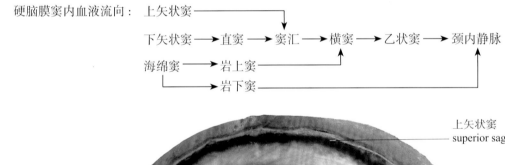

硬脑膜窦内血液流向：

上矢状窦 ⟶ 窦汇

下矢状窦 ⟶ 直窦 ⟶ 窦汇 ⟶ 横窦 ⟶ 乙状窦 ⟶ 颈内静脉

海绵窦 ⟶ 岩上窦

海绵窦 ⟶ 岩下窦

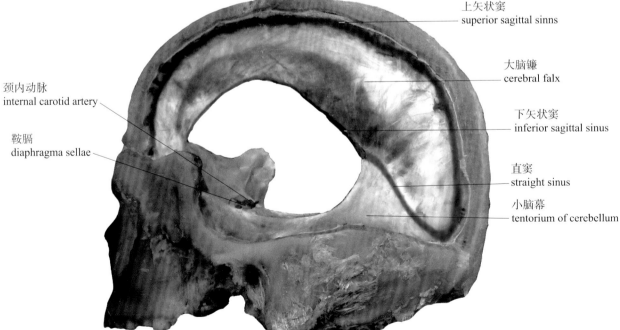

上矢状窦
superior sagittal sinns

大脑镰
cerebral falx

颈内动脉
internal carotid artery

下矢状窦
inferior sagittal sinus

鞍膈
diaphragma sellae

直窦
straight sinus

小脑幕
tentorium of cerebellum

图 13-78　硬脑膜及其静脉窦
Cerebral dura mater and venous sinus

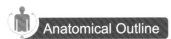

Anatomical Outline

The direction of the blood flow inside the dural sinuses:

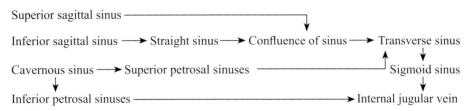

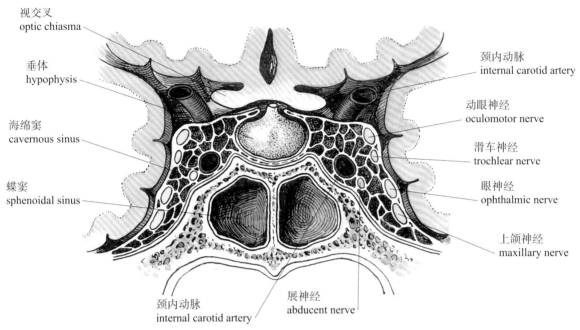

图 13-79　海绵窦（额状切面）
Cavernous sinuses (coronal section)

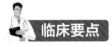

临床要点

1. 海绵窦位于颅中窝蝶骨体两侧，窦的外侧壁有动眼神经、滑车神经、眼神经及上颌神经；内侧壁有颈内动脉和展神经。海绵窦与其周围的静脉有广泛的交通。海绵窦外侧壁肿瘤或海绵窦血栓形成等原因可能导致海绵窦综合征，又称 Foix 氏综合征。若引起眼眶静脉回流障碍，可出现眶周、眼睑、结膜水肿和眼球突出。若动眼神经、滑车神经、外展神经和三叉神经第 1、2 支受损，可导致瞳孔散大，光反射消失，眼睑下垂，复视，眼球各方运动受限或固定，三叉神经第 1、2 支分布区痛觉减退，角膜反射消失等。

2. 颅脑疾病引发脑脊液循环通路障碍或脑脊液分泌过多，导致脑积水和颅内压增高，可压迫脑实质或出现脑组织移位，引发脑疝危及生命。

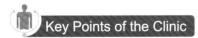

Key Points of the Clinic

1. The cavernous sinus is located on both sides of the sphenoid body of the middle cranial fossa. The internal carotid artery and abducent nerve are located on the medial wall, and the oculomotor nerve, trochlear nerve, ophthalmic nerve, and maxillary nerve are located on the lateral wall of the cavernous sinus. There are extensive communications between the cavernous sinus and the surrounding veins. Cavernous sinus syndrome, also known as Foix's syndrome, can be caused

by tumor or cavernous sinus thrombosis. If the orbital venous is affected, periorbital tissue, eyelid and conjunctival edema, and eyeball protrusion can be found. If oculomotor nerve, trochlear nerve, abducent nerve and the 1st and 2nd branches of trigeminal nerve are involved, pupil dilation, light reflex disappearance, eyelid droop, double vision, eye movement restriction or fixation, loss of sensation of the distribution area of the 1st and 2nd branches of trigeminal nerve and disability of corneal reflex will appear.

2. The craniocerebral disease can cause a disturbance in the circulation of the cerebrospinal fluid or excessive secretion of the cerebrospinal fluid, which can lead to hydrocephalus and increased intracranial pressure, resulting in compression of brain or displacement of brain tissue, called cerebral hernia. The cerebral hernia is life-threatening.

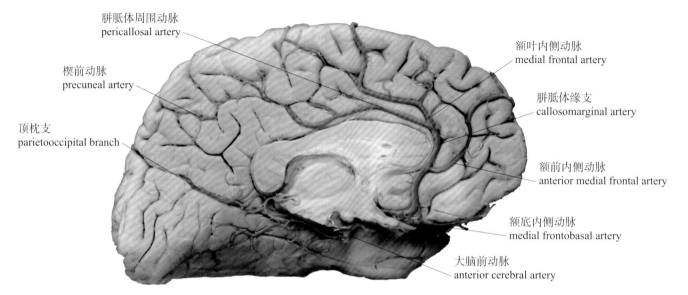

胼胝体周围动脉
pericallosal artery

楔前动脉
precuneal artery

顶枕支
parietooccipital branch

额叶内侧动脉
medial frontal artery

胼胝体缘支
callosomarginal artery

额前内侧动脉
anterior medial frontal artery

额底内侧动脉
medial frontobasal artery

大脑前动脉
anterior cerebral artery

图 13-80 大脑前动脉（内侧面观）
Anterior cerebral artery (medial view)

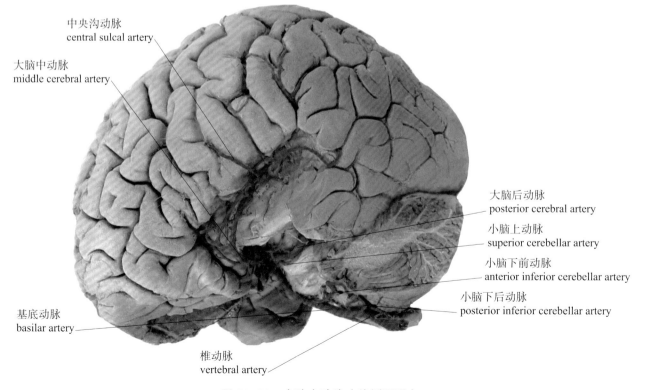

中央沟动脉
central sulcal artery

大脑中动脉
middle cerebral artery

基底动脉
basilar artery

椎动脉
vertebral artery

大脑后动脉
posterior cerebral artery

小脑上动脉
superior cerebellar artery

小脑下前动脉
anterior inferior cerebellar artery

小脑下后动脉
posterior inferior cerebellar artery

图 13-81 大脑中动脉（外侧面观）
Middle cerebral artery (lateral view)

解剖纲要

大脑动脉环（Willis 环）：由前交通动脉、两侧大脑前动脉、两侧颈内动脉末端、两侧后交通动脉和两侧大脑后动脉共同构成。

Anatomical Outline

Cerebral artery circle (Willis circle) : Willis ring is formed by anterior communicating artery, bilateral anterior cerebral arteries, the terminal part of bilateral internal carotid arteries, bilateral posterior communicating arteries and bilateral posterior cerebral arteries.

 临床要点

大脑动脉环为脑血管的潜在代偿装置，正常情况下可均衡血流，在病理情况下可使血液重新分配发挥代偿作用。

 Key Points of the Clinic

Willis circle is the potential compensatory structure for cerebral blood supply. At normal conditions, the ring can balance the cerebral blood supply, while under pathological conditions, it can redistribute the blood in the brain.

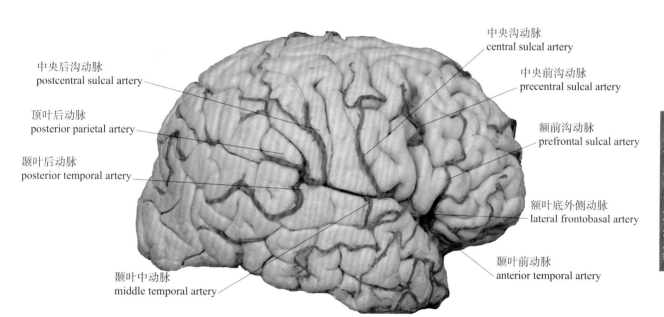

图 13-82　大脑半球动脉（外侧面观）
Arteries of the cerebral hemisphere (lateral view)

第五篇　神经与内分泌系统
Part 5 Nervous and Endocrine System

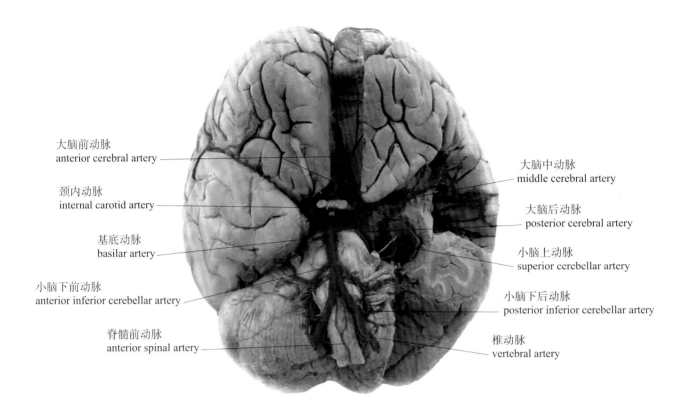

图 13-83 大脑前、中、后动脉（底面观）
Anterior, middle and posterior cerebral artery (basilar view)

大脑前动脉
anterior cerebral artery

颈内动脉
internal carotid artery

基底动脉
basilar artery

小脑下前动脉
anterior inferior cerebellar artery

脊髓前动脉
anterior spinal artery

大脑中动脉
middle cerebral artery

大脑后动脉
posterior cerebral artery

小脑上动脉
superior cerebellar artery

小脑下后动脉
posterior inferior cerebellar artery

椎动脉
vertebral artery

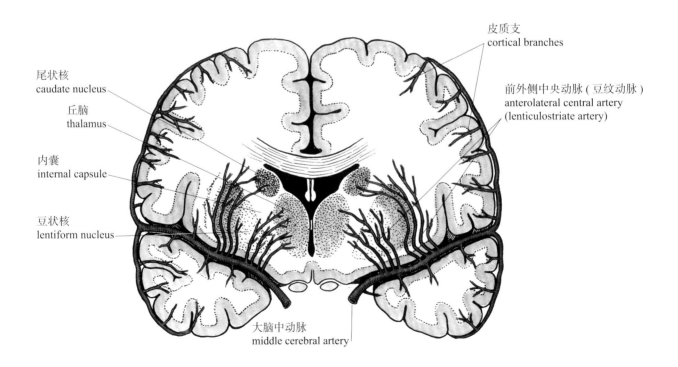

图 13-84 大脑中动脉的中央支
Central branches of the middle cerebral artery

皮质支
cortical branches

前外侧中央动脉（豆纹动脉）
anterolateral central artery
(lenticulostriate artery)

尾状核
caudate nucleus

丘脑
thalamus

内囊
internal capsule

豆状核
lentiform nucleus

大脑中动脉
middle cerebral artery

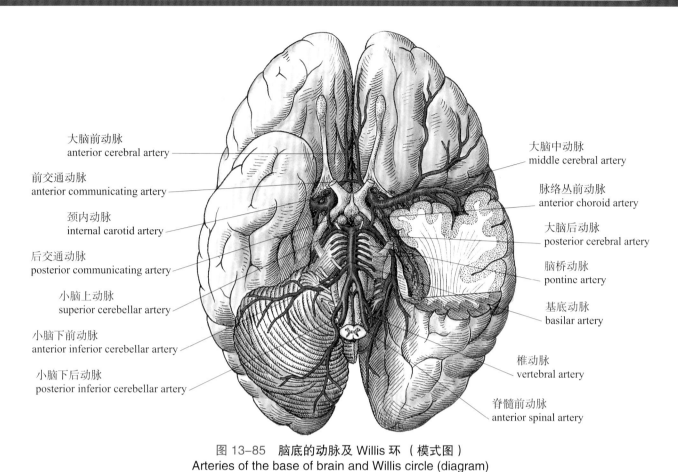

大脑前动脉
anterior cerebral artery

前交通动脉
anterior communicating artery

颈内动脉
internal carotid artery

后交通动脉
posterior communicating artery

小脑上动脉
superior cerebellar artery

小脑下前动脉
anterior inferior cerebellar artery

小脑下后动脉
posterior inferior cerebellar artery

大脑中动脉
middle cerebral artery

脉络丛前动脉
anterior choroid artery

大脑后动脉
posterior cerebral artery

脑桥动脉
pontine artery

基底动脉
basilar artery

椎动脉
vertebral artery

脊髓前动脉
anterior spinal artery

图 13-85　脑底的动脉及 Willis 环（模式图）
Arteries of the base of brain and Willis circle (diagram)

大脑前动脉
anterior cerebral artery

大脑后动脉
posterior cerebral artery

小脑上动脉
superior cerebellar artery

三叉神经
trigeminal nerve

椎动脉
vertebral artery

舌咽神经
glossopharyngeal nerve

迷走神经
vagus nerve

舌下神经
hypoglossal nerve

副神经
accessory nerve

前交通动脉
anterior communicating artery

颈内动脉
internal carotid artery

大脑中动脉
middle cerebral artery

后交通动脉
posterior communicating artery

动眼神经
oculomotor nerve

基底动脉
basilar artery

展神经
abducent nerve

面神经
facial nerve

前庭蜗神经
vestibulocochlear nerve

图 13-86　脑底的动脉及 Willis 环
Arteries of the base of brain and Willis circle

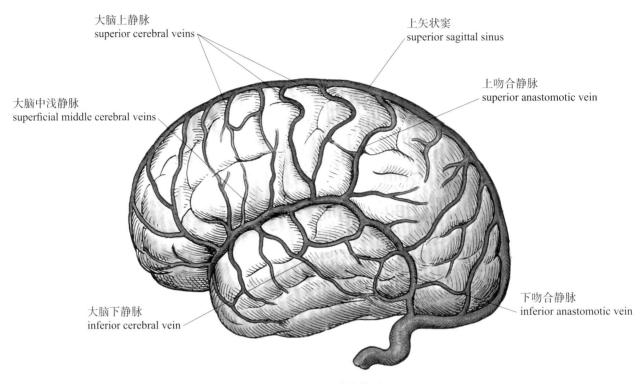

图 13-87　大脑浅静脉
Superficial cerebral veins

大脑上静脉
superior cerebral veins

上矢状窦
superior sagittal sinus

大脑中浅静脉
superficial middle cerebral veins

上吻合静脉
superior anastomotic vein

大脑下静脉
inferior cerebral vein

下吻合静脉
inferior anastomotic vein

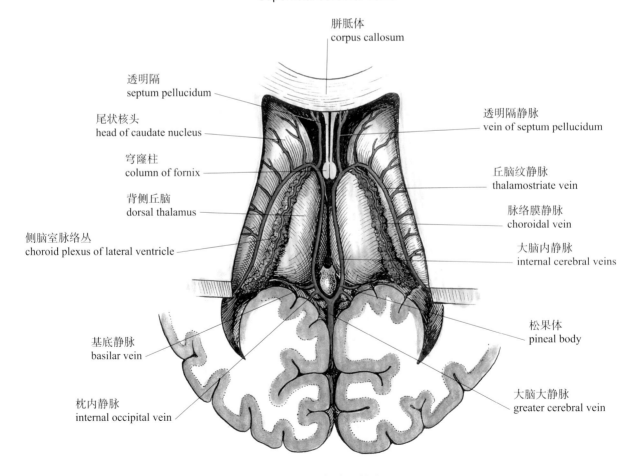

胼胝体
corpus callosum

透明隔
septum pellucidum

透明隔静脉
vein of septum pellucidum

尾状核头
head of caudate nucleus

丘脑纹静脉
thalamostriate vein

穹窿柱
column of fornix

脉络膜静脉
choroidal vein

背侧丘脑
dorsal thalamus

大脑内静脉
internal cerebral veins

侧脑室脉络丛
choroid plexus of lateral ventricle

基底静脉
basilar vein

松果体
pineal body

枕内静脉
internal occipital vein

大脑大静脉
greater cerebral vein

图 13-88　大脑深静脉
Deep cerebral veins

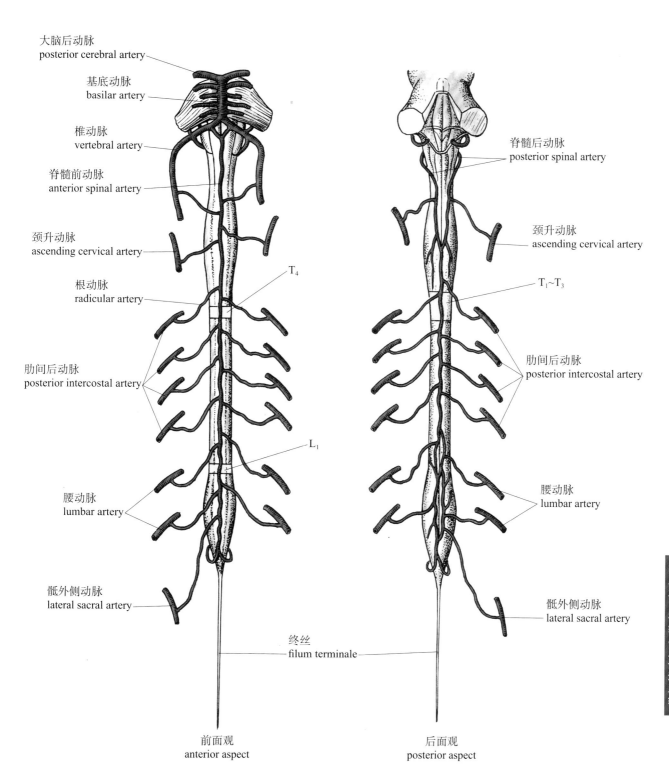

大脑后动脉
posterior cerebral artery

基底动脉
basilar artery

椎动脉
vertebral artery

脊髓前动脉
anterior spinal artery

颈升动脉
ascending cervical artery

根动脉
radicular artery

肋间后动脉
posterior intercostal artery

腰动脉
lumbar artery

骶外侧动脉
lateral sacral artery

脊髓后动脉
posterior spinal artery

颈升动脉
ascending cervical artery

肋间后动脉
posterior intercostal artery

腰动脉
lumbar artery

骶外侧动脉
lateral sacral artery

终丝
filum terminale

T_4

L_1

$T_1 \sim T_3$

前面观
anterior aspect

后面观
posterior aspect

图 13-89　脊髓的动脉
Arteries of spinal cord

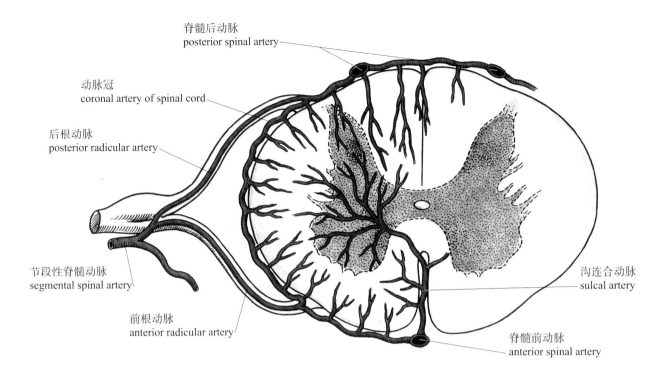

脊髓后动脉
posterior spinal artery

动脉冠
coronal artery of spinal cord

后根动脉
posterior radicular artery

节段性脊髓动脉
segmental spinal artery

前根动脉
anterior radicular artery

沟连合动脉
sulcal artery

脊髓前动脉
anterior spinal artery

图 13-90　脊髓内部的动脉分布
Arterial distribution in spinal cord

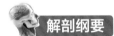 解剖纲要

脑脊液产自各脑室的脉络丛。

脑脊液的循环流向为：

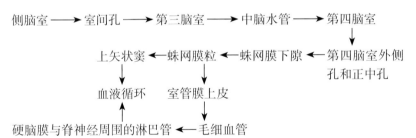

侧脑室 ⟶ 室间孔 ⟶ 第三脑室 ⟶ 中脑水管 ⟶ 第四脑室

上矢状窦 ⟵ 蛛网膜粒 ⟵ 蛛网膜下隙 ⟵ 第四脑室外侧
孔和正中孔

血液循环　　室管膜上皮

硬脑膜与脊神经周围的淋巴管 ⟵ 毛细血管

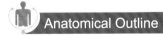 Anatomical Outline

The cerebral spinal fluid is produced by the choroid plexus in the cerebral ventricles.

The circulation direction of cerebrospinal fluid is as follows:

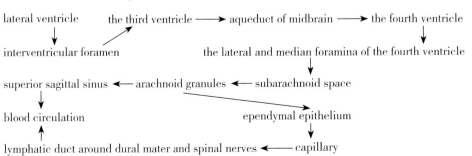

lateral ventricle　　the third ventricle ⟶ aqueduct of midbrain ⟶ the fourth ventricle

interventricular foramen　　the lateral and median foramina of the fourth ventricle

superior sagittal sinus ⟵ arachnoid granules ⟵ subarachnoid space

blood circulation　　ependymal epithelium

lymphatic duct around dural mater and spinal nerves ⟵ capillary

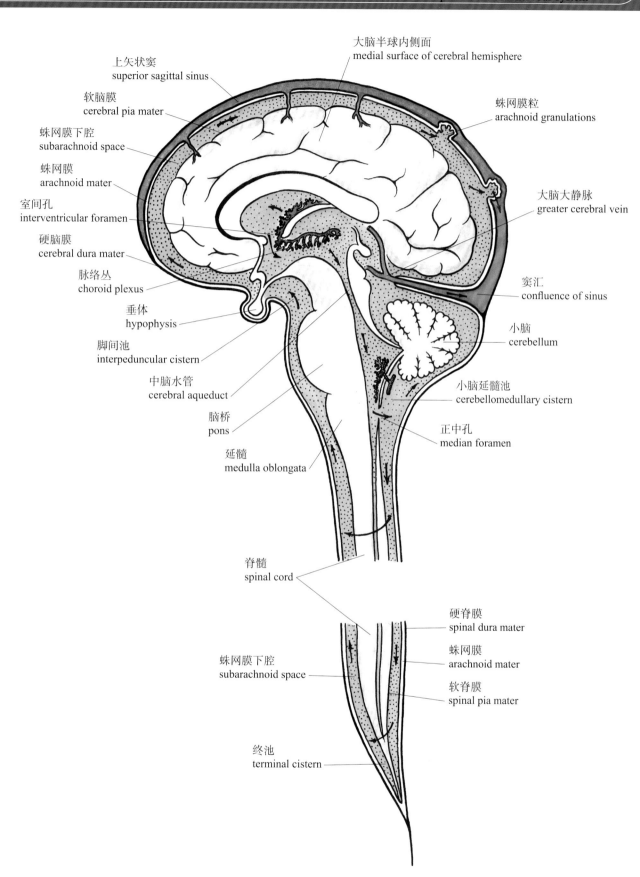

上矢状窦
superior sagittal sinus

大脑半球内侧面
medial surface of cerebral hemisphere

软脑膜
cerebral pia mater

蛛网膜粒
arachnoid granulations

蛛网膜下腔
subarachnoid space

蛛网膜
arachnoid mater

大脑大静脉
greater cerebral vein

室间孔
interventricular foramen

硬脑膜
cerebral dura mater

窦汇
confluence of sinus

脉络丛
choroid plexus

小脑
cerebellum

垂体
hypophysis

脚间池
interpeduncular cistern

小脑延髓池
cerebellomedullary cistern

中脑水管
cerebral aqueduct

脑桥
pons

正中孔
median foramen

延髓
medulla oblongata

脊髓
spinal cord

硬脊膜
spinal dura mater

蛛网膜
arachnoid mater

蛛网膜下腔
subarachnoid space

软脊膜
spinal pia mater

终池
terminal cistern

图 13-91 脑脊液及其循环
Cerebral spinal fluid and its circulation

第五篇 神经与内分泌系统 Part 5 Nervous and Endocrine System

第十四章 周围神经系统
Chapter 14 Peripheral nervous system

第一节 脊神经 Section 1 Spinal nerve

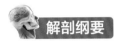 **解剖纲要**

脊神经：连接于脊髓的周围神经，共 31 对。脊神经含有四种纤维成分：躯体感觉纤维、内脏感觉纤维、躯体运动纤维和内脏运动纤维。脊神经的典型分支有：前支、后支、交通支和脊膜支。

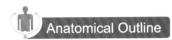 **Anatomical Outline**

Spinal nerve: The spinal nerves are the nerves arising from the spinal cord. The total number of spinal nerves is 31 pairs. There are four kinds of fibers inside each spinal nerve: somatic sensory fiber, motor fiber, somatic visceral sensory fiber, and visceral motor fiber. The typical branches of the spinal nerve include anterior, posterior, communicating and meningeal branches.

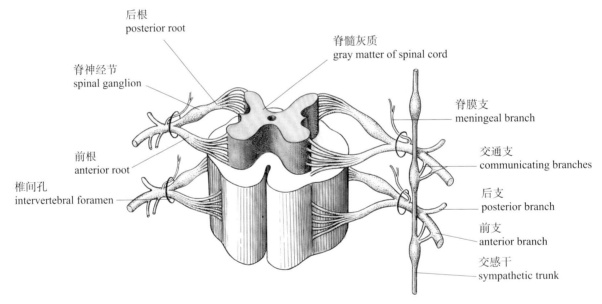

图 14-1 脊神经的典型分支
Typical branches of spinal nerve

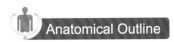 **解剖纲要**

颈丛：由 C_1~C_4 前支组成，位于胸锁乳突肌上部深面，中斜角肌及肩胛提肌起点前方，主要分支有分布于颈部的皮支和肌支，膈神经是其最重要的分支之一。

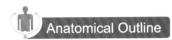 **Anatomical Outline**

Cervical plexus: It is composed of C_1-C_4 anterior ramus, and lies deep to the upper part of the sternocleidomastoid and anterior to the origins of the scalenus medialis and the levator scapularis. The major branches of cervical plexus include the cutaneous branches in the neck and muscular branches. The phrenic nerve is one of the important branches of the cervical plexus.

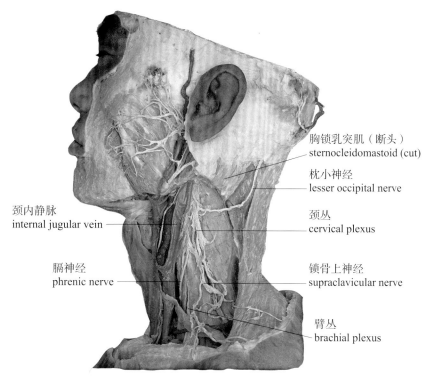

胸锁乳突肌（断头）
sternocleidomastoid (cut)

枕小神经
lesser occipital nerve

颈内静脉
internal jugular vein

颈丛
cervical plexus

膈神经
phrenic nerve

锁骨上神经
supraclavicular nerve

臂丛
brachial plexus

图 14-2 颈丛
Cervical plexus

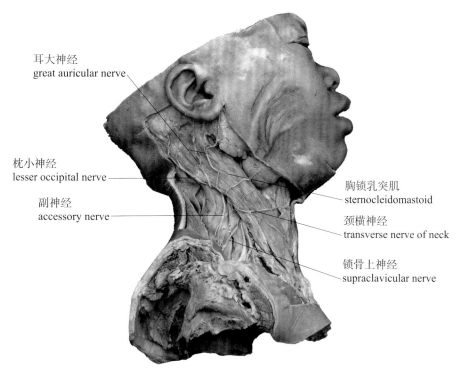

耳大神经
great auricular nerve

枕小神经
lesser occipital nerve

副神经
accessory nerve

胸锁乳突肌
sternocleidomastoid

颈横神经
transverse nerve of neck

锁骨上神经
supraclavicular nerve

图 14-3 颈丛皮支
Cutaneous branches of cervical plexus

第五篇 神经与内分泌系统 Part 5 Nervous and Endocrine System

临床要点

　　胸锁乳突肌后缘中点是颈丛皮支浅出的部位，也是颈部浅层结构浸润麻醉的阻滞点，临床又将其称为神经点，邻近中医的扶突穴。

　　膈神经的运动纤维支配膈肌的运动，感觉纤维分布于胸膜、心包。一般认为，右膈神经的感觉纤维还分布于肝、胆囊和肝外胆道的浆膜。

　　膈神经受到损伤后，表现为腹式呼吸减弱或消失，严重者有窒息感。膈神经受到刺激时可发生呃逆。

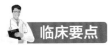 Key Points of the Clinic

　　The middle point of the posterior margin of the sternocleidomastoid is the site where the cutaneous branches of the cervical plexus emerge. It is also the block point of infitration anesthesia in the superficial structure of neck and is known as the nerve point in the clinic. In Chinese medicine, it is adjacent to FuTu acupoint.

　　The motor fiber of phrenic nerve innervates diaphragm, and the sensory fiber of the phrenic nerve controls the sensation of the pleura and pericardium. The sensory fibers of the right phrenic nerve are also distributed in the serous menbrance of the liver, gallbladder and extrahepatic biliary duct.

　　The injury of the phrenic nerve can cause weak or disappear of abdominal respiration and even asphyxia. Stimulation of the phrenic nerve can induce hiccup.

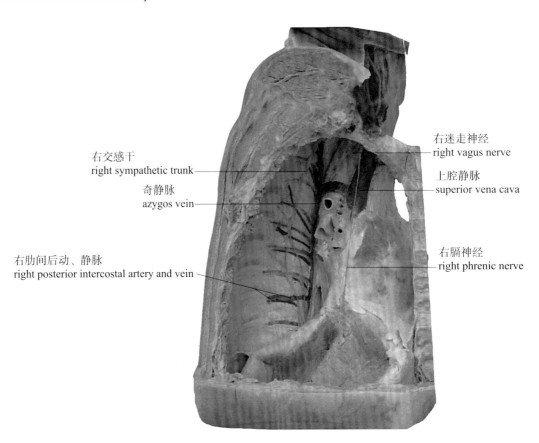

右交感干
right sympathetic trunk

奇静脉
azygos vein

右肋间后动、静脉
right posterior intercostal artery and vein

右迷走神经
right vagus nerve

上腔静脉
superior vena cava

右膈神经
right phrenic nerve

图 14-4　右膈神经
Right phrenic nerve

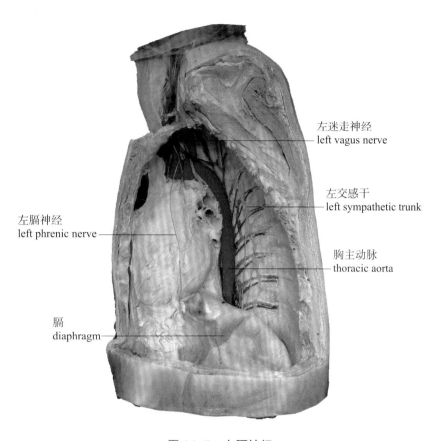

图 14-5 左膈神经
Left phrenic nerve

左迷走神经
left vagus nerve

左交感干
left sympathetic trunk

胸主动脉
thoracic aorta

左膈神经
left phrenic nerve

膈
diaphragm

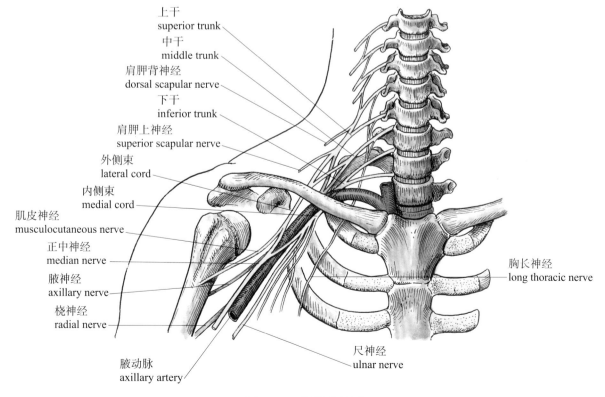

上干
superior trunk

中干
middle trunk

肩胛背神经
dorsal scapular nerve

下干
inferior trunk

肩胛上神经
superior scapular nerve

外侧束
lateral cord

内侧束
medial cord

肌皮神经
musculocutaneous nerve

正中神经
median nerve

腋神经
axillary nerve

桡神经
radial nerve

腋动脉
axillary artery

胸长神经
long thoracic nerve

尺神经
ulnar nerve

图 14-6 臂丛的位置
Location of brachial plexus

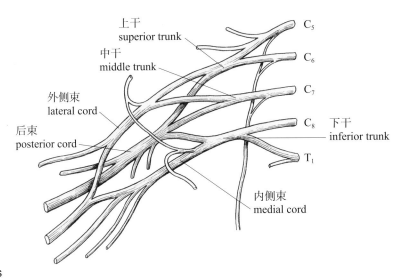

图 14-7　臂丛模式图
Diagram of brachial plexus

解剖纲要

臂丛：由 $C_5 \sim C_8 + T_1$ 前支交织形成，分为锁骨上、下两部，锁骨上部位于斜角间隙，锁骨下部位于腋窝内，分支支配上肢及胸前外侧壁皮肤和肌肉。臂丛重要分支包括正中神经、肌皮神经、尺神经、桡神经、腋神经。

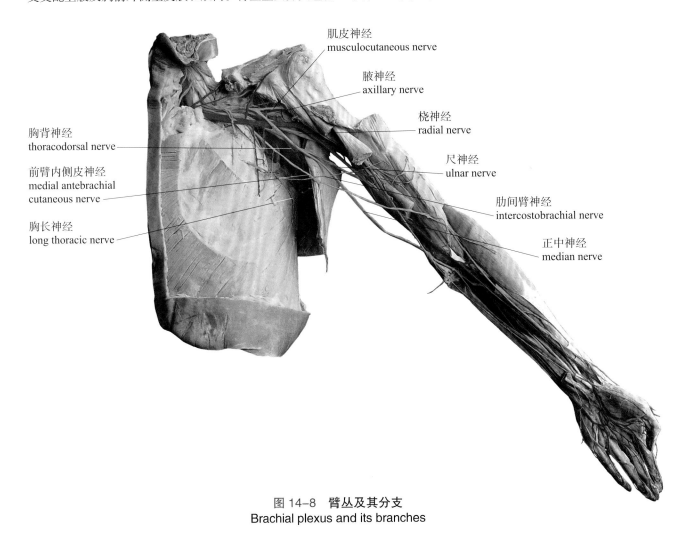

图 14-8　臂丛及其分支
Brachial plexus and its branches

Brachial plexus: The anterior ramus of C_5-C_8 and T_1 interweave and form the brachial plexus. It is divided into two parts: supraclavicular and infraclavicular parts. The supraclavicular part is located in the scalene fissure, and the infraclavicular part is located in the axillary fossa. The branches innervate the skin and muscles of the upper limb and the anterolateral thoracic wall. The important branches of brachial plexus include median nerve, musculocutaneous nerve, ulnar nerve, radial nerve and axillary nerve.

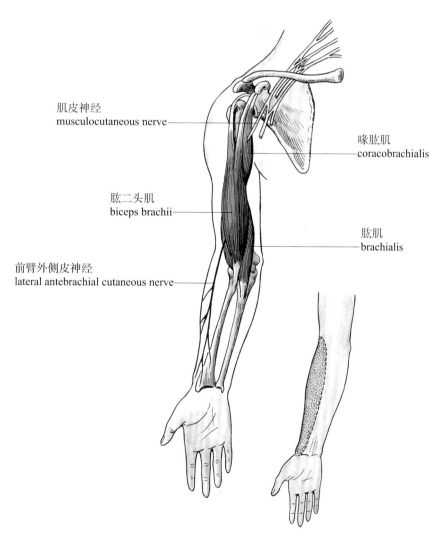

肌皮神经
musculocutaneous nerve

喙肱肌
coracobrachialis

肱二头肌
biceps brachii

肱肌
brachialis

前臂外侧皮神经
lateral antebrachial cutaneous nerve

图 14-9 肌皮神经
Musculocutaneous nerve

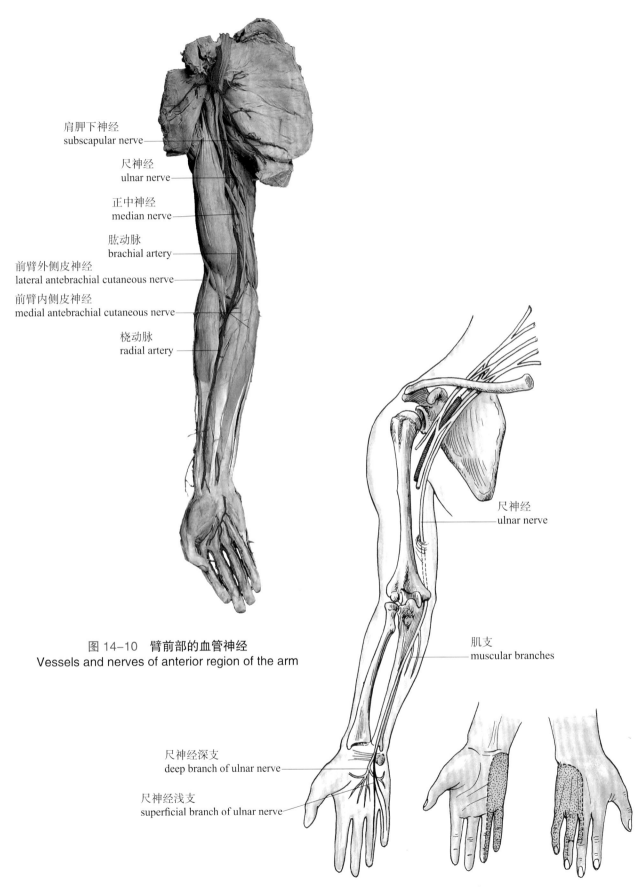

肩胛下神经
subscapular nerve

尺神经
ulnar nerve

正中神经
median nerve

肱动脉
brachial artery

前臂外侧皮神经
lateral antebrachial cutaneous nerve

前臂内侧皮神经
medial antebrachial cutaneous nerve

桡动脉
radial artery

图 14-10 臂前部的血管神经
Vessels and nerves of anterior region of the arm

尺神经
ulnar nerve

肌支
muscular branches

尺神经深支
deep branch of ulnar nerve

尺神经浅支
superficial branch of ulnar nerve

图 14-11 尺神经
Ulnar nerve

临床要点

尺神经损伤的表现：屈腕力减弱，拇指不能内收，环指和小指远节不能屈，各指不能内收和屈，呈"爪形手"。

正中神经损伤表现：前臂不能旋前，屈腕力减弱，拇、食指不能屈，拇指不能对掌，呈"猿手"。

 Key Points of the Clinic

Injury of ulnar nerve results in weak wrist flexion, disability of thumb adduction, disability flexion of the distal segment of ring and little fingers, disability of adduction of all fingers and presents a"claw"hand.

Injury of median nerve results in disabled pronation of the forearm, weak wrist flexion, disability of flexion of thumb and index finger a loss of opposition of thun, and presents "ape's hand".

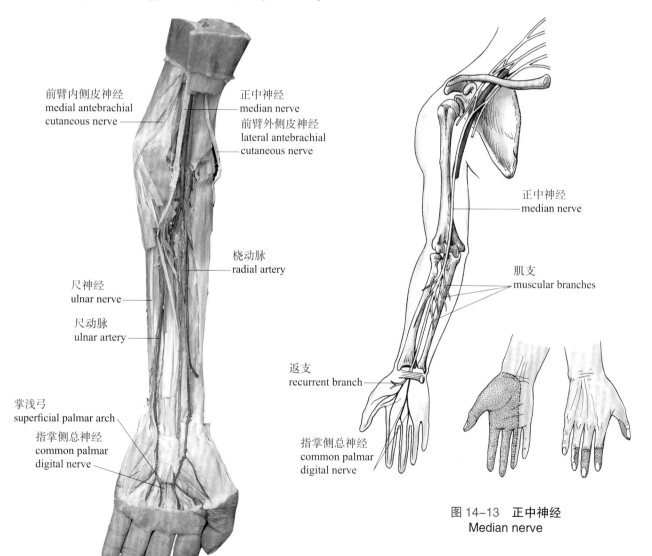

图 14-12　前臂前部的血管神经
Vessels and nerves of anterior
region of the forearm

图 14-13　正中神经
Median nerve

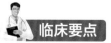 **临床要点**

桡神经损伤的表现：主要表现为伸腕伸指无力，抬前臂时呈"垂腕"状。

第五篇　神经与内分泌系统
Part 5 Nervous and Endocrine System

Injury of radial nerve results in the inability of wrist and finger extension, "wrist drop" is presented when the patients are asked to lift their forearm.

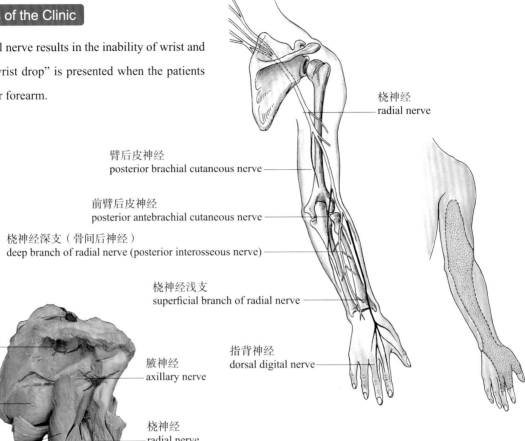

桡神经
radial nerve

臂后皮神经
posterior brachial cutaneous nerve

前臂后皮神经
posterior antebrachial cutaneous nerve

桡神经深支（骨间后神经）
deep branch of radial nerve (posterior interosseous nerve)

桡神经浅支
superficial branch of radial nerve

指背神经
dorsal digital nerve

图 14-14　桡神经
Radial nerve

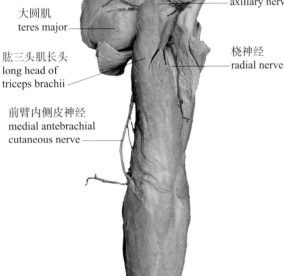

肩胛上神经
suprascapular nerve

大圆肌
teres major

肱三头肌长头
long head of
triceps brachii

前臂内侧皮神经
medial antebrachial
cutaneous nerve

腋神经
axillary nerve

桡神经
radial nerve

尺神经
ulnar nerve

桡神经浅支
superficial branch
of radial nerve

图 14-15　上肢背面的神经
Nerves of posterior region of upper limb

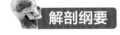

解剖纲要

胸神经皮支节段性分布

脊神经	分布部位
T_2	胸骨角平面
T_4	乳头平面
T_6	剑突平面
T_8	肋弓平面
T_{10}	脐平面
T_{12}	耻骨联合与脐连线中点平面

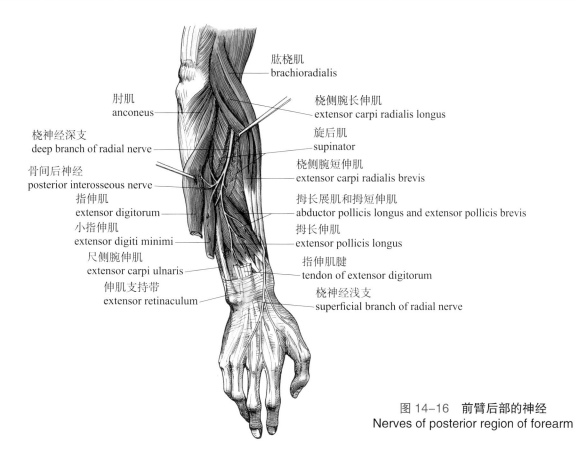

肘肌
anconeus

桡神经深支
deep branch of radial nerve

骨间后神经
posterior interosseous nerve

指伸肌
extensor digitorum

小指伸肌
extensor digiti minimi

尺侧腕伸肌
extensor carpi ulnaris

伸肌支持带
extensor retinaculum

肱桡肌
brachioradialis

桡侧腕长伸肌
extensor carpi radialis longus

旋后肌
supinator

桡侧腕短伸肌
extensor carpi radialis brevis

拇长展肌和拇短伸肌
abductor pollicis longus and extensor pollicis brevis

拇长伸肌
extensor pollicis longus

指伸肌腱
tendon of extensor digitorum

桡神经浅支
superficial branch of radial nerve

图 14-16　前臂后部的神经
Nerves of posterior region of forearm

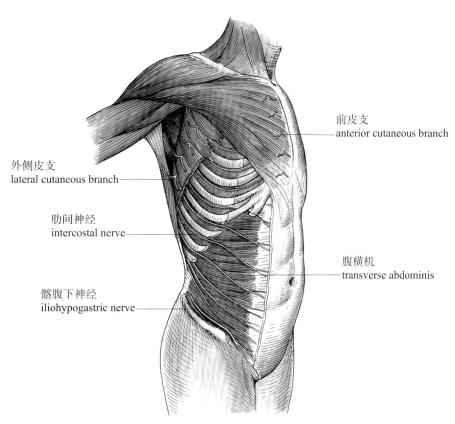

外侧皮支
lateral cutaneous branch

肋间神经
intercostal nerve

髂腹下神经
iliohypogastric nerve

前皮支
anterior cutaneous branch

腹横机
transverse abdominis

图 14-17　胸神经前支
Anterior branches of thoracic nerve

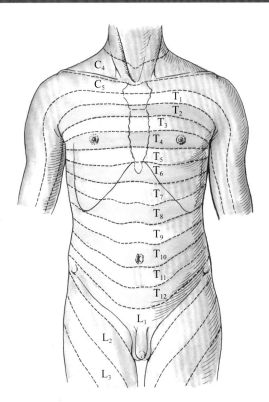

图 14-18　胸神经前支的分布
Distribution of anterior branches of thoracic nerve

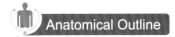

Anatomical Outline

Segmental distribution of cutaneous branches of thoracic nerves

Spinal nerve	Distribution of anatomical site
T_2	Sternal angle level
T_4	Nipple level
T_6	Xiphoid process level
T_8	Costal arch level
T_{10}	Umbilical level
T_{12}	The level at the midpoint between the umbilicus and pubic symphysis

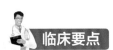

临床要点

根据胸神经前支在胸、腹壁皮肤分布的节段性特性，临床工作中可以依据躯体皮肤感觉障碍的发生区域来分析和推断受损的胸神经。此外，手术前患者的麻醉也可以根据感觉丧失的区域来判断。

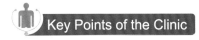

Key Points of the Clinic

According to the segmental distribution pattern on thoracic and abdominal wall of the thoracic nerves, the doctor can identify the injured thoracic nerve from the skin sensation loss of the patient. In addition, doctor can judge the anesthetic range from the sensation loss of the skin.

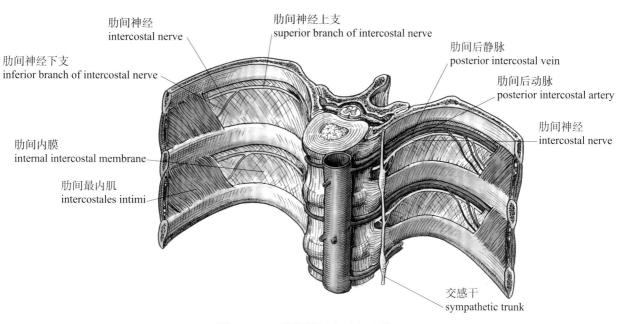

图 14-19　肋间神经和肋间血管
Intercostal nerves and intercostal vessels

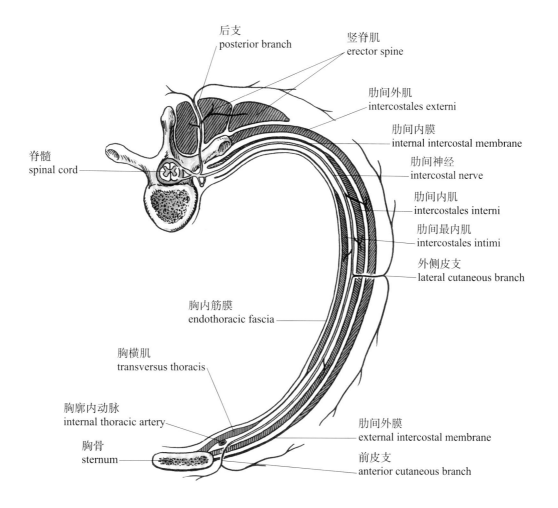

图 14-20　肋间神经（水平切面示意图）
Intercostal nerves (diagram of horizontal section)

第五篇　神经与内分泌系统

Part 5 Nervous and Endocrine System

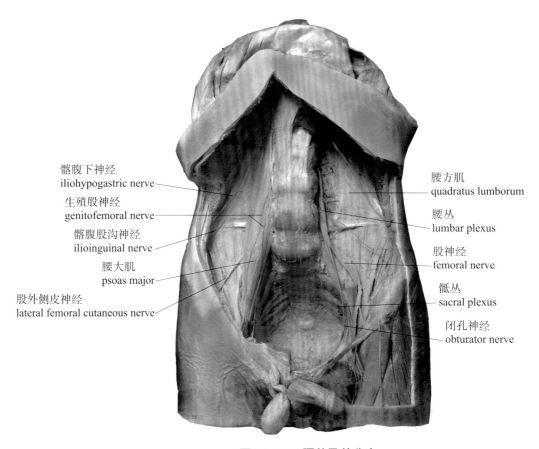

髂腹下神经
iliohypogastric nerve

生殖股神经
genitofemoral nerve

髂腹股沟神经
ilioinguinal nerve

腰大肌
psoas major

股外侧皮神经
lateral femoral cutaneous nerve

腰方肌
quadratus lumborum

腰丛
lumbar plexus

股神经
femoral nerve

骶丛
sacral plexus

闭孔神经
obturator nerve

图 14-21　**腰丛及其分支**
Lumbar plexus and its branches

解剖纲要

腰丛：由 T_{12} 前支一部分、L_1~L_3 前支和 L_4 前支一部分组成，位于腰大肌深面、腰椎横突之前，主要分支有股神经、闭孔神经等。

股神经：腰丛分支。肌支支配缝匠肌、股四头肌和耻骨肌；皮支分布于大腿前内侧皮肤，其中，隐神经分布于髌下、小腿内侧面及足内侧缘皮肤。

Anatomical Outline

Lumbar plexus: Lumbar plexus consists of part of T_{12} anterior ramus, L_1~L_3 anterior ramus and part of L_4 anterior ramus. It is located before the transverse process of lumbar vertebra and deep to the psoas major. Its main braches include femoral nerve and obturator nerve.

Femoral nerve：It is coming from the lumbar plexus. Its muscular branches innervate sartorius, quadriceps femoris, and pectineus and the cutaneous branches innervate the skin of anterior and medial part of the thigh and the medial part of the leg and foot.

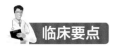 临床要点

股神经损伤表现为屈髋无力，坐位时不能伸小腿，行走困难，膝跳反射消失，大腿前面和小腿内侧面皮肤感觉障碍。

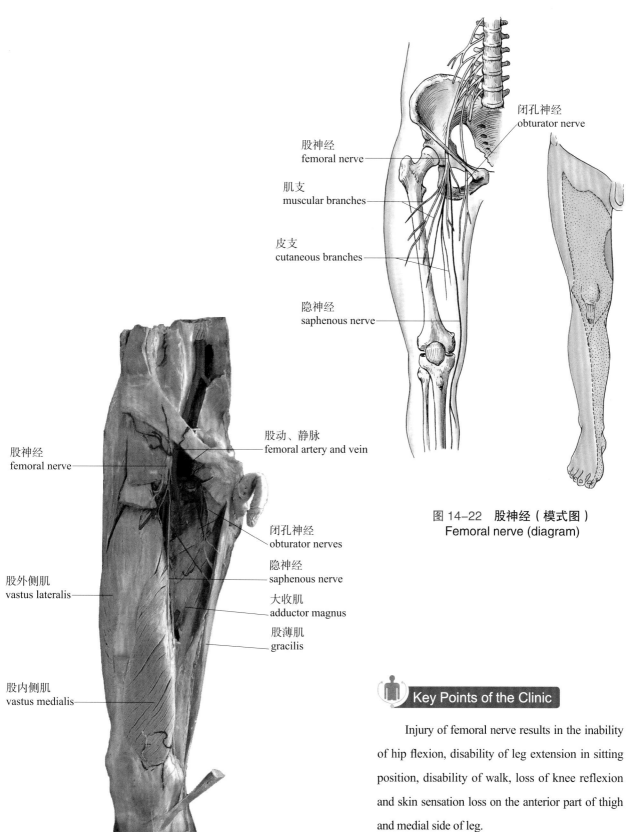

闭孔神经
obturator nerve

股神经
femoral nerve

肌支
muscular branches

皮支
cutaneous branches

隐神经
saphenous nerve

图 14-22　股神经（模式图）
Femoral nerve (diagram)

股神经
femoral nerve

股动、静脉
femoral artery and vein

闭孔神经
obturator nerves

隐神经
saphenous nerve

股外侧肌
vastus lateralis

大收肌
adductor magnus

股薄肌
gracilis

股内侧肌
vastus medialis

图 14-23　股前部的血管神经
Vessels and nerves of anterior region of the thigh

Key Points of the Clinic

Injury of femoral nerve results in the inability of hip flexion, disability of leg extension in sitting position, disability of walk, loss of knee reflexion and skin sensation loss on the anterior part of thigh and medial side of leg.

第五篇　神经与内分泌系统　Part 5 Nervous and Endocrine System

解剖纲要

骶丛：由腰骶干（L$_4$、L$_5$前支合成）和全部骶、尾神经前支组成，位于骶骨和梨状肌前面，分支包括阴部神经及坐骨神经等。

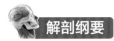 Anatomical Outline

Sacral plexus: It is composed of the lumbosacral trunk (formed by L$_4$, L$_5$ anterior ramus) and all anterior ramus of sacral and coccygeal nerves, and is located in front of the sacrum and piriformis. Its branches include the sciatic nerve, pudendal nerve, etc.

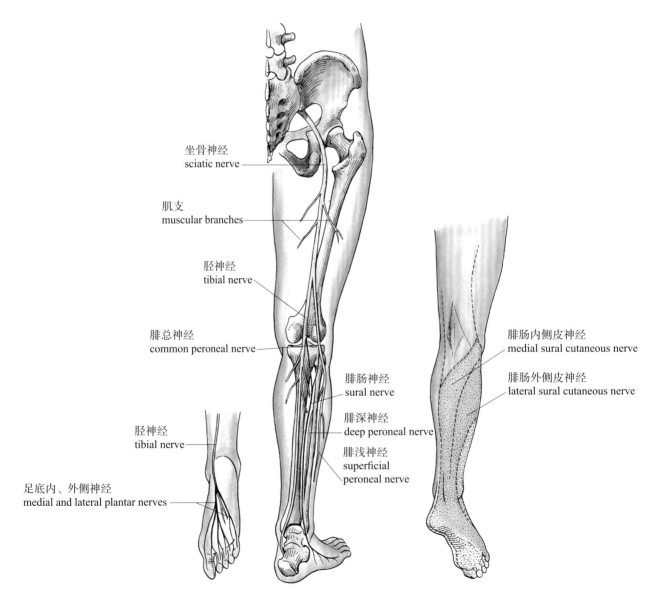

图 14-24　坐骨神经（模式图）
Sciatic nerve (diagram)

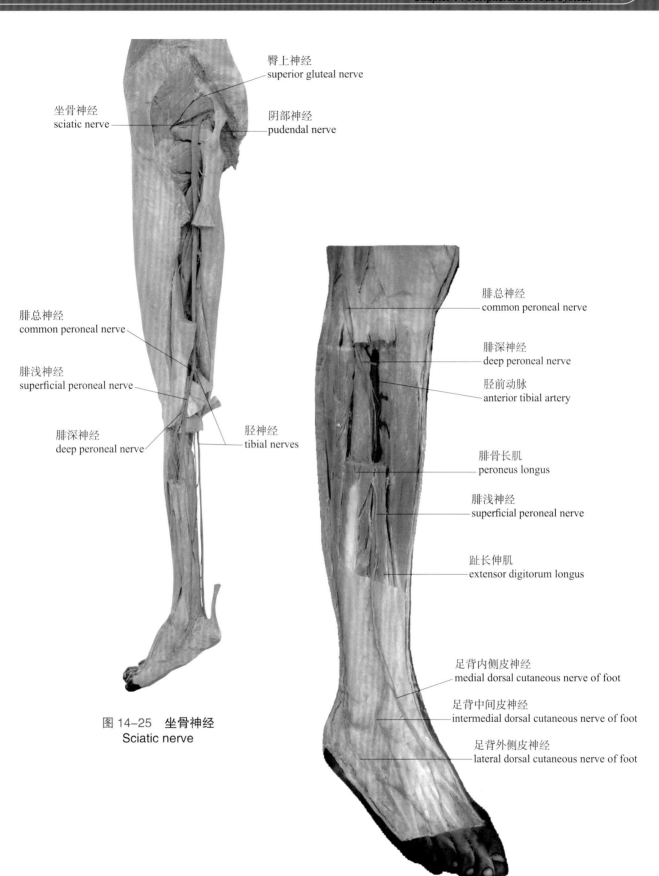

臀上神经
superior gluteal nerve

坐骨神经
sciatic nerve

阴部神经
pudendal nerve

腓总神经
common peroneal nerve

腓浅神经
superficial peroneal nerve

腓深神经
deep peroneal nerve

胫神经
tibial nerves

图 14-25 坐骨神经
Sciatic nerve

腓总神经
common peroneal nerve

腓深神经
deep peroneal nerve

胫前动脉
anterior tibial artery

腓骨长肌
peroneus longus

腓浅神经
superficial peroneal nerve

趾长伸肌
extensor digitorum longus

足背内侧皮神经
medial dorsal cutaneous nerve of foot

足背中间皮神经
intermedial dorsal cutaneous nerve of foot

足背外侧皮神经
lateral dorsal cutaneous nerve of foot

图 14-26 小腿前部的血管神经
Vessels and nerves of anterior region of the leg

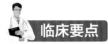

坐骨神经损伤：若损伤部位发生在坐骨神经上端，则股后群肌、小腿肌及足肌全部瘫痪，使膝关节不能屈曲、足与足趾的运动完全丧失，行走困难，小腿后外侧和足的大部分感觉消失，跟腱反射及跖反射消失；若损伤部位发生在坐骨神经下端，股后肌群不受影响，则膝关节仍能屈曲。

胫神经损伤：足不能跖屈内翻，而呈背屈外翻状态，出现所谓"仰趾足"（钩形足）畸形。

腓总神经损伤：运动障碍表现为足不能背屈和外翻，不能伸趾，呈"马蹄内翻足"畸形，行走时呈"跨阈步态"。

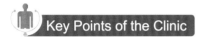

Injury of sciatic nerve: The upper part injury results in paralysis of posterior group muscles of the thigh and all muscles of the leg and foot and leads to disability of knee flexion, loss of movement of leg and foot, difficulty in walking, loss of sensation of the posterolateral portion of leg and most part of the foot, loss of achilles tendon reflex and plantar reflex. If the injury happened at the lower part, the posterior group muscles of the thigh are not affected and flexion ability of the knee joint will be reserved.

Injury of tibial nerve: It can cause disability of plantar flexion and varus and the foot presents dorsal flexion and eversion position which is the so-called "hooked feet".

Injury of common peroneal nerve: It can cause disability of dorsal flexion, eversion and flexion of the toes and the foot presents plantar flexion and varus position and the patients present "steppage gait" when they try to walk.

第二节 脑神经 Section 2 Cranial nerve

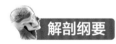

脑神经是与脑相连的周围神经，共 12 对。脑神经的纤维成分包括 7 种：一般躯体感觉纤维、特殊躯体感觉纤维、一般内脏感觉纤维、特殊内脏感觉纤维、一般躯体运动纤维、一般内脏运动纤维和特殊内脏运动纤维。

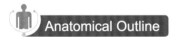

The cranial nerve is the peripheral nerve contacting with the brain. There are 12 pairs in total. Cranial nerves include 7 kinds of fiber: general somatic sensory fiber, special somatic sensory fiber, general visceral sensory fiber, special visceral sensory fiber, general somatic motor fiber, general visceral motor fiber and special visceral motor fiber.

解剖纲要

每一对脑神经用罗马数字表示如下：Ⅰ嗅Ⅱ视Ⅲ动眼，Ⅳ滑Ⅴ叉Ⅵ外展，Ⅶ面Ⅷ听Ⅸ舌咽，迷副舌下顺序全。

Anatomical Outline

Each pair of cranial nerves is represented in Roman numerals as follows: Ⅰ olfactory nerve, Ⅱ optic nerve, Ⅲ oculomotor nerve, Ⅳ trochlear nerve, Ⅴ trigeminal nerve, Ⅵ abducent nerve, Ⅶ facial nerve, Ⅷ vestibulocochlear nerve, Ⅸ glossopharyngeal nerve, Ⅹ vagus nerve, Ⅺ accessory nerve, Ⅻ hypoglossal nerve order complete.

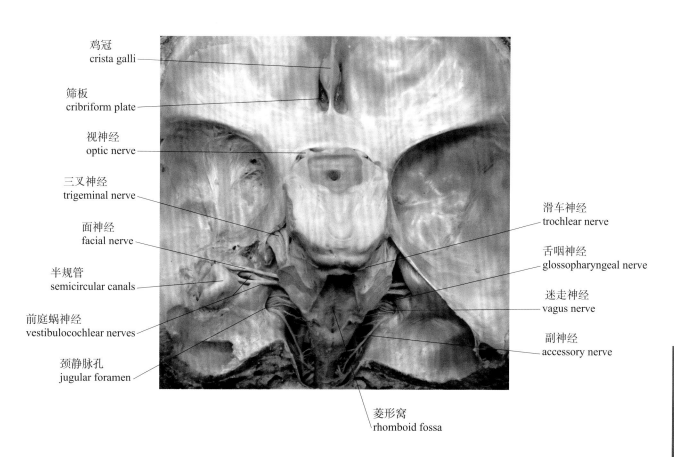

图 14-27 原位脑神经连脑部位
Locations of cranial nerves connecting with brain in situ

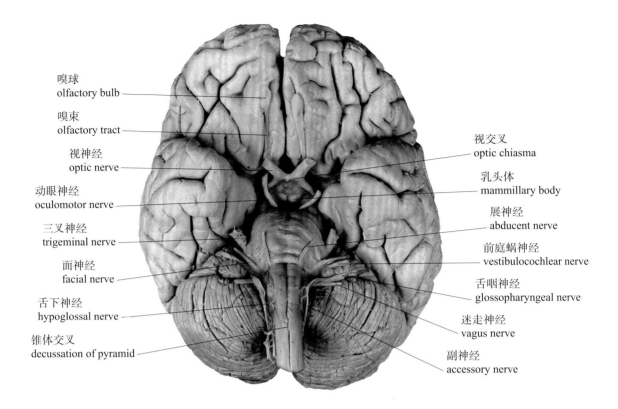

嗅球
olfactory bulb

嗅束
olfactory tract

视神经
optic nerve

动眼神经
oculomotor nerve

三叉神经
trigeminal nerve

面神经
facial nerve

舌下神经
hypoglossal nerve

锥体交叉
decussation of pyramid

视交叉
optic chiasma

乳头体
mammillary body

展神经
abducent nerve

前庭蜗神经
vestibulocochlear nerve

舌咽神经
glossopharyngeal nerve

迷走神经
vagus nerve

副神经
accessory nerve

图 14-28　脑神经连脑部位（底面观）
Locations of cranial nerves connecting with brain (inferior view)

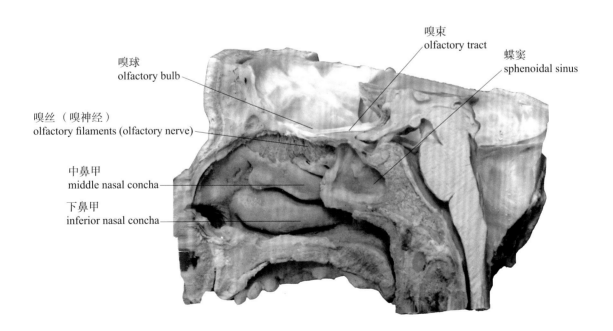

嗅束
olfactory tract

蝶窦
sphenoidal sinus

嗅球
olfactory bulb

嗅丝（嗅神经）
olfactory filaments (olfactory nerve)

中鼻甲
middle nasal concha

下鼻甲
inferior nasal concha

图 14-29　嗅神经
Olfactory nerve

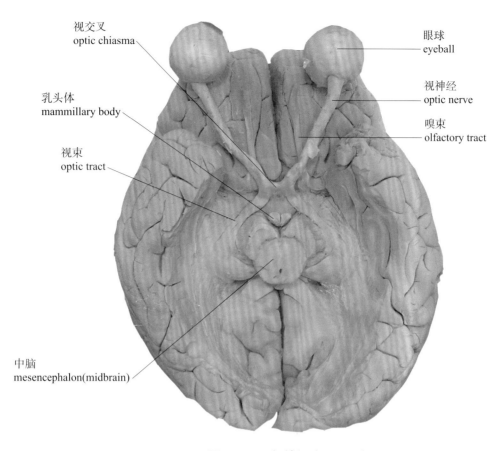

图 14-30 视神经（下面观）
Optic nerve (inferior view)

视交叉 optic chiasma
眼球 eyeball
视神经 optic nerve
乳头体 mammillary body
嗅束 olfactory tract
视束 optic tract
中脑 mesencephalon(midbrain)

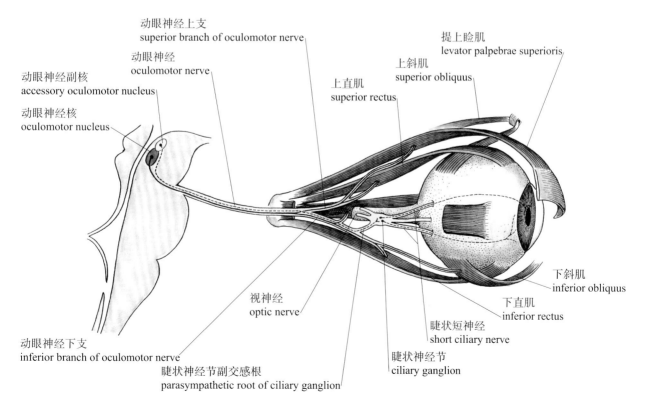

图 14-31 动眼神经
Oculomotor nerve

动眼神经上支 superior branch of oculomotor nerve
动眼神经 oculomotor nerve
提上睑肌 levator palpebrae superioris
上斜肌 superior obliquus
动眼神经副核 accessory oculomotor nucleus
上直肌 superior rectus
动眼神经核 oculomotor nucleus
视神经 optic nerve
下斜肌 inferior obliquus
下直肌 inferior rectus
睫状短神经 short ciliary nerve
动眼神经下支 inferior branch of oculomotor nerve
睫状神经节 ciliary ganglion
睫状神经节副交感根 parasympathetic root of ciliary ganglion

第五篇 神经与内分泌系统
Part 5 Nervous and Endocrine System

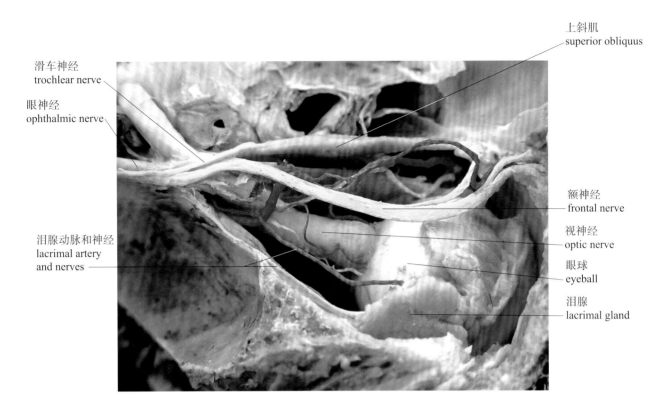

上斜肌
superior obliquus

滑车神经
trochlear nerve

眼神经
ophthalmic nerve

额神经
frontal nerve

视神经
optic nerve

泪腺动脉和神经
lacrimal artery
and nerves

眼球
eyeball

泪腺
lacrimal gland

图 14-32 滑车神经（上面观）
Trochlear nerve (superior view)

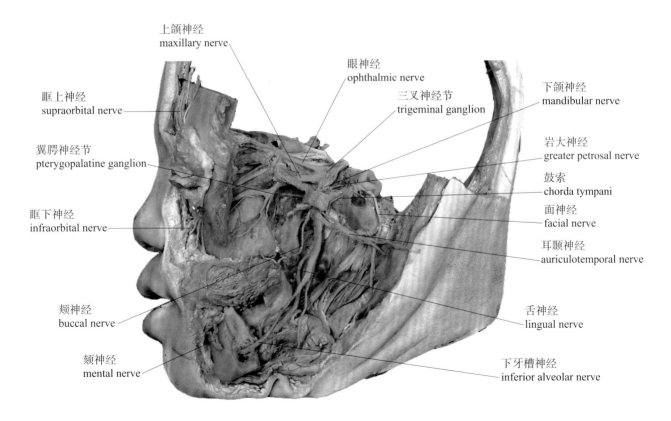

上颌神经
maxillary nerve

眼神经
ophthalmic nerve

三叉神经节
trigeminal ganglion

下颌神经
mandibular nerve

眶上神经
supraorbital nerve

岩大神经
greater petrosal nerve

翼腭神经节
pterygopalatine ganglion

鼓索
chorda tympani

面神经
facial nerve

眶下神经
infraorbital nerve

耳颞神经
auriculotemporal nerve

颊神经
buccal nerve

舌神经
lingual nerve

颏神经
mental nerve

下牙槽神经
inferior alveolar nerve

图 14-33 三叉神经
Trigeminal nerve

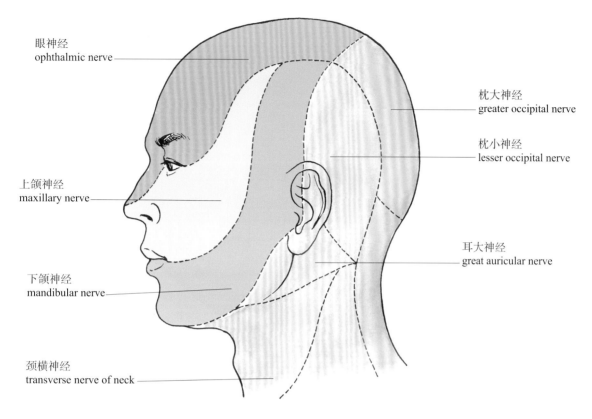

图 14-34　头面部皮神经分布
Cutaneous innervation of head and face

眼神经
ophthalmic nerve

枕大神经
greater occipital nerve

枕小神经
lesser occipital nerve

上颌神经
maxillary nerve

耳大神经
great auricular nerve

下颌神经
mandibular nerve

颈横神经
transverse nerve of neck

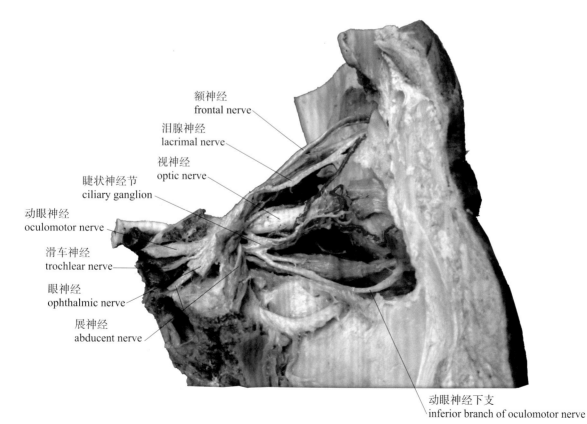

额神经
frontal nerve

泪腺神经
lacrimal nerve

视神经
optic nerve

睫状神经节
ciliary ganglion

动眼神经
oculomotor nerve

滑车神经
trochlear nerve

眼神经
ophthalmic nerve

展神经
abducent nerve

动眼神经下支
inferior branch of oculomotor nerve

图 14-35　展神经
Abducent nerve

第五篇　神经与内分泌系统
Part 5 Nervous and Endocrine System

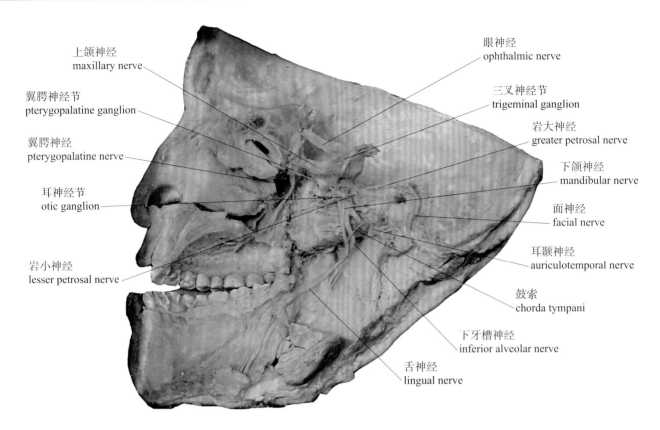

上颌神经
maxillary nerve

翼腭神经节
pterygopalatine ganglion

翼腭神经
pterygopalatine nerve

耳神经节
otic ganglion

岩小神经
lesser petrosal nerve

眼神经
ophthalmic nerve

三叉神经节
trigeminal ganglion

岩大神经
greater petrosal nerve

下颌神经
mandibular nerve

面神经
facial nerve

耳颞神经
auriculotemporal nerve

鼓索
chorda tympani

下牙槽神经
inferior alveolar nerve

舌神经
lingual nerve

图 14-36　面神经与三叉神经（内侧面观）
Facial nerve and trigeminal nerve (medial view)

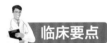 临床要点

三叉神经痛是三叉神经的常见病变。临床上检查三叉神经时，常在眶上切迹、眶下孔和颏孔部位按压。

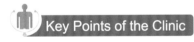 Key Points of the Clinic

Prosopalgia is a common disease of the trigeminal nerve. The trigeminal nerve can be examined by pressing at the supraorbital notch, infraorbital foramen and mental foramen in clinic.

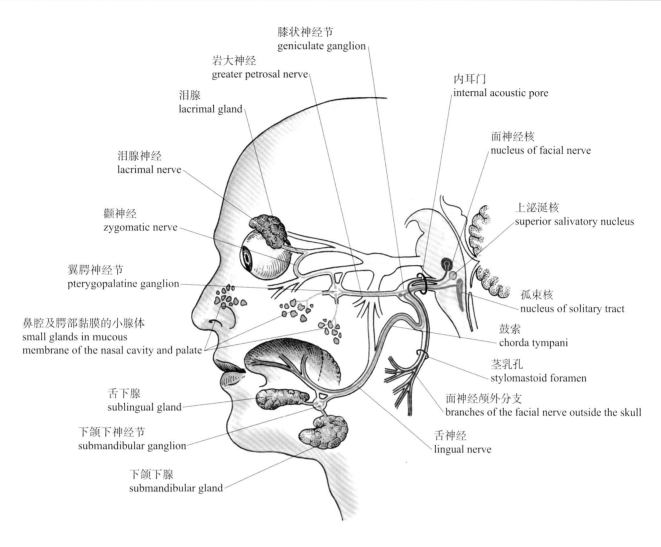

图 14-37 面神经及其分布示意图
Diagram of the facial nerve and its distribution

解剖纲要

翼腭神经节：为副交感神经节，位于翼腭窝上部，其上方通过几条短的翼腭神经（感觉根）与上颌神经相连，来自岩大神经的副交感纤维在节内换元后，节后纤维分布于泪腺、鼻、腭部的小腺体。

下颌下神经节：为副交感神经节，位于下颌下腺与舌神经之间，来自鼓索的副交感纤维在此节内换元，节后纤维分布于下颌下腺和舌下腺。

睫状神经节：为副交感神经节，位于视神经和外直肌之间，来自动眼神经的副交感纤维在此节交换神经元，节后纤维支配瞳孔括约肌和睫状肌。

Anatomical Outline

The pterygopalatine ganglion: It is the parasympathetic ganglion and located in the superior part of the pterygopalatine fossa. Superiorly, it connects with maxillary nerve through several short pterygopalatine nerves (sensory roots of the ganglion). The parasympathetic fibers coming from the greater petrosal nerve enter the ganglion and make relay. Then the postganglionic fibers are distributed in the lacrimal gland, small glands in the nose and palatine.

The submandibular ganglion: It is the parasympathetic ganglion and located between the submandibular gland and the lingual nerve. The parasympathetic fibers coming from chorda tympani enter the ganglion and make relay. Then the postganglionic fibers are distributed in the submandibular gland and the sublingual gland.

Ciliary ganglion: It is the parasympathetic ganglion and located between the optic nerve and the external rectus muscle. The parasympathetic fibers coming from the oculomotor nerve enter the ganglion and make relay. The postganglionic fibers innervate the pupil sphincter and ciliary muscles.

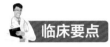 临床要点

面神经炎又称特发性面神经麻痹或 Bell 麻痹，系因茎乳孔内面神经非特异性炎症所致的周围性面瘫。常见的激发因素有头面部受冷或病毒感染等，这些因素使局部的血液循环障碍引起面神经缺血、水肿和受压而发病。

Key Points of the Clinic

The inflammation of the facial nerve, also named idiopathic facial paralysis or Bell's palsy, is a peripheral facial paralysis resulting from the inflammation of facial nerve in stylomastoid foramen. The head and face are subjected to cold and virus infection and so on, which cause local blood circulation disorder, leading to facial nerve ischemia, edema and compression onset.

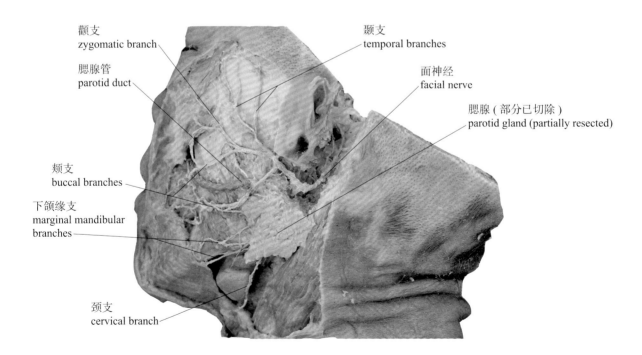

图 14-38　面神经颅外分支
Branches of the facial nerve outside of skull

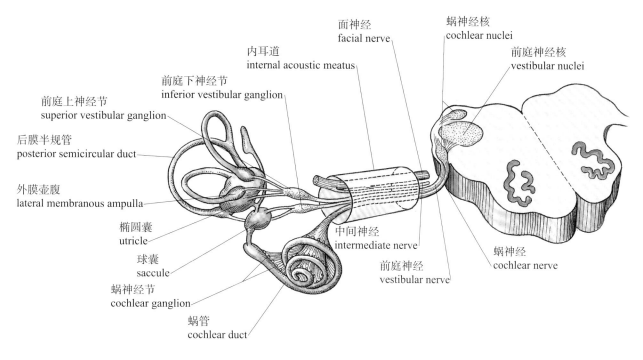

图 14-39 前庭蜗神经（模式图）
Vestibulocochlear nerve (diagram)

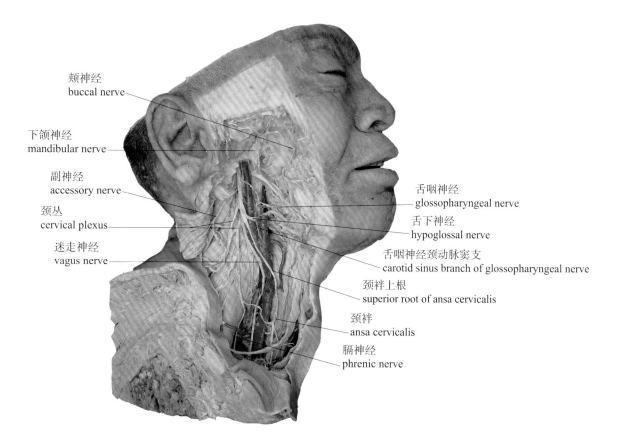

图 14-40 面侧深区和颈部的脑神经
Cranial nerves in lateral deep region of face and neck

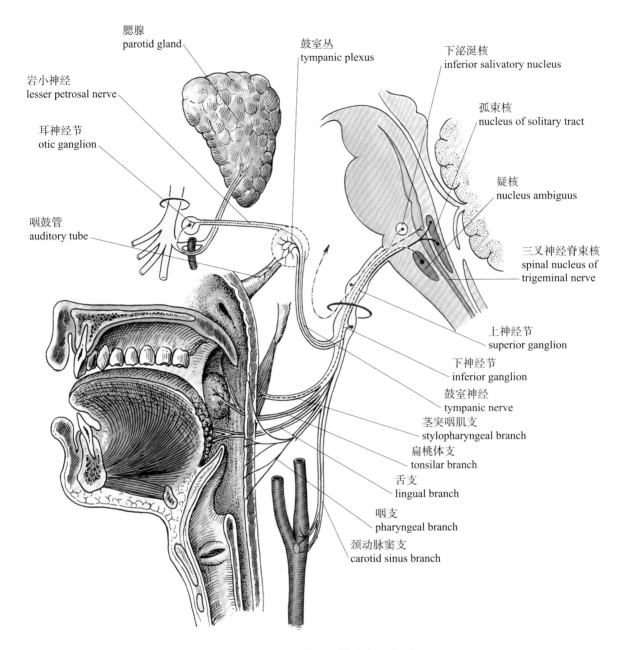

腮腺
parotid gland

鼓室丛
tympanic plexus

下泌涎核
inferior salivatory nucleus

岩小神经
lesser petrosal nerve

孤束核
nucleus of solitary tract

耳神经节
otic ganglion

疑核
nucleus ambiguus

咽鼓管
auditory tube

三叉神经脊束核
spinal nucleus of trigeminal nerve

上神经节
superior ganglion

下神经节
inferior ganglion

鼓室神经
tympanic nerve

茎突咽肌支
stylopharyngeal branch

扁桃体支
tonsilar branch

舌支
lingual branch

咽支
pharyngeal branch

颈动脉窦支
carotid sinus branch

图 14-41　舌咽神经及其分布示意图
Diagram of glossopharyngeal nerve and its distribution

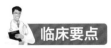 临床要点

　　舌咽神经痛是一种局限于舌咽神经分布区（扁桃体、舌根、咽、耳道深部）的发作性剧烈疼痛。吞咽、谈话、打哈欠、咳嗽等咽部运动常可诱发。

Key Points of the Clinic

　　Glossopharyngeal neuralgia is a paroxysmal severe pain that is localized in the distribution areas of the glossopharyngeal nerve such as tonsil, the root of tongue, pharynx, and the deep part of external acoustic meatus. It is usually evoked by swallowing, talking, yawning, coughing, and other pharyngeal movements.

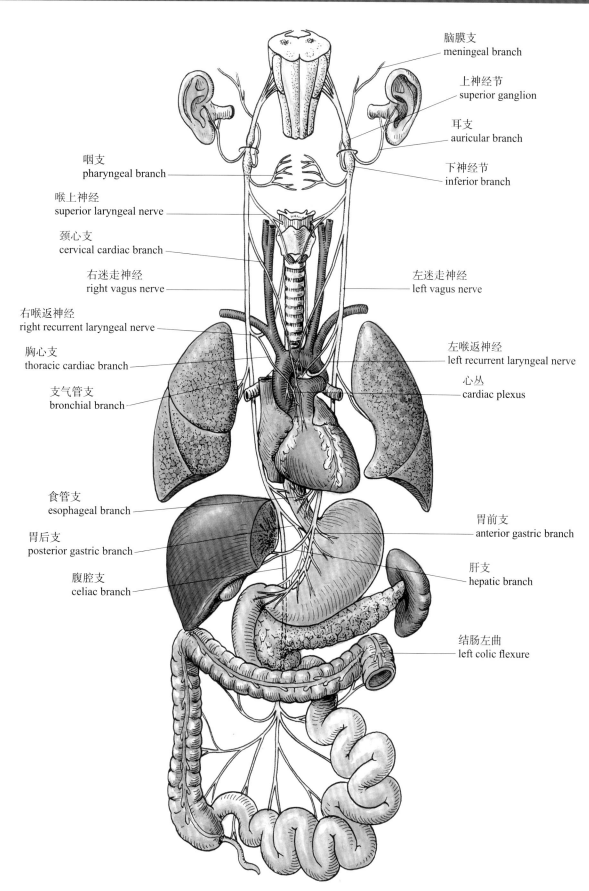

脑膜支
meningeal branch

上神经节
superior ganglion

耳支
auricular branch

下神经节
inferior branch

咽支
pharyngeal branch

喉上神经
superior laryngeal nerve

颈心支
cervical cardiac branch

右迷走神经
right vagus nerve

左迷走神经
left vagus nerve

右喉返神经
right recurrent laryngeal nerve

左喉返神经
left recurrent laryngeal nerve

胸心支
thoracic cardiac branch

支气管支
bronchial branch

心丛
cardiac plexus

食管支
esophageal branch

胃前支
anterior gastric branch

胃后支
posterior gastric branch

肝支
hepatic branch

腹腔支
celiac branch

结肠左曲
left colic flexure

图 14-42　迷走神经
Vagus nerve

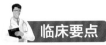 临床要点

迷走神经的喉上神经和喉返神经在抵达喉以前与甲状腺和甲状腺的血管毗邻，因此甲状腺手术时如不小心损伤上述神经可造成发音障碍、吞咽困难等。

 Key Points of the Clinic

The superior laryngeal nerve and recurrent laryngeal nerve of vagus nerve are adjacent to the thyroid gland and the vessels of the gland before they reach the larynx. The dysphonia and dysphagia may happen in case of the damage of the nerves at the surgery of the thyroid gland.

第三节　内脏神经系统　Section 3　Visceral nervous system

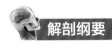 解剖纲要

内脏神经包含内脏运动和内脏感觉两种纤维成分。内脏运动神经调节内脏、心血管的运动和腺体的分泌，通常不受人的意志控制，又称之为自主神经系统或植物神经系统。内脏运动神经包括交感神经和副交感神经两部分。

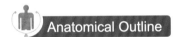 Anatomical Outline

The visceral nerve contains visceral motor and visceral sensory two kinds of fibers. The visceral motor nerve also named autonomic or vegetative nervous system because it mediates the unconsious function of viscera, controls the movement of visceral organs, angiocarpy and the secretion of glands. The visceral motor nerve is subdivided into two parts: sympathetic nerves and parasympathetic nerves.

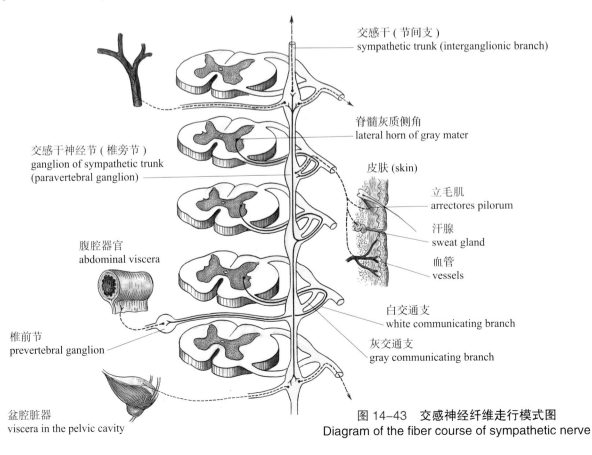

图 14-43　交感神经纤维走行模式图
Diagram of the fiber course of sympathetic nerve

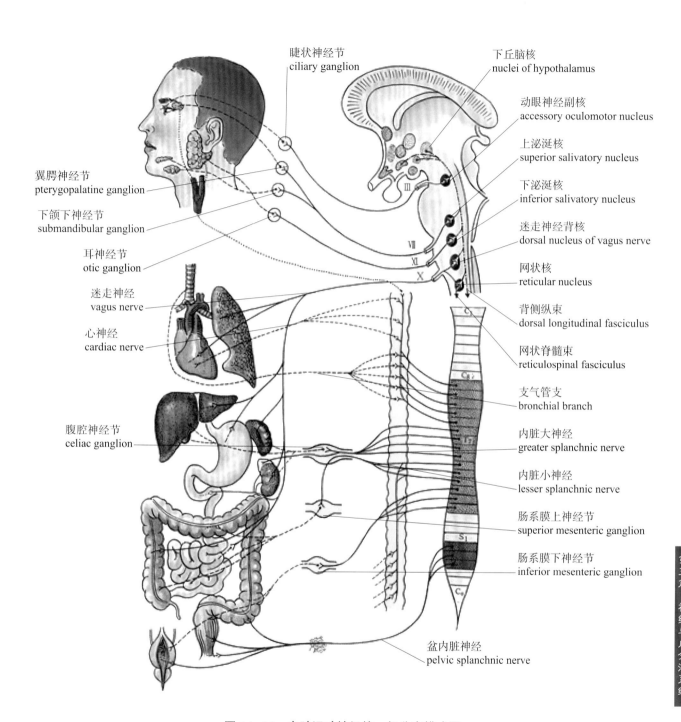

睫状神经节
ciliary ganglion

下丘脑核
nuclei of hypothalamus

动眼神经副核
accessory oculomotor nucleus

上泌涎核
superior salivatory nucleus

下泌涎核
inferior salivatory nucleus

迷走神经背核
dorsal nucleus of vagus nerve

网状核
reticular nucleus

背侧纵束
dorsal longitudinal fasciculus

网状脊髓束
reticulospinal fasciculus

支气管支
bronchial branch

内脏大神经
greater splanchnic nerve

内脏小神经
lesser splanchnic nerve

肠系膜上神经节
superior mesenteric ganglion

肠系膜下神经节
inferior mesenteric ganglion

翼腭神经节
pterygopalatine ganglion

下颌下神经节
submandibular ganglion

耳神经节
otic ganglion

迷走神经
vagus nerve

心神经
cardiac nerve

腹腔神经节
celiac ganglion

盆内脏神经
pelvic splanchnic nerve

图 14-44　内脏运动神经的一般分布模式图
Diagram showing general arrangement of the visceral motor nerves

第五篇　神经与内分泌系统
Part 5 Nervous and Endocrine System

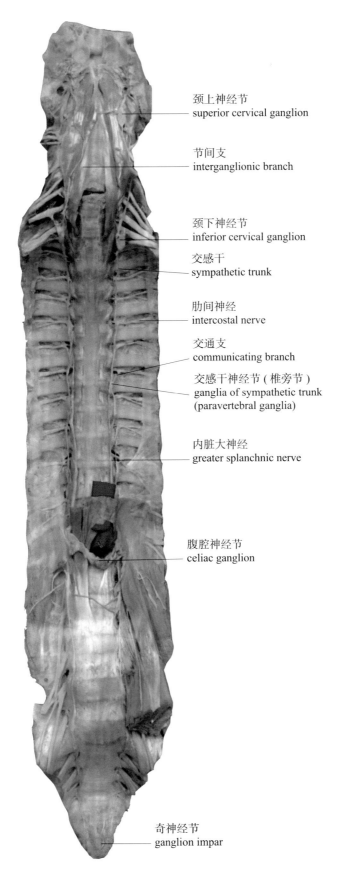

颈上神经节
superior cervical ganglion

节间支
interganglionic branch

颈下神经节
inferior cervical ganglion

交感干
sympathetic trunk

肋间神经
intercostal nerve

交通支
communicating branch

交感干神经节（椎旁节）
ganglia of sympathetic trunk
(paravertebral ganglia)

内脏大神经
greater splanchnic nerve

腹腔神经节
celiac ganglion

奇神经节
ganglion impar

图 14-45　交感干
Sympathetic trunk

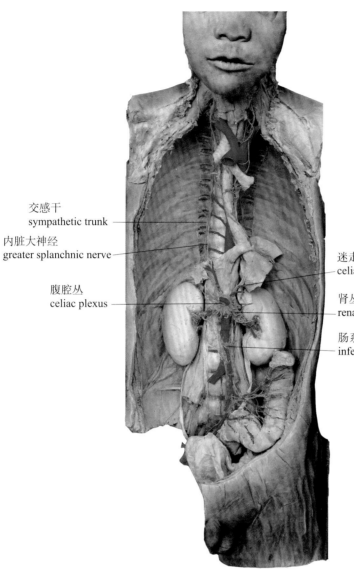

交感干
sympathetic trunk

内脏大神经
greater splanchnic nerve

腹腔丛
celiac plexus

迷走神经腹腔支
celiac branch of vagus nerve

肾丛
renal plexus

肠系膜下丛
inferior mesenteric plexus

图 14-46　交感干和神经丛
Sympathetic trunk and plexuses

第五篇　神经与内分泌系统

Part 5 Nervous and Endocrine System

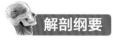 解剖纲要

内脏大神经：由穿过第 5 或第 6~9 胸交感干神经节的节前纤维组成，向前下方行走中合成一干，穿过膈脚，主要终于腹腔神经节。

内脏小神经：由穿过第 10~12 胸交感干神经节的节前纤维组成，下行穿过膈脚，主要终于主动脉肾神经节。

腰内脏神经：由穿过腰神经节的节前纤维组成，终于腹主动脉丛和肠系膜下丛内的椎前神经节。

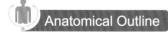 Anatomical Outline

The greater splanchnic nerve: It is formed by the preganglionic fibers from T_5 or T_6–T_9 ganglia, and terminates in the celiac ganglion after passing through the diaphragmatic crus.

The lesser splanchnic nerve: It is formed by the preganglionic fibers from T_{10}–T_{12} ganglia, and terminates in the aorticorenal ganglion after passing through the diaphragmatic crus.

The lumbar splanchnic nerve: It is formed by the preganglionic fibers from lumbar ganglia, and terminates in the prevertebral ganglia in the abdominal aortic plexus and inferior mesenteric plexus.

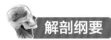 解剖纲要

内脏神经丛：交感神经、副交感神经和内脏感觉神经在分布到相应脏器的过程中，常相互交织形成内脏神经丛，有的位于脏器附近，有的攀附在动脉的周围，由这些丛发出的分支常随动脉分支到达支配的器官。主要的内脏神经丛有心丛、肺丛、腹腔丛、腹主动脉丛、上腹下丛和下腹下丛等。

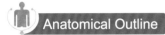 Anatomical Outline

The visceral nerve plexuses: They are formed by the combination of branches from sympathetic, parasympathetic and visceral sensory nerves along their travel to organs. Some of the visceral nerve plexuses are around the target organs, some twine in the root of arteries, traveling along the artery to pass to the organs. The main visceral nerve plexuses include cardiac plexus, pulmonary plexus, celiac plexus, abdominal aortic plexus, superior and inferior hypogastric plexuses, etc.

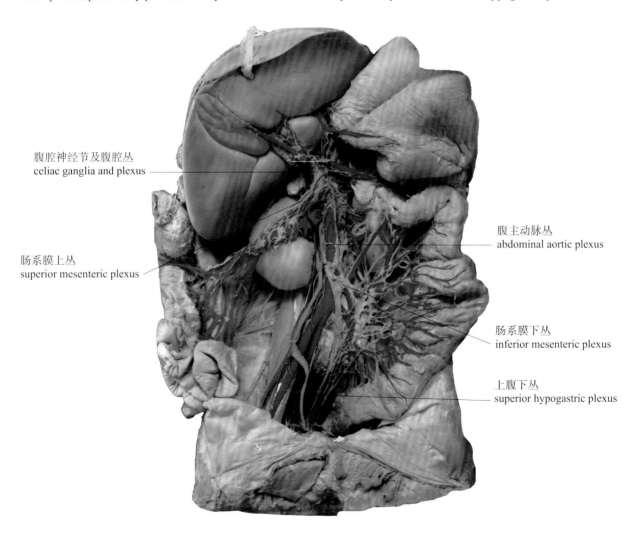

图 14-47　交感神经丛
Sympathetic plexuses

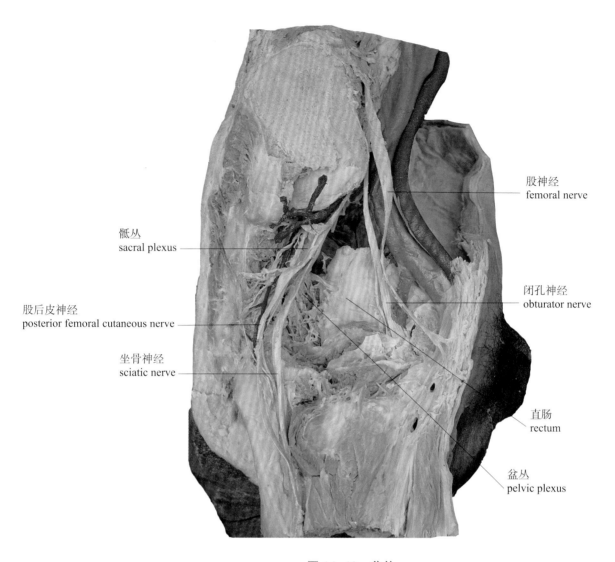

股神经
femoral nerve

骶丛
sacral plexus

闭孔神经
obturator nerve

股后皮神经
posterior femoral cutaneous nerve

坐骨神经
sciatic nerve

直肠
rectum

盆丛
pelvic plexus

图 14-48 **盆丛**
Pelvic plexus

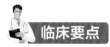 **临床要点**

多汗症主要症状为自幼出现不明原因的两侧手掌、腋窝及足底多汗。胸交感神经链切断术（切除胸 4 交感神经节）是治疗多汗症的有效手段。

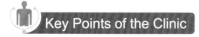 **Key Points of the Clinic**

The principal symptom of ephidrosis is unexplained sweating in the palms, axillary fossae, and soles since young. The thoracic sympathectomy (cutting the T_4 sympathetic ganglions) is a valid method to treat the ephidrosis.

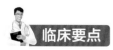 **临床要点**

当某些内脏器官发生病变时，常在体表一定区域产生感觉过敏或痛觉，为内脏性牵涉痛。例如，有肝胆疾患时，常在右肩部感到疼痛，根据牵涉痛的特征，有助于临床某些疾病的诊断。

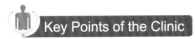 **Key Points of the Clinic**

When some visceral organs have lesions, a certain area of the surface of the body often produce algesia or pain, referred to as visceral pain. This is referred pain. For example, when suffering from hepatobiliary diseases, pain is often felt in the right shoulder, which is helpful for clinical diagnosis of some diseases according to the characteristics of referred pain.

交感神经与副交感神经的区别

区别点　　　　　结构	交感神经	副交感神经
低级中枢	脊髓 T_1 ~ L_3 节段侧角	脑干内和脊髓 S_2 ~ S_4 节段内副交感神经核
神经节	椎旁节、椎前节	器官旁节、器官内节
节前纤维和节后纤维	节前纤维短，节后纤维长 一个节前神经元可以与许多节后神经元形成突触	节前纤维长，节后纤维短 节前神经元只能与少数节后神经元形成突触
分布范围	广泛。全身的血管、腺体和立毛肌以及头颈、胸、腹、盆的脏器	较为局限。只分布于脏器和一般腺体，而大部分血管、汗腺、立毛肌和肾上腺髓质无副交感神经分布
功能	兴奋、应激状态，耗能	安静、休息状态，储能

The difference between sympathetic nerve and parasympathetic nerve

Structure Difference	Sympathetic nerve	Parasympathetic nerve
Lower center	The lateral horn of the T_1-L_3 segments of spinal cord	Parasympathetic nuclei in the brain stem and S_2-S_4 segments of spinal cord
Ganglia	Prevertebral and paravertebral ganglia	Para-organ and intra-organ ganglia
Preganglionic and postganglionic fibers	Preganglionic fibers are shorter than postganglionic fibers. One preganglionic neuron can synapse with many postganglionic neurons	Preganglionic fibers are long, postganglionic fibers are short. One preganglionic neuron can synapse with several postganglionic neurons
Distribution	Widely: the blood, glands and arrector pili muscle in whole body; organs in head, neck, thorax, abdomen, and pelvis	Limitations. It is only distributed in viscera and general glands, but most of the blood vessels, sweat glands, arrector pili muscle, and adrenal medulla have no parasympathetic distribution
Function	State of excitement, stress, energy consumption	Quiet, rest state, energy storage

第十五章　神经系统的传导通路
Chapter 15　Conductive pathways of nervous system

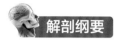 **解剖纲要**

感觉（上行）传导通路的特点：3（三级神经元）；2（两次突触换元）；1（一次交叉）。

 Anatomical Outline

The characteristics of the sensory (ascending) pathway include 3 orders of neurons; 2 synapses; 1 time of decussation.

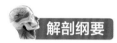 **解剖纲要**

重要上行传导通路概要列表

传导通路名称	第 1 级神经元	第 2 级神经元	第 3 级神经元
躯干、四肢本体（深）感觉	脊神经节	薄束核、楔束核	丘脑腹后外侧核
躯干、四肢浅感觉	脊神经节	脊髓第 Ⅰ、Ⅳ~Ⅶ层	丘脑腹后外侧核
头面部浅感觉	三叉神经节	三叉神经脊束核、脑桥核	丘脑腹后内侧核
视觉	双极细胞	节细胞	外侧膝状体

 Anatomical Outline

The general description of main ascending pathway

Pathway	1st neuron	2nd neuron	3rd neuron
Deep sensory (proprioception) pathway of trunk and limbs	Spinal ganglion	Gracile nucleus，cuneate nucleus	Ventral posterolateral nucleus
Superficial sensory pathway of trunk and limbs	Spinal ganglion	Spinal cord laminae Ⅰ，Ⅳ–Ⅶ	Ventral posterolateral nucleus
Superficial sensory pathway of head and face	Trigeminal ganglion	Pontine and spinal nuclei of the trigeminal nerve	Ventral posteromedial nucleus
Visual pathway	Bipolar cell	Ganglion cell	Lateral geniculate body

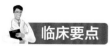 **临床要点**

脊髓后索综合征：它是脊髓不完全损伤的特有的表现，主要伤及脊髓后部，造成薄束、楔束受损，即涉及了躯干、四肢意识性本体感觉和精细触觉传导通路。损伤平面以下本体感觉丧失，而运动和痛、温觉存在。主要表现：可出现闭目站立时身体倾斜、摇晃、易跌倒，同时精细触觉和振动觉丧失。若疑为脊髓楔束受损，常进行指鼻试验。

指鼻试验：嘱患者将前臂外旋、伸直，以示指触自己的鼻尖，先慢后快，先睁眼后闭眼，反复上述运动，称指鼻试验。指鼻试验阳性表示脊髓楔束可能受损。

第五篇　神经与内分泌系统　Part 5 Nervous and Endocrine System

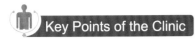 Key Points of the Clinic

Posterior cord syndrome: It is a unique manifestation of incomplete spinal cord injury, which mainly involves the posterior part of the spinal cord and causes damage to the fasciculus gracilis and fasciculus cuneatus, namely, it involves the conscious proprioception and fine tactile pathway of the trunk and limbs. Loss of proprioception and the presence of movement and pain and warmth below the injury level. Main performance: can appear when standing with eyes closed tilt, shaking, easy to fall, while the loss of fine touch and vibration sense. If fasciculus cuneatus is suspected to be damaged, finger-nose test is often performed.

The finger-nose test: the patient is asked to turn the forearm outward and straighten it, and touch the tip of his nose with index, first slowly and then quickly, first open and then close his or her eyes, and repeat the above movements, called finger-nose test. A positive finger-nose test indicates possible damage of fasciculus cuneatus.

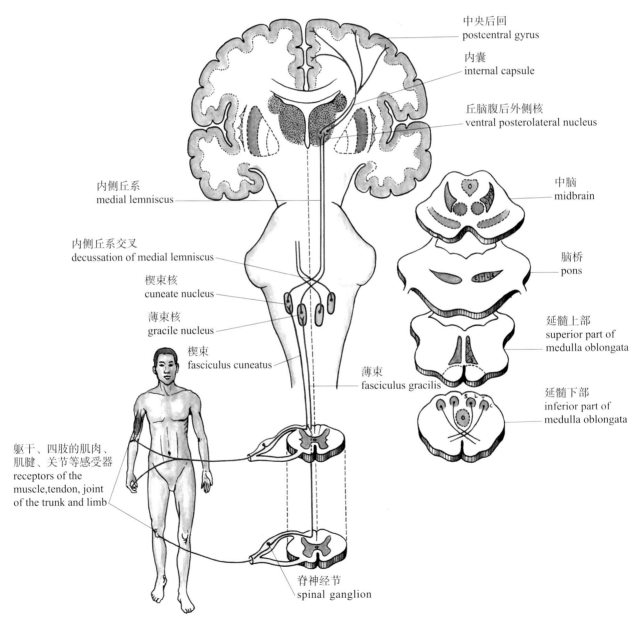

图 15-1 躯干、四肢意识性本体感觉和精细触觉传导通路
Pathway of the conscious proprioceptive sensibility and fine touch of trunk and limbs

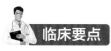

临床要点

一侧脊髓丘脑侧束损伤，表现为对侧损伤平面以下痛、温觉障碍，因后索完好，故粗触觉无明显障碍。

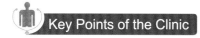

The injury of one side of the lateral spinothalamic tract presents pain, sensation and thermal disturbances below the injured plane at the opposite side, while the influence of rough tactile is not obvious for the intact posterior funiculus.

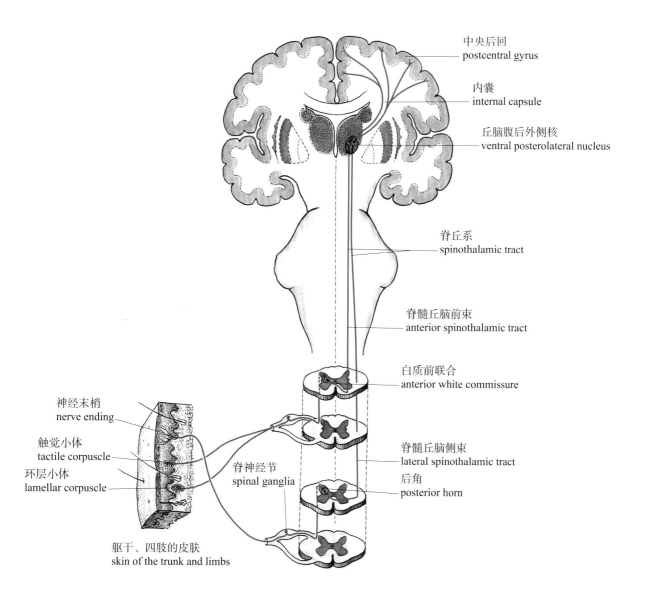

中央后回
postcentral gyrus

内囊
internal capsule

丘脑腹后外侧核
ventral posterolateral nucleus

脊丘系
spinothalamic tract

脊髓丘脑前束
anterior spinothalamic tract

白质前联合
anterior white commissure

神经末梢
nerve ending

触觉小体
tactile corpuscle

环层小体
lamellar corpuscle

脊神经节
spinal ganglia

脊髓丘脑侧束
lateral spinothalamic tract

后角
posterior horn

躯干、四肢的皮肤
skin of the trunk and limbs

图 15-2　躯干、四肢浅感觉传导通路
Superficial sensory pathways of trunk and limbs

第五篇　神经与内分泌系统
Part 5 Nervous and Endocrine System

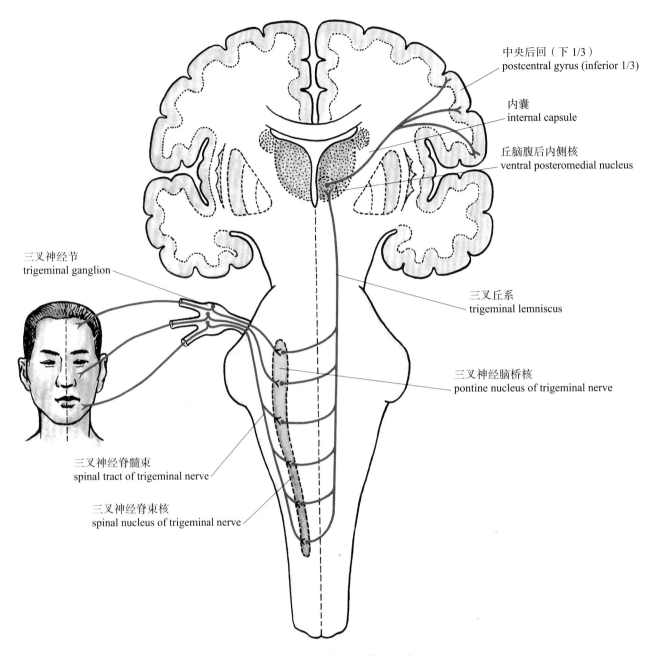

中央后回（下 1/3）
postcentral gyrus (inferior 1/3)

内囊
internal capsule

丘脑腹后内侧核
ventral posteromedial nucleus

三叉神经节
trigeminal ganglion

三叉丘系
trigeminal lemniscus

三叉神经脑桥核
pontine nucleus of trigeminal nerve

三叉神经脊髓束
spinal tract of trigeminal nerve

三叉神经脊束核
spinal nucleus of trigeminal nerve

图 15-3 头面部浅感觉传导通路
Superficial sensory pathways of head and face

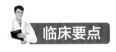 临床要点

视觉传导通路损伤后的表现

损伤部位	临床表现
一侧视神经	该眼视野全盲
视交叉中央部	双眼视野颞侧半偏盲（管状视野）
视交叉外侧部	患侧视野鼻侧半偏盲
一侧视束（视辐射、视区）	双眼病灶对侧视野同向性偏盲

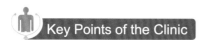

Key Points of the Clinic

Manifestations of the injured visual pathway

Lesion	Clinical features
Optic nerve on one side	Bindness of vision of the affected eye
Center part of the optic chiasma	Temporal hemianopia of both eyes (barrel vision)
Lateral part of the optic chiasma	Nasal hemianopia of the affected eye
Optic tract (optic radiation and visual cortex) on one side	Contralateral homonymous hemianopia of both eyes at opposite sides lesion

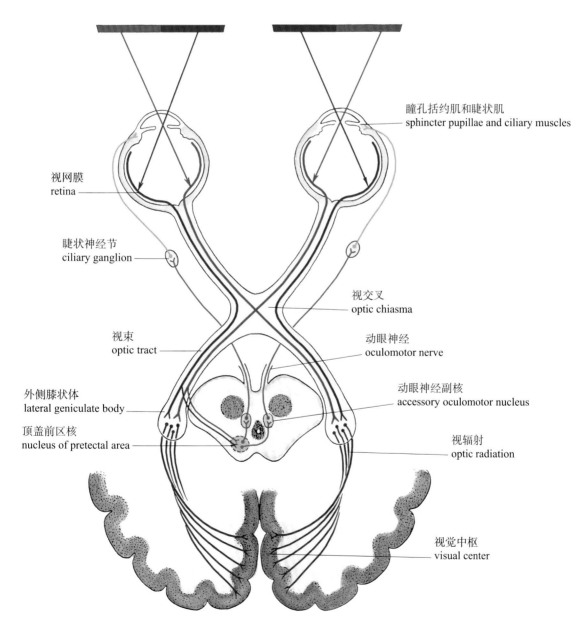

图 15-4 视觉和瞳孔对光反射传导通路
Visual and pupillary reflexes pathways

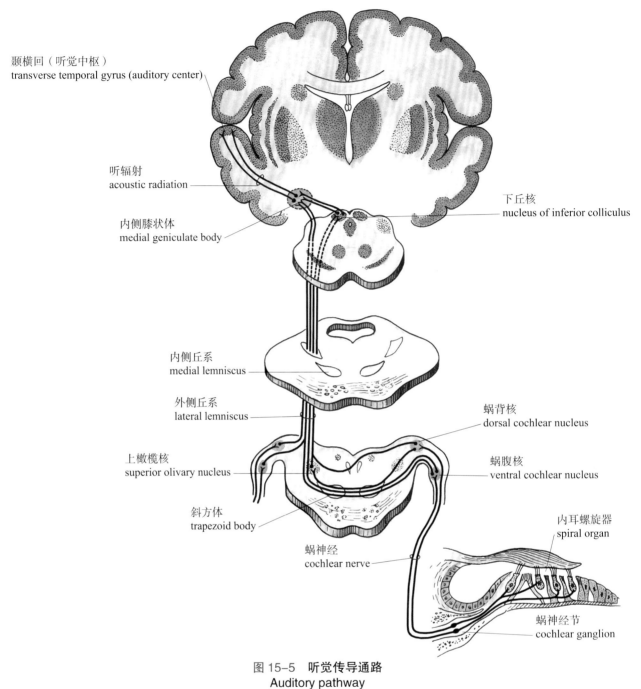

颞横回（听觉中枢）
transverse temporal gyrus (auditory center)

听辐射
acoustic radiation

内侧膝状体
medial geniculate body

下丘核
nucleus of inferior colliculus

内侧丘系
medial lemniscus

外侧丘系
lateral lemniscus

蜗背核
dorsal cochlear nucleus

上橄榄核
superior olivary nucleus

蜗腹核
ventral cochlear nucleus

斜方体
trapezoid body

内耳螺旋器
spiral organ

蜗神经
cochlear nerve

蜗神经节
cochlear ganglion

图 15-5 听觉传导通路
Auditory pathway

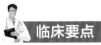 临床要点

听觉障碍俗称耳聋。临床上耳聋分为以外耳和中耳病变引起的传导性耳聋，以内耳和听神经病变引起的神经性耳聋，以外中耳病变和中耳听神经共同病变引起的混合性耳聋。

Key Points of the Clinic

Hearing impairment is commonly known as deafness. Clinically, the conductive deafness is caused by lesions in the middle and outer ear; the neuropathic deafness is caused by lesions in the inner ear and auditory nerve. The lesions in the middle and outer ear as well as in the auditory nerve together can result in mixed deafness.

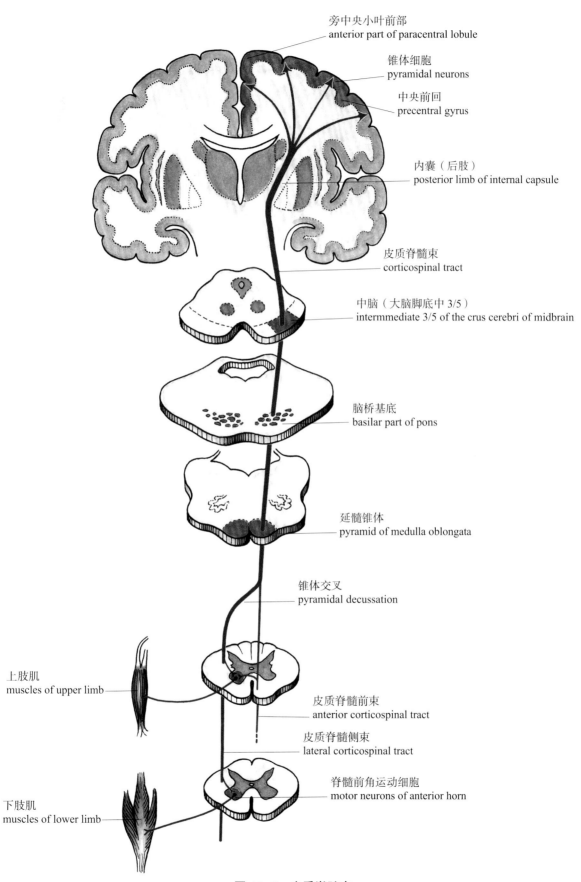

旁中央小叶前部
anterior part of paracentral lobule

锥体细胞
pyramidal neurons

中央前回
precentral gyrus

内囊（后肢）
posterior limb of internal capsule

皮质脊髓束
corticospinal tract

中脑（大脑脚底中 3/5）
intermmediate 3/5 of the crus cerebri of midbrain

脑桥基底
basilar part of pons

延髓锥体
pyramid of medulla oblongata

锥体交叉
pyramidal decussation

上肢肌
muscles of upper limb

皮质脊髓前束
anterior corticospinal tract

皮质脊髓侧束
lateral corticospinal tract

脊髓前角运动细胞
motor neurons of anterior horn

下肢肌
muscles of lower limb

图 15-6　皮质脊髓束
Corticospinal tract

第五篇　神经与内分泌系统
Part 5 Nervous and Endocrine System

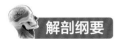 解剖纲要

锥体系上、下运动神经元

传导路	上运动神经元	下运动神经元
皮质脊髓束	中央前回中上部、中央旁小叶前部锥体细胞及其轴突	脊髓前角运动细胞及其轴突
皮质核束	中央前回下部锥体细胞及其轴突	脑干内的一般躯体和特殊内脏运动脑神经核及其轴突

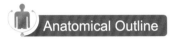 Anatomical Outline

The upper and lower motor neurons of the pyramidal tract

Pathway	Upper motor neuron	Lower motor neuron
Corticospinal tract	Giant pyramidal cells of the superior and middle parts of the precentral gyrus and anterior part of the paracentral lobule and its axons	Motor cells in anterior horn of the spinal cord and its axons
Corticonuclear tract	Giant pyramidal cells of the inferior part of the precentral gyrus and its axons	General somatic motor and special visceral motor nuclei of the brain stem and its axons

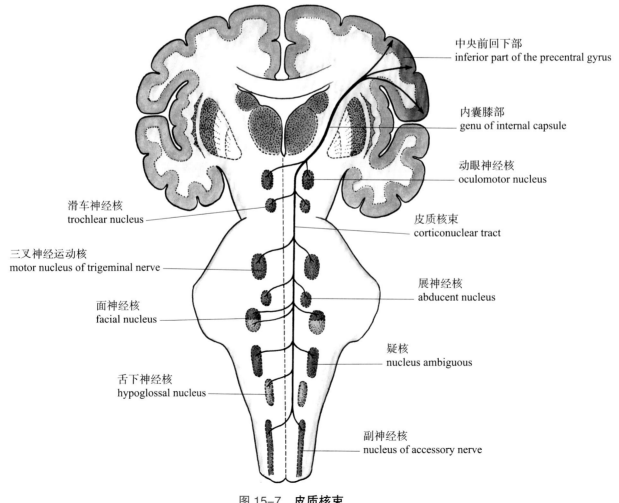

图 15-7 皮质核束
Corticonuclear tract

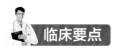

上、下运动神经元损伤后的比较

临床表现	上运动神经元损伤（核上瘫）	下运动神经元损伤（核下瘫）
瘫痪特点	痉挛性瘫痪（硬瘫）	弛缓性瘫痪（软瘫）
肌张力	增高	降低
深反射	亢进	消失
浅反射	减弱或消失	消失
病理反射	阳性（＋）（如 Babinski 征）	阴性（－）
肌萎缩	不明显或出现较晚	明显
肌电	正常	失神经电位

Key Points of the Clinic

Comparison of the upper and lower motor neurons lesion

clinical feature	Upper motor neuron lesion (supranuclear paralysis)	Lower motor neuron lesion (subnuclear paralysis)
Characteristics of paralysis	Spastic paralysis (stiff paralysis)	Flaccid (soft) paralysis
Muscle tension	Increase	Decrease
Deep reflex	Hyperactivity	Disappear
Superficial reflex	Weakened or disappear	Disappear
Pathological reflex	Positive（＋）（such as Babinski sign）	Negative（－）
Amyotrophy	Not obvious or appearing later	Obvious
Myoelectricity	Normal	Denervated potential

第十六章 内分泌系统

Chapter 16 Endocrine system

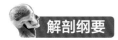 解剖纲要

内分泌系统概述

项目 组成	内分泌腺	内分泌组织
特点	无排泄管，分泌激素直接入血液，作用于特定靶器官	以细胞团分散于其他器官或组织
结构	脑垂体、松果体、甲状腺、甲状旁腺、胸腺、肾上腺	胰岛、睾丸内间质细胞、卵巢内的卵泡与黄体

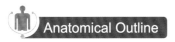 Anatomical Outline

Introduction of endocrine system

Composition / Item	Endocrine gland	Endocrine tissue
Traits	Endocrine glands don't have excretory tubes and their hormones secret directly into the bloodstream, which acts on specific target organs	Endocrine tissue is dispersed by cell aggregates among other organs or tissues
structure	Hypophysis/pituitary gland, pineal gland, thyroid gland, parathyroid gland, thymus gland, suprarenal gland	Islets of pancreas, stromal cells in the testis, follicles and corpus luteum in the ovary

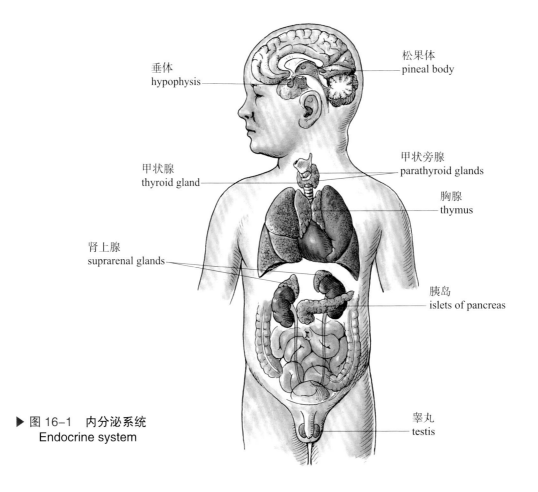

▶ 图 16-1 内分泌系统
Endocrine system

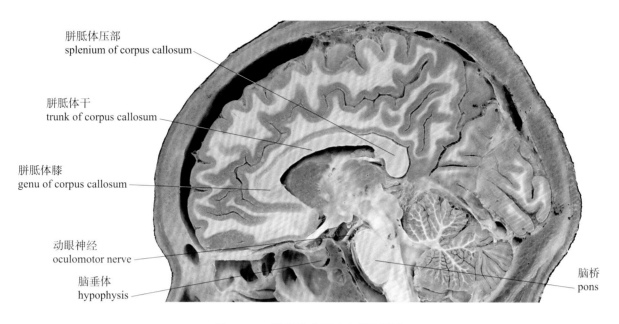

胼胝体压部
splenium of corpus callosum

胼胝体干
trunk of corpus callosum

胼胝体膝
genu of corpus callosum

动眼神经
oculomotor nerve

脑垂体
hypophysis

脑桥
pons

图 16-2 脑垂体（正中矢状切面）
Hypophysis (median sagittal section)

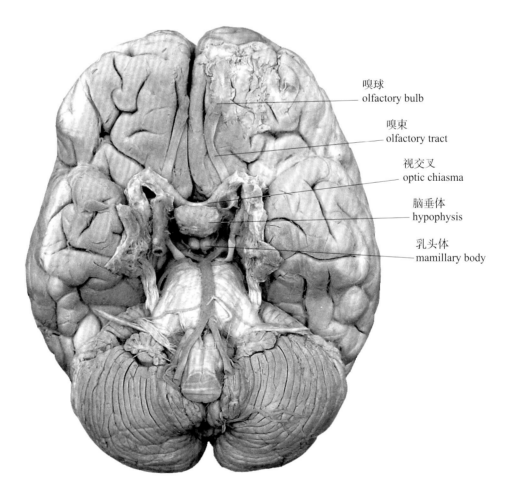

嗅球
olfactory bulb

嗅束
olfactory tract

视交叉
optic chiasma

脑垂体
hypophysis

乳头体
mamillary body

图 16-3 脑垂体（下面观）
Hypophysis (inferior view)

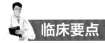
临床要点

1.脑垂体:脑垂体包括腺垂体和神经垂体两部分。腺垂体细胞分泌的激素主要有 7 种,它们分别为生长激素、催乳素、促甲状腺激素、促性腺激素(黄体生成素和卵泡刺激素)、促肾上腺皮质激素和黑色细胞刺激素。神经垂体本身不分泌激素,有贮存激素的功能。垂体疾病最多见的是垂体肿瘤。若为生长激素瘤,幼年表现为巨人症,成人表现为肢端肥大症。

2.松果体:松果体分泌褪黑素,具有抑制性成熟和抗衰老作用。松果体肿瘤可导致性早熟或第二性征的异常发育。

3.结节性甲状腺肿:是一种最常见的甲状腺疾病。其病因不是十分清楚,可能与内分泌紊乱、高碘饮食、环境因素、遗传因素和放射线接触史等有关。

Key Points of the Clinic

1. Hypophysis: the hypophysis consists of two parts: the adenohypophysis and the neurohypophysis. There are seven main hormones secreted by adenohypophysis, which are growth hormone, prolactin, thyroid-stimulating hormone, gonadotropin (luteinizing hormone and follicle stimulating hormone) , adrenocorticotropic hormone and melanocyte-stimulating hormone. The neurohypophysis itself does not secrete hormones and has the function of storing hormones. The most common pituitary diseases are pituitary tumors. In the case of somato trophinoma, gigantism occurs in childhood and acromegaly in adults.

2. The pineal body: the pineal body secretes melatonin, which inhibits sexual maturation and has anti-aging effects. Pineal tumors can lead to early puberty or abnormal development of secondary sexual characteristics.

3. Nodular goiter: one of the most common thyroid diseases. Its etiology is not very clear and may be related to endocrine disorders, high iodine diet, environmental factors, genetic factors and history of radiation exposure.

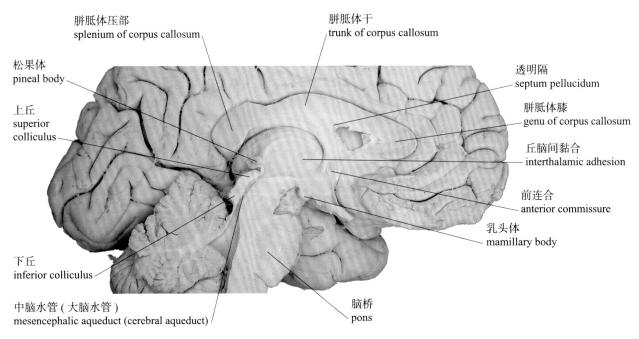

图 16-4 松果体(正中矢状切面)
Pineal body (median sagittal section)

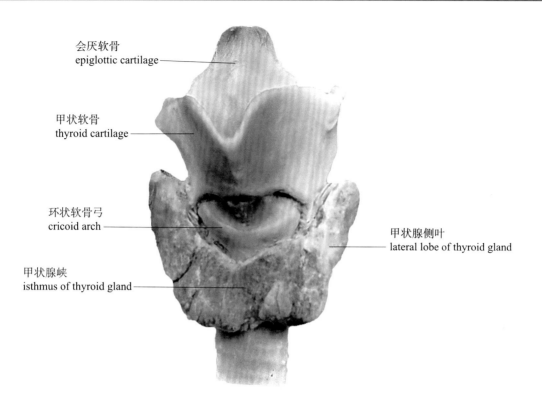

会厌软骨
epiglottic cartilage

甲状软骨
thyroid cartilage

环状软骨弓
cricoid arch

甲状腺侧叶
lateral lobe of thyroid gland

甲状腺峡
isthmus of thyroid gland

图 16-5 甲状腺（前面观）
Thyroid gland（anterior view）

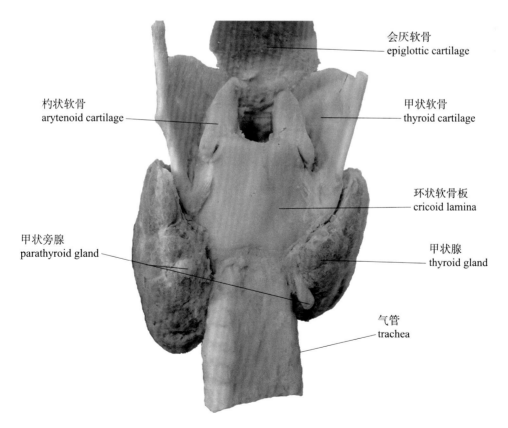

会厌软骨
epiglottic cartilage

杓状软骨
arytenoid cartilage

甲状软骨
thyroid cartilage

环状软骨板
cricoid lamina

甲状旁腺
parathyroid gland

甲状腺
thyroid gland

气管
trachea

图 16-6 甲状旁腺（后面观）
Parathyroid gland (posterior view)

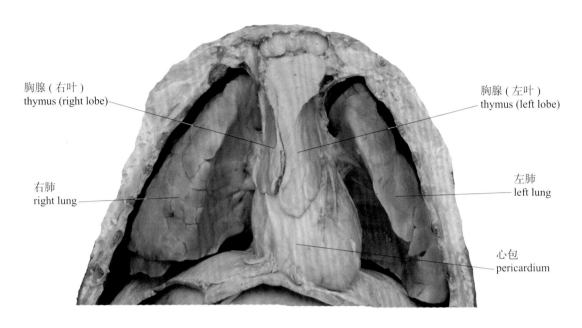

胸腺（右叶）thymus (right lobe)

胸腺（左叶）thymus (left lobe)

右肺 right lung

左肺 left lung

心包 pericardium

图 16-7　胸腺（前面观）
Thymus (anterior view)

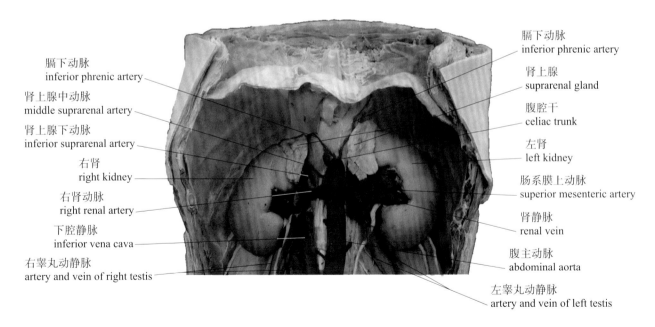

膈下动脉 inferior phrenic artery

肾上腺中动脉 middle suprarenal artery

肾上腺下动脉 inferior suprarenal artery

右肾 right kidney

右肾动脉 right renal artery

下腔静脉 inferior vena cava

右睾丸动静脉 artery and vein of right testis

膈下动脉 inferior phrenic artery

肾上腺 suprarenal gland

腹腔干 celiac trunk

左肾 left kidney

肠系膜上动脉 superior mesenteric artery

肾静脉 renal vein

腹主动脉 abdominal aorta

左睾丸动静脉 artery and vein of left testis

图 16-8　肾上腺（显示腹膜后隙脏器）
Suprarenal gland (showing visceral organs in retroperitoneal space)

附 录

典型磁共振成像图（MRI）

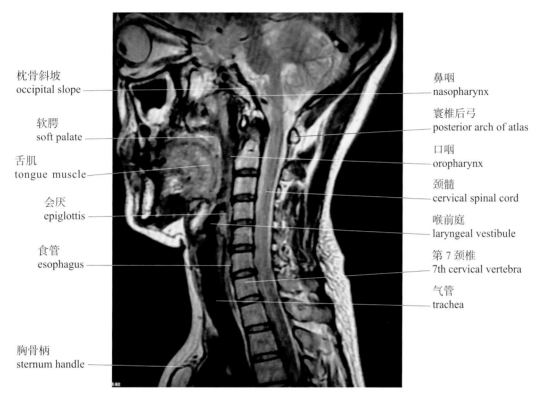

枕骨斜坡
occipital slope

软腭
soft palate

舌肌
tongue muscle

会厌
epiglottis

食管
esophagus

胸骨柄
sternum handle

鼻咽
nasopharynx

寰椎后弓
posterior arch of atlas

口咽
oropharynx

颈髓
cervical spinal cord

喉前庭
laryngeal vestibule

第 7 颈椎
7th cervical vertebra

气管
trachea

附图 1　颈部矢状位 MRI
MRI of neck (sagittal section)

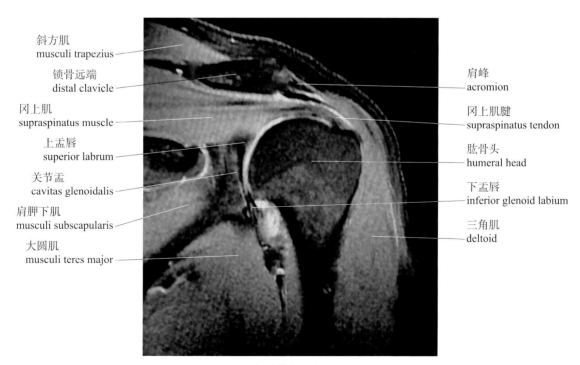

斜方肌
musculi trapezius

锁骨远端
distal clavicle

冈上肌
supraspinatus muscle

上盂唇
superior labrum

关节盂
cavitas glenoidalis

肩胛下肌
musculi subscapularis

大圆肌
musculi teres major

肩峰
acromion

冈上肌腱
supraspinatus tendon

肱骨头
humeral head

下盂唇
inferior glenoid labium

三角肌
deltoid

附图 2　肩关节斜冠状位 MRI
MRI of shoulder joint (oblique coronal section)

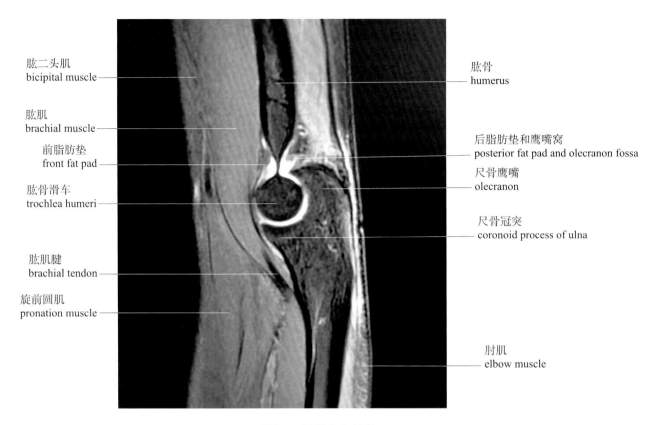

肱二头肌
bicipital muscle

肱肌
brachial muscle

前脂肪垫
front fat pad

肱骨滑车
trochlea humeri

肱肌腱
brachial tendon

旋前圆肌
pronation muscle

肱骨
humerus

后脂肪垫和鹰嘴窝
posterior fat pad and olecranon fossa

尺骨鹰嘴
olecranon

尺骨冠突
coronoid process of ulna

肘肌
elbow muscle

附图 3　肘关节矢状位 MRI
MRI of elbow joint (sagittal section)

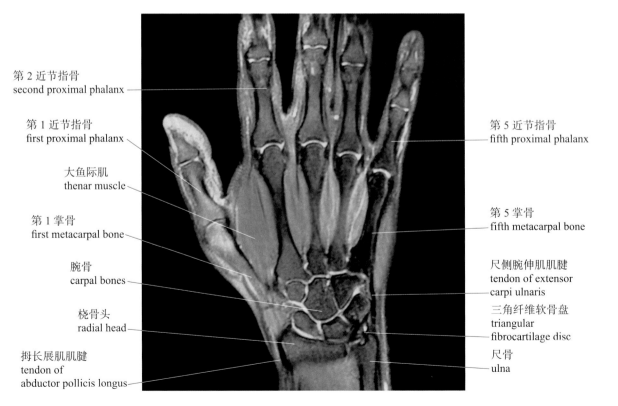

第 2 近节指骨
second proximal phalanx

第 1 近节指骨
first proximal phalanx

大鱼际肌
thenar muscle

第 1 掌骨
first metacarpal bone

腕骨
carpal bones

桡骨头
radial head

拇长展肌肌腱
tendon of
abductor pollicis longus

第 5 近节指骨
fifth proximal phalanx

第 5 掌骨
fifth metacarpal bone

尺侧腕伸肌肌腱
tendon of extensor
carpi ulnaris

三角纤维软骨盘
triangular
fibrocartilage disc

尺骨
ulna

附图 4　腕关节冠状位 MRI
MRI of wrist joint (coronal section)

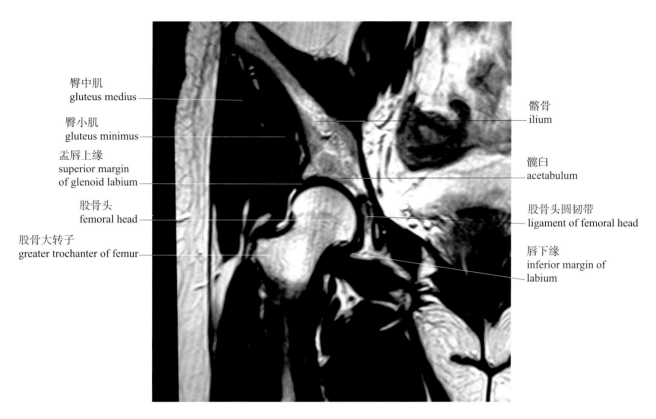

臀中肌
gluteus medius

臀小肌
gluteus minimus

盂唇上缘
superior margin
of glenoid labium

股骨头
femoral head

股骨大转子
greater trochanter of femur

髂骨
ilium

髋臼
acetabulum

股骨头圆韧带
ligament of femoral head

唇下缘
inferior margin of
labium

附图 5　髋关节冠状位 MRI
MRI of hip joint (coronal section)

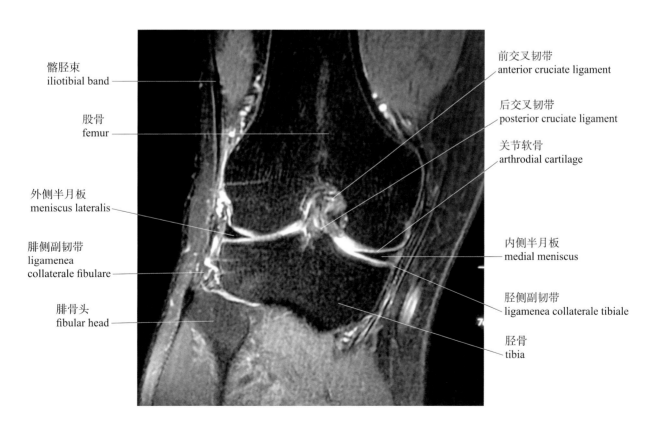

髂胫束
iliotibial band

股骨
femur

外侧半月板
meniscus lateralis

腓侧副韧带
ligamenea
collaterale fibulare

腓骨头
fibular head

前交叉韧带
anterior cruciate ligament

后交叉韧带
posterior cruciate ligament

关节软骨
arthrodial cartilage

内侧半月板
medial meniscus

胫侧副韧带
ligamenea collaterale tibiale

胫骨
tibia

附图 6　膝关节冠状位 MRI
MRI of knee joint (coronal section)

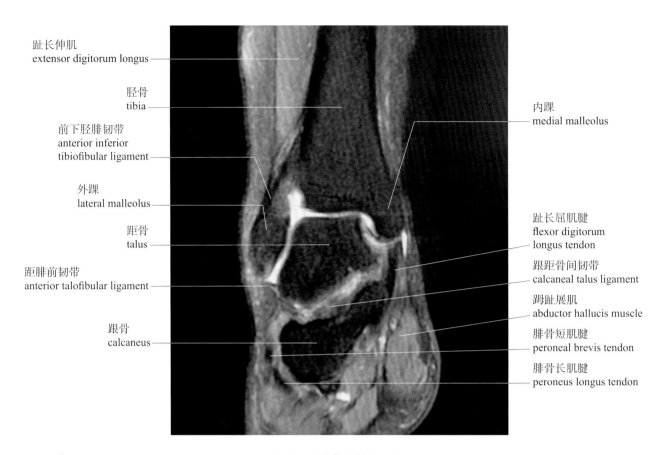

趾长伸肌
extensor digitorum longus

胫骨
tibia

前下胫腓韧带
anterior inferior
tibiofibular ligament

外踝
lateral malleolus

距骨
talus

距腓前韧带
anterior talofibular ligament

跟骨
calcaneus

内踝
medial malleolus

趾长屈肌腱
flexor digitorum
longus tendon

跟距骨间韧带
calcaneal talus ligament

姆趾展肌
abductor hallucis muscle

腓骨短肌腱
peroneal brevis tendon

腓骨长肌腱
peroneus longus tendon

附图 7　踝关节冠状位 MRI
MRI of ankle joint (coronal section)

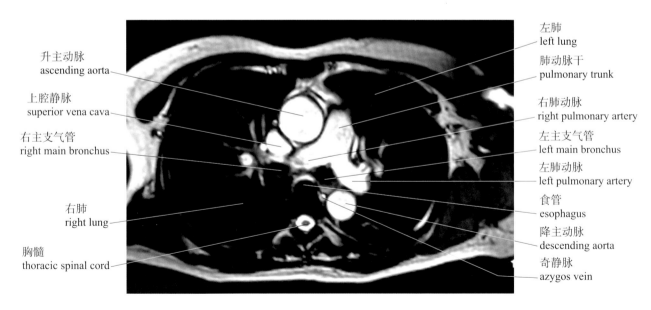

升主动脉
ascending aorta

上腔静脉
superior vena cava

右主支气管
right main bronchus

右肺
right lung

胸髓
thoracic spinal cord

左肺
left lung

肺动脉干
pulmonary trunk

右肺动脉
right pulmonary artery

左主支气管
left main bronchus

左肺动脉
left pulmonary artery

食管
esophagus

降主动脉
descending aorta

奇静脉
azygos vein

附图 8　经升主动脉胸部横切面 MRI
MRI of transverse section of the thorax (passing the ascending aorta)

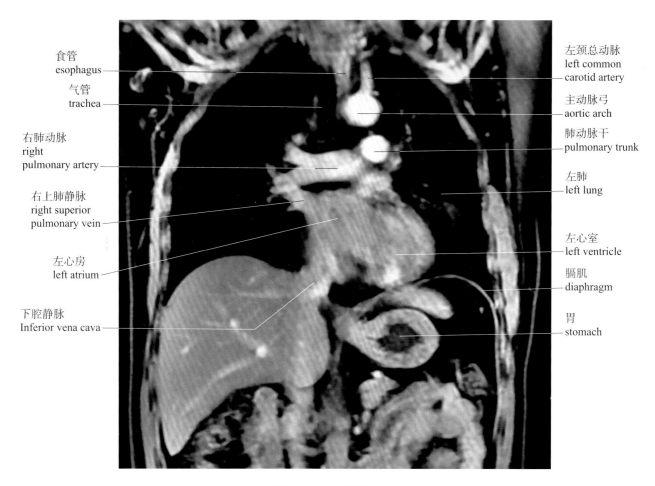

食管
esophagus

气管
trachea

右肺动脉
right
pulmonary artery

右上肺静脉
right superior
pulmonary vein

左心房
left atrium

下腔静脉
Inferior vena cava

左颈总动脉
left common
carotid artery

主动脉弓
aortic arch

肺动脉干
pulmonary trunk

左肺
left lung

左心室
left ventricle

膈肌
diaphragm

胃
stomach

附图 9　胸部冠状位 MRI
MRI of thorax (coronal section)

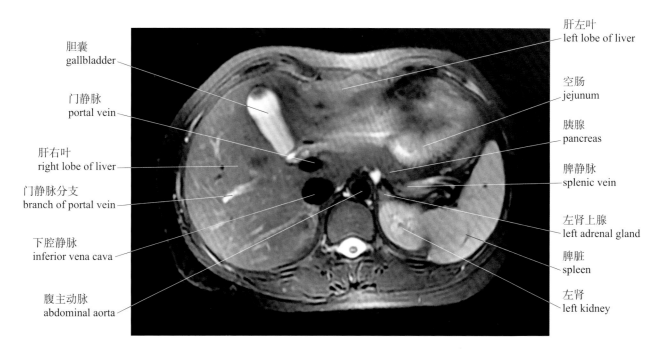

胆囊
gallbladder

门静脉
portal vein

肝右叶
right lobe of liver

门静脉分支
branch of portal vein

下腔静脉
inferior vena cava

腹主动脉
abdominal aorta

肝左叶
left lobe of liver

空肠
jejunum

胰腺
pancreas

脾静脉
splenic vein

左肾上腺
left adrenal gland

脾脏
spleen

左肾
left kidney

附图 10　经门静脉腹部横切面 MRI
MRI of transverse section of the abdomen (passing the portal vein)

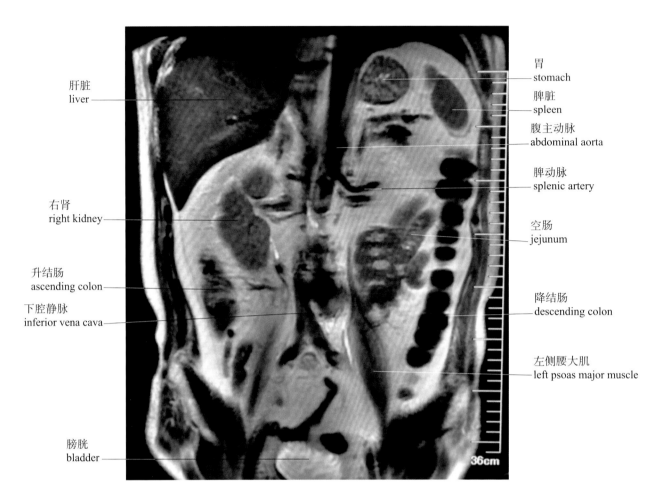

肝脏
liver

右肾
right kidney

升结肠
ascending colon

下腔静脉
inferior vena cava

膀胱
bladder

胃
stomach

脾脏
spleen

腹主动脉
abdominal aorta

脾动脉
splenic artery

空肠
jejunum

降结肠
descending colon

左侧腰大肌
left psoas major muscle

36cm

附图 11　腹部冠状位 MRI
MRI of the abdomen (coronal section)

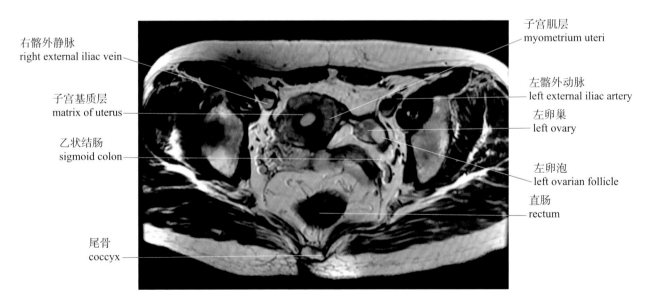

右髂外静脉
right external iliac vein

子宫基质层
matrix of uterus

乙状结肠
sigmoid colon

尾骨
coccyx

子宫肌层
myometrium uteri

左髂外动脉
left external iliac artery

左卵巢
left ovary

左卵泡
left ovarian follicle

直肠
rectum

附图 12　盆腔横切面 MRI（女性）
MRI of transverse section of the pelvic cavity (in female)

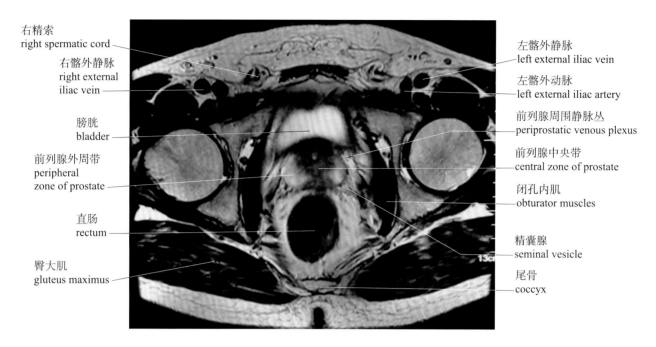

右精索
right spermatic cord

右髂外静脉
right external
iliac vein

膀胱
bladder

前列腺外周带
peripheral
zone of prostate

直肠
rectum

臀大肌
gluteus maximus

左髂外静脉
left external iliac vein

左髂外动脉
left external iliac artery

前列腺周围静脉丛
periprostatic venous plexus

前列腺中央带
central zone of prostate

闭孔内肌
obturator muscles

精囊腺
seminal vesicle

尾骨
coccyx

附图 13　盆腔横切面 MRI（男性）
MRI of transverse section of the pelvic cavity (in male)

弥散张量成像（DTI）白质纤维束图

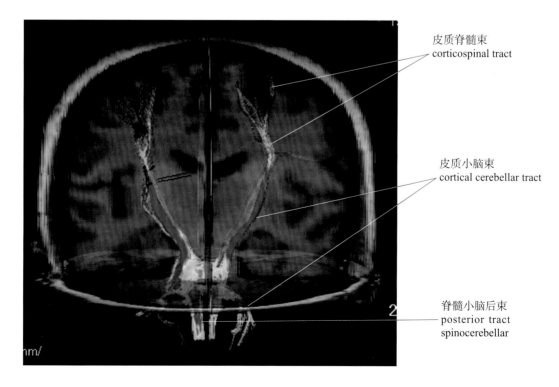

皮质脊髓束
corticospinal tract

皮质小脑束
cortical cerebellar tract

脊髓小脑后束
posterior tract
spinocerebellar

附图 14　皮质脊髓束（DTI）
Corticospinal tract (DTI)

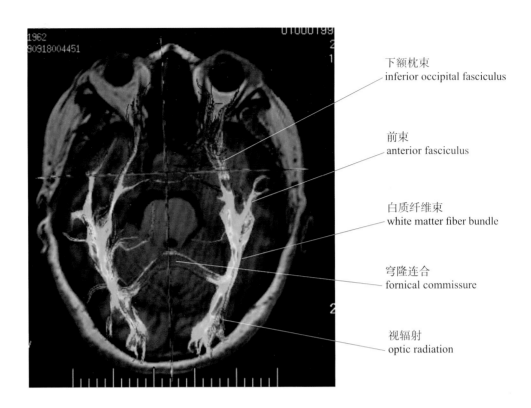

下额枕束
inferior occipital fasciculus

前束
anterior fasciculus

白质纤维束
white matter fiber bundle

穹隆连合
fornical commissure

视辐射
optic radiation

附图 15　下纵束（DTI）
Inferior longitudinal fasciculus (DTI)

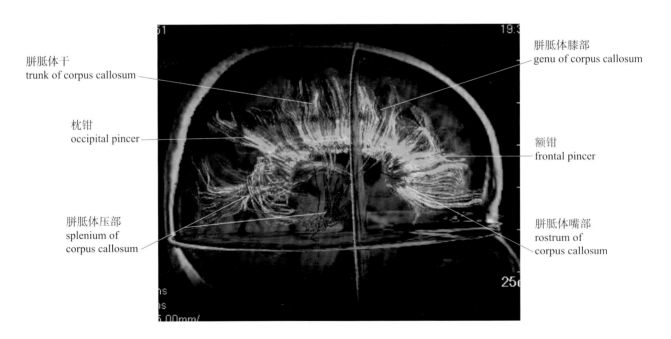

胼胝体干
trunk of corpus callosum

枕钳
occipital pincer

胼胝体压部
splenium of
corpus callosum

胼胝体膝部
genu of corpus callosum

额钳
frontal pincer

胼胝体嘴部
rostrum of
corpus callosum

附图 16　胼胝体纤维束（DTI）
Fasciculus of corpus callosum (DTI)